Building on Women's Strengths

A Social Work Agenda for the Twenty-First Century

Second Edition

Building on Women's Strengths

A Social Work Agenda for the Twenty-First Century

Second Edition

K. Jean Peterson, DSW
Alice A. Lieberman, PhD
Editors

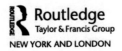

Routledge
Taylor & Francis Group
NEW YORK AND LONDON

First Published by

The Haworth Social Work Practice Press, an imprint of The Haworth Press, Inc., 10 Alice Street, Binghamton, NY 13904-1580.

Transferred to Digital Printing 2010 by Routledge
270 Madison Ave, New York NY 10016
2 Park Square, Milton Park, Abingdon, Oxon, OX14 4RN

Quotation from C. Meyer, A feminist perspective on foster family care: A redefinition of the categories, *Child Welfare, 64,* pp. 249-258. Reprinted by permission of the Child Welfare League of America, 440 First Street, NW, Washington, DC.

Quotation from M. A. Jiminez, A feminist analysis of welfare reform, *Affilia: Journal of Women & Social Work, 14*(3), pp. 290-291. Copyright © 1999 by *Affilia.* Reprinted by permission of Sage Publications.

Quotation from S. Anderson and B. Sussex, Resilience in lesbians: An exploratory study, from *Lesbians & Lesbian Families: Reflections on Theory and Practice,* ed. Joan Laird. © 1999 Columbia University Press. Reprinted by permission of the publisher.

Quotation from Joan Laird, Women's Secrets—Women's Silences from *Secrets in Families and Family Therapy,* edited by Evan Imber-Black. Copyright © 1993 by Evan Imber-Black. Reprinted by permission of W. W. Norton & Co.

Cover design by Anastasia Litwak.

Library of Congress Cataloging-in-Publication Data

Building on women's strengths: a social work agenda for the twenty-first century / K. Jean Peterson, Alice A. Lieberman, editors—2nd ed.

    p. cm.
Some chapters rewritten, some completely new chapters added for this ed.
Includes bibliographical references and index.
ISBN 0-7890-0869-6 (alk. paper)—ISBN 0-7890-1616-8 (soft : alk. paper)
    1. Social work with women—United States. 2. Women—United States—Social conditions.
I. Peterson, K. Jean. II. Lieberman, Alice A.

HV1445 .B85 2001
362.83´0973—dc21

00-069608

CONTENTS

ABOUT THE EDITORS

K. Jean Peterson, DSW, is Associate Professor and Director of Practicum at the University of Kansas School of Social Welfare. She writes in the areas of gay and lesbian health and issues affecting women and edited the book *Health Care for Lesbians and Gay Men: Confronting Homophobia and Sexism.*

Alice A. Lieberman, PhD, MSW, is Associate Professor and Director of the BSW Program at the University of Kansas School of Social Welfare. She has written and studied in the fields of child welfare, health care, and reproductive issues for women.

CONTRIBUTORS

Faye Y. Abram, MSW, PhD, is Associate Professor in the School of Social Service at Saint Louis University.

Sandra C. Anderson, MSW, PhD, Professor in the Graduate School of Social Work at Portland State University, has written extensively in the area of women and alcoholism, and more recently about clinical issues in working with gay men and lesbians.

Rosemary Chapin, MSW, PhD, Associate Professor in the School of Social Welfare at the University of Kansas, and Director of the Office of Aging, has written extensively in the area of policy practice issues for older adults.

Leanne W. Charlesworth, MSW, PhD, is a member of the Welfare Research Group at the University of Maryland at Baltimore, School of Social Work.

Liane V. Davis, MSW, PhD, was Professor and Associate Dean for Academic Programs at the University of Kansas School of Social Welfare before her death in 1995. She published on practice and policy issues affecting women as clients and women in the social work profession.

Jan L. Hagen, MSW, PhD, is Professor, School of Social Welfare, the State University of New York at Albany. Her areas of expertise include the impact of welfare policy on female recipients. She co-authored numerous articles with Dr. Davis.

Elizabeth D. Hutchison, MSW, PhD, Associate Professor at the School of Social Work, Virginia Commonwealth University, writes in the areas of child welfare and human behavior.

Joan Laird, MSW, Professor Emeritus at Smith College School for Social Work, writes in the areas of family work and gay and lesbian issues. She is the co-author with Ann Hartman of the widely used text, *Family Centered Social Work Practice.*

Dorothy C. Miller, MSW, DSW, is Associate Professor in the Center for Women's Studies at Wichita State University. She is the author of *Women and Social Welfare: A Feminist Analysis.*

Patricia O'Brien, MSW, PhD, Assistant Professor in the Jane Addams School of Social Work, University of Illinois, Chicago, has worked with and written about women in the correctional system.

Jeanette Mott Oxford, MDiv, is the Executive Director of the Reform Organization of Welfare in St. Louis, Missouri.

Angela H. Roffle, MSW, is a social work practitioner in St. Louis, Missouri.

Margaret E. Severson, MSW, JD, Associate Professor in the School of Social Welfare at the University of Kansas, consults, and writes about mental health evaluation and treatment systems in jails.

Barbara Levy Simon, MSW, PhD, Associate Professor at Columbia University School of Social Work, has written on various issues affecting women and their multiple roles as workers and caregivers.

Ann Weick, MSW, PhD, Dean and Professor at the University of Kansas School of Social Welfare, has written extensively on women's issues as well as on the philosophical underpinnings of the profession.

Preface to the First Edition

This book represents the unique collaboration of twelve strong women. We have a shared commitment to our chosen profession: social work. We have a shared commitment to discover and develop the unique strengths in the women who are and have always been the majority of clients. We also have our differences. Some of us are Caucasians; some of us are women of color. Some of us are heterosexual; some of us are lesbians. We are Catholic, Jewish, Protestant, and atheist. Some of us proudly call ourselves feminists; some of us are uncomfortable with that label.

We came together as a group for two days at the University of Kansas for a special experience: to engage one another in a dialogue and, out of that dialogue, to build a social work agenda for women for the twenty-first century. Because we are all academics, we had put much thought into the papers we brought to share. But rather than being unchangeable pillars of stone into which we had poured our fragile egos, our papers were works in progress. Our instructions were clear: come with an openness to share ideas and hear other voices.

None of us was fully prepared for the impact of those two days. Something unusual was going on—something few of us had experienced within the context of our academic lives. We knew what was different, but it took awhile for us to feel free enough to express it: we were all women. Although the conference was open to interested fac-

---

The second edition of this book reflects the changes that have occurred in the past decade that have affected the lives of women. We began this project by critically examining the first edition and asking: "How do we reconstruct this book to reflect the changes of the last decade, while honoring those ideas that have served us well?" The result was that most of the original contributors to the first edition who wrote about social policy radically rewrote their original chapters, while other chapters remained virtually unchanged. Completely new chapters were also added to the book that reflected the concerns of specific populations of women. Finally, the organization of the book was changed to accommodate these new perspectives.

ulty, students, and community professionals, the few who joined us were almost all women. One man, a doctoral student, sat silently through one day of our meeting. He later commented in private that he felt he was an intruder, yet he was learning too much to leave. A second man, a faculty member, joined us briefly to hear a former colleague speak.

But mostly we were women. As we sat and talked in the small, homey conference room nestled in the library, we became increasingly aware of our shared gender and the comfort we felt in being able to speak in our own voices without having to explain ourselves, without having to worry about hurting others' feelings, and without fearing that we would become invisible or be discounted if we said something too radical or too feminist. We rejoiced in being able to hear the voices of different women and were enriched by our diversity.

Throughout the two days, we kept returning to the uniqueness of the experience. We were engaged in a dialogue. This was why we had come into academia—to think, to be challenged, to expand our own parochial views. Instead, we often found ourselves in settings in which people performed and most of us felt obligated to join the game. For once, we were in an environment in which we could be ourselves. An important part of being ourselves was letting down the barriers we often erected between our professional, scholarly, and private selves. We talked as women to women.

Lest you get the wrong impression, we were not engaged in male bashing. To the contrary, we were unapologetically celebrating the strengths of women, without much concern for men. For those two days, some of us implicitly understood the appeal of separatism, although few of us would choose that either for our personal, political, or professional lives.

The chapters in this volume were enhanced by this process. We all went home, enriched by the lively discussions, and looked anew at what we had written. In some cases, we made minor changes. In others, we wrote entirely new papers.

The papers address issues we believe are central to transforming women's lives as we approach the new century. We could not address everything relevant to improving the lives of women in the twenty-first century. In fact, as we thought about it, little is not relevant to improving the lives of women. In deciding whom to invite, more concern was for *who* the women were than the specific expertise they brought. We wanted a group of women who were able to have a conversation with one another, a group of women committed to enhancing a women's agenda rather than their own. We also wanted social workers who could speak about issues of social work practice and social policy and who understood the common ground that lay beneath them.

Although many themes frame this book, two interconnected ones are central. Throughout history, women have been taught to see the world through the eyes of those who are more powerful (who happen to be men) and to accept that world as *reality*. A major aspect of that world has been the definition of women as incomplete, defective, and weak. There have always been voices to challenge men's hegemony over reality making, but those voices have become louder over the past few decades. If it has achieved nothing else, the women's movement (if we can still call it that) has fueled the construction of alternative, highly credible realities. The newer realities validate the strengths that women have always had but too often have kept hidden. The first theme of this book, then, is that any agenda for women must be built on their already present strengths.

Reality making extends beyond women's conception of themselves. It encompasses making sense of the world in which we all live. This dual focus on self and society is the second theme of this book.

Emily Grosholz (1988), in writing about feminist historians, asks: "Why are we feminists?" Her response reflects our hope for this book. We are feminists, she says,

> Because we want to change social reality in accord with our perception of certain kinds of inequalities; and part of this change is that women take a broader, more active role in the construction of social reality. We want to criticize the world as it stands, in accord with certain moral principles, and we want people (including ourselves) to act differently in the future. (p. 174)

This book represents our efforts as women and as social workers to actively construct a new agenda for our profession, an agenda whose aim is to redress the continuing inequalities that women face, that is built on the strengths of women, that is firmly grounded in the values of our profession, and that guides us to act differently as we enter a new century.

Liane V. Davis
University of Kansas
School of Social Welfare
Lawrence, Kansas

REFERENCE

Grosholz, E. (1988). Women, history, and practical deliberation. In M. M. Gergen (Ed.), *Feminist thought and the structure of knowledge*. New York: New York University Press.

Preface to the Second Edition

DO WE STILL NEED A WOMEN'S AGENDA FOR THE TWENTY-FIRST CENTURY?

It is, to us, a great irony that on the day we are putting the final touches to this manuscript, the U.S. Supreme Court has ruled against the State of Nebraska's efforts to legislate a ban on a certain type of late-term abortion (*Stenberg v. Carhart*, 99-830). Under the law as it was written, the state would have been allowed to ban the procedure regardless of the consequences to the mother's life or health. The narrowness with which this case was decided underscores the tenuousness of what constitutes an undue burden on a woman's right to choose. Regardless of one's opinion on this particular issue, we think it is a good idea to use this occasion to reflect on our collective progress and how we might reshape and refine the agenda for the women of tomorrow. In other words, we think the answer to the question that opened this preface is a resounding "yes," and that this book represents one group's contribution to that dialogue.

This book is a tribute to our friend, mentor, and colleague, Liane Davis. Her untimely death in 1995 occurred just as the first edition of this book was receiving its first warm reviews. Although she lived long enough to see one of them, in *The Women's Review of Books*, she was unable to enjoy the impact that the book had in the feminist scholarly community. We are privileged to continue her mission with this second edition of her book.

We have tried to remain true to the original overarching theme of this book: how do we take the strengths women have—have always had—and use them to build a world that is validating, liberating, and inclusive? This is the question that Liane devoted herself to, with her enthusiasm, her joy, and her formidable intellect.

As social workers, we have much to contribute. Our professional work with women provides us with the unique opportunity to see precisely how our clients strive, survive, and thrive—or not—and the social policies that influenced that outcome. As scholars, we can contribute to the construction of knowledge about policies and practices that are most likely to result in the good outcomes (a primary goal of this book). Finally, our skills in the social change arena can be used to contribute to positive policy and practice changes resulting in increased decision making, choice, and independence for all women.

We began this project by critically examining the first edition and asking ourselves the basic question, "How do we reconstruct this book to reflect the changes of the past decade, while honoring those ideas that have served us well?" It seemed clear to us, for example, that the legislation popularly know as "welfare reform" had changed the landscape in social policy: its influence is felt far beyond the narrow confines of income maintenance. Thus, most of the original contributors to the first edition who wrote about social policy either had to rewrite their old chapters radically or submit completely new ones (Miller; Hutchison and Charlesworth). We remain indebted to them for these new contributions.

Other chapters, however, stood the test of time. Davis, Simon, Weick, and Laird each wrote chapters which, taken together, analyze the struggle of this predominantly female profession to find its place and its voice, from Henry Street to our state and national capitols, from modernism to postmodernism in our ways of knowing. Completely new additions to this book include the works of Severson, Hagen, O'Brien, Chapin, Abram and colleagues, and Anderson. Each has taken a female population of concern, and expounded upon the policy and practice issues that affect them.

Reading the final draft, we were struck by how much has changed in this decade for women, both for good and ill. It reinforced for us the idea that, not only do we need an agenda, we also need to keep returning to it to measure our progress, to add new items, and maybe even to remove old ones. It is important work. It must continue.

This book would never have become a reality were it not for the generosity of several people. Carlton E. Munson, Senior Editor at The Haworth Press, has been forbearing in his tolerance of missed deadlines, and The Haworth Press has been financially generous to the scholarship fund endowed in Liane's memory; David Brown, Liane's husband, relinquished his rights to royalties from this edition, thereby allowing us to channel the proceeds to this fund; our very special colleagues at the University of Kansas who provide collegial support and humor every day, including our librarian, Channette Kirby, who assisted with editing; and the fine contributors to this book. Some of them knew Liane personally, some did not, but they all embraced her vision. For this we are deeply grateful.

K. Jean Peterson
Alice A. Lieberman
University of Kansas
School of Social Welfare
Lawrence, Kansas

Chapter 1

Why We Still Need a Women's Agenda for Social Work

Liane V. Davis

INTRODUCTION

Social work has a unique perspective on "women's issues." From the beginning, women have been the major players on both sides of the profession: as workers and as clients (see Vandiver, 1980, for a brief "herstory" of women in social work). We have powerful foremothers, women such as Jane Addams, Bertha Capen Reynolds, and Mary Richmond, who, from the earliest days, provided strong leadership to develop strategies for meeting the needs of persons who were oppressed, most of whom were women and their children. Today, we have a professional code of ethics that provides us with an ongoing reminder of our commitment to actively work for a society in which all persons, irrespective of personal characteristics, condition, or status, have equal opportunity (NASW, 1990).

And yet despite (or perhaps because of) our roots as a profession primarily of and for women, and despite our historic commitments to equal opportunity for all persons, social work is only now recognizing the pervasiveness and persistence of discrimination against women and the damage done to women (and to society) by their systematic exclusion from society's major institutions.

The authors of this book examine some of the major social issues affecting the lives of women clients and how these issues can be addressed by both policymakers and practitioners. The individual chapters, built on the theme of "building on women's strengths," challenge the readers to look anew at major areas of women's lives, and how they, as social workers, can engage in practice that is empowering for women. Understanding where we are to go in the twenty-first century and how we are to get there, however, requires knowing where we have come from. It also requires understanding where we are at present. This first chapter seeks to ground the reader in the immediate past and present of women's struggle to be included as an equal participant in U.S. society.

It begins with a brief history of twentieth-century political changes that were attempted and achieved in the fight to gain equality for women. It concludes with a more troubling discussion of the changes that are still needed if women's voices are to be heard throughout social institutions. The first is a discussion of political battles that touch on deep interpersonal and personal issues. The second is a discussion of the very foundations of our knowledge and reality-making enterprise. Understanding both is necessary if we, as social workers, are to effectively participate in the future struggles to achieve equality for women.

THE WOMEN'S MOVEMENT
AND POLITICAL CHANGE

It has been more than a century since women first came together in any mobilized way to fight for women's rights. It took this "first wave" of feminists, as they have since been called, some forty years to achieve their overarching goal: securing for women the right to vote. It would be another forty or so years before women once again mobilized. This "second wave" of feminists had a far broader call—the liberation of women. Women's liberation, or "women's lib" as its critics disparagingly called the movement, conjured up, for many, images of combat-boot-wearing lesbians and bra-burning hippies—as threatening to the social order as the draft-card burners of the Vietnam protests. The public perception, or the media-inspired perception, was that these women wanted a social revolution and had little need or tolerance for men in their new society. Needless to say, there was much resistance to what was perceived as a call for radical action.

As with any social movement, there are multiple views of what went right and what went wrong with the women's movement. Some perceive that women have achieved a tremendous amount since the early 1970s. They talk about the choices now open to young women, the growing numbers of women in schools of law and medicine and the military, and the increasing involvement of men in arenas traditionally reserved for women, such as child rearing. Others perceive that little of importance has changed. They talk about the impoverishment of women or the feminization of poverty (see Abramovitz [1991] for a stimulating discussion of how labels affect social workers' perception of issues affecting women), the violence against women, single-mother families, and the glass ceiling that prevents women from rising to positions of leadership. Some perceive that feminism is no longer either a necessary or viable political philosophy (see, for example, Davidson, 1988); some perceive that feminism is as much needed and as viable today as it was 100 years ago (see, for example, Davis, 1991; Hawkesworth, 1990).

How there can be such divergent views of where we are and where we are to go is a part of this chapter. Two major political battles illustrate these differing perceptions. The first centers around achieving equality under the law; the second centers around reproductive rights.

The Equal Rights Amendment: An Unfinished Story

With much hope and hoopla, both houses of Congress overwhelmingly passed the Equal Rights Amendment in 1972 and sent it to the states where its ratification was believed likely. And yet, as we all know, the ERA failed to achieve approval by the thirty-eight states needed for it to be enacted into law. The story of its demise provides an important lesson for future change efforts in this country's women's agenda. It is fitting that the discussion of history begins here.

What exactly was the Equal Rights Amendment? Although it was the banner carried by the women's movement of the 1970s, the Equal Rights Amendment was not created by the second wave of feminists. It was first proposed in 1923 by the National Women's Party specifically because post–Civil War court decisions continued to hold that sex, unlike race or national origin or religion, was a legitimate basis for discrimination (Freeman, 1975). The original amendment, which read: "Men and women shall have equal rights throughout the United States and every place subject to its jurisdiction," first introduced in Congress in 1923, was reintroduced in various forms in almost every Congress until its final passage in 1972 (Boles, 1979). The Amendment that finally passed was brief. It had three provisions:

Section 1. Equality of rights under the law shall not be denied or abridged by the United States or by any State on account of sex.

Section 2. The Congress shall have the power to enforce, by appropriate legislation, the provisions of this article.

Section 3. This amendment shall take effect two years after the date of ratification.

To its supporters, "the ERA was to be an important but benign implement for removing the legal barriers to female equality" (Boles, 1979, p. 7). To its opponents, it was a tool so powerful that it would undermine family life as we know it and weaken our nation's ability to defend our country. Its demise is due, in large part, to the success of the opponents in convincing state legislators of the truth of their version of the story (Boles, 1979; Davis, 1991).

As with much legislation, it is difficult to know exactly what its framers intended and impossible to predict how it would have been interpreted subsequently. The evidence suggests, however, that the intent of the ERA was far less revolutionary than portrayed by its opponents.

This amendment to the Constitution was designed to make it illegal to discriminate on the basis of gender just as the Fourteenth Amendment had made it illegal to discriminate on the basis of race. According to contemporary legal scholars, the ERA was expected to affect four major arenas: education, employment, military service, and family law (Boles, 1979). It was designed to eliminate all forms of discrimination against women in publicly supported schools. This included eliminating sex discrimination from admissions and scholarship decisions and from employment policies. It was designed to eliminate gender discrimination from employment—for example, barring policies that forbade women from certain occupations just because of their gender. It was intended to enable women to join the armed forces and to obtain postservice military benefits under the same conditions as their male peers. It was also designed to eliminate gender discrimination from family law. This meant that alimony and child-support provisions would be gender neutral. Such decisions could take into account the circumstances of the individual, but not the gender of the parties (Boles, 1979; Davis, 1991).

Despite the opponents' claims, the original framers did not intend that pregnant women or mothers would be drafted into the armed forces. There have always been exemptions from the draft for specific groups of persons; the ERA would have made such exemptions gender neutral. For example, all expectant parents or custodial parents of children under the age of two could have been exempted. They did not intend to eliminate gender itself from family law. The intent was to eliminate disparities based on gender. Thus, states could prohibit marriages between same-sex persons as long as they applied the provisions equally to women and men. There was no intent to bar the separation of persons of different genders under appropriate circumstances. For example, it would be all right to have same-sex bathrooms or same-sex dormitories to assure persons the constitutional right to privacy. Nor was the law intended to prevent policies that protected women in employment as long as those policies could also be extended to men (Boles, 1979; Davis, 1991).

The failure of the ERA has been widely debated (see, for example, Boles, 1979; Conover and Gray, 1983; Davidson, 1988; Davis, 1991; Gelb and Palley, 1987). A common belief is that the ERA failed largely because its supporters were white, middle-class, liberal women blinded to the realities of other women's lives. In their blindness, they failed to see that their desire to achieve equality in the labor market was not shared by two other significant groups of women: those who enjoyed and wanted to retain their protected status as homemakers and mothers and those who, thrust by necessity into the low-paid labor market, wanted nothing more than the opportunity to come home to care for their children and families. Yet evidence exists that feminists were not misreading public sentiment. A 1972 Roper poll had found that 49 percent of men and 48 percent of women were in favor of efforts to strengthen or change women's status in society. By 1974, 63 percent of men and 57 percent of women were in favor of such changes (Boles, 1979, p. 52). Perhaps the ERA's failure was due less to feminist myopia than to poor timing. Public sentiment had not yet reached the halls of the state houses (Boles, 1979). Or perhaps, although a majority of both women and men favored unspecified changes in the status of women, they were not yet ready for the radical overthrow of traditional societal and family values that the opponents of the ERA kept vividly in public view.

Gelb and Palley (1987) suggest that a major factor in women winning some battles and losing others is whether an issue is seen to produce role equity or role change.

> Role equity issues are those policies which extend rights now enjoyed by other groups (men, other minorities) to women and which appear to be relatively delineated or narrow in their implications. . . . In contrast, role change issues appear to produce change in the dependent female role of wife, mother, and homemaker, holding out the potential of greater sexual freedom and independence in a variety of contexts. (p. 6)

Although the intent of the pro-ERA forces was to give equity to women, opponents played into the fear that the entire fabric of society as we know it would be radically transformed. They portrayed a world in which women and men shared the same public rest rooms and prisons, pregnant women and mothers were forced to go to war, and homosexuals could marry and adopt children. They played on women's fears that gender-neutral laws would no longer grant them alimony or custody of their children following divorce or that they would be forced to enter the labor market to share the financial burden of caring for their families even if they were married (Davis, 1991). In fighting the ERA, the New Right, as it was soon to be called, developed a "pro-family" agenda that successfully energized those wanting to maintain the status quo.

Although the commonly held belief is that the ERA was lost by feminists who failed to take into account the interests of women different from them, perhaps this is just another instance of blaming the victim. To assume that feminists lost the fight is to assume they had the power to win it. But while women, both feminist and nonfeminist, were most audible in defining and lobbying the issues, they were largely absent where it really mattered: in the state legislatures. In the states that failed to ratify the amendment, women legislators were overwhelmingly in favor of its passage; men were not (Davis, 1991). Had women been equitably represented in the legislatures, which they were not, the ERA would have passed. A more credible view, therefore, is that the ERA was not lost by feminists, but was defeated by those who stood to lose the most: the white privileged men who cast the votes in state legislatures across the country.

Piecemeal Change Is Easier Than Global Change

The ERA represented the hopes of what were labeled "liberal feminists" (see Jagger and Struhl, 1978, for a discussion of the political spectrum of feminists). Liberal feminists wanted to have an equal share of the U.S. pie and believed that the way to obtain their fair share was through federal action. In their idealism, they had hoped that the ERA would lay a foundation for broad social change. But as the death of the ERA taught them, they were going to have to achieve their share of the pie one small piece at a time. And they succeeded to some extent.

Not surprisingly, many of their successes related to equality in the workplace, the most pressing concern to the millions of women who were finding themselves, both by choice and necessity, in the paid labor market. The Civil Rights Act of 1964 was a major vehicle for such change. Title VII, the Equal Employment Opportunity section of the Civil Rights Act, prohibited private employers as well as state and local governments from discriminating on the basis of race, color, religion, and national origin. Feminists achieved a surprising victory when gender was added to the list. The Civil Rights Act also created a new federal agency, the Equal Employment Opportunity Commission (EEOC), whose duty it was to interpret and enforce the legislation. In 1980, the EEOC took a major step when it issued guidelines making sexual harassment a form of sex discrimination covered under Title VII of the Civil Rights Act (Hazou, 1990). Other important changes occurred. Title IX of the Education Amendments Act of 1972 prohibited any school that obtained federal monies from discriminating on the basis of gender (Gelb and Palley, 1987). The Pregnancy Discrimination Act of 1978, an amendment to Title VII of the Civil Rights Act, gave guarantees to women that pregnancy would not threaten their employment, while giving them qualified guarantees that they could return to their jobs after a reasonable unpaid maternity leave (Hazou, 1990). Changes that had a profound effect on women's lives occurred in other arenas as well. For example, the Equal Credit Opportunity Act, passed in 1974, made it illegal to discriminate on the basis of gender in the granting of credit (Gelb and Palley, 1987). This was vital for the economic well-being of the growing numbers of never-married and no-longer-married women. By small steps, women were achieving some degree of equality under the law. Many of these successes can be credited to the ongoing battle for the ERA, which called attention to the widespread discrimination against women (Davis, 1991). As history was to reveal, however, constant vigilance was needed to maintain the successes.

Reproductive Rights: A Major Battle

Nowhere has the need for vigilance been clearer than in the ongoing battle to secure for women the right to control their own reproductive systems. In 1973, feminists achieved a major victory when the Supreme Court extended the right to privacy to include women's right to decide for themselves whether to bear a child. It is important to understand the depth of that victory.

The most unalterable difference between women and men is that women are the bearers of society's children. For society to continue, women, as a group, must continue to fulfill that function. For individual women to achieve equality with men, however, they must have the right to make their own decisions about whether and when they will reproduce, and they must have access to the safest, most effective, and most affordable means to carry out their decisions. For feminists, women's right to choose abortion (as well as access to safe contraceptives) makes bearing children a choice that each individual woman can make, not a social mandate that she must fulfill. When only one alternative is available and publicly supported, regardless of whether that alternative is pronatal or proabortion, the right of individual women to determine their own lives is sacrificed in the interest of the social good.

When framed in this way, the emotional energy involved in the battle to maintain women's reproductive rights becomes understandable. When women are fighting to achieve equality in the classroom, equality in employment, and equality under the law, it is deeply threatening to be told that, despite all these achievements, they still cannot make the most personal decision, whether to bear a child. The passions (and inconsistencies) of the antichoice forces are also understandable. Although their public rhetoric is about the rights of the unborn children, (and while many deeply hold these beliefs), they too are energized by the far-reaching implications of giving women the right to control their own reproduction. George Gilder, a conservative author widely cited by the New Right, expressed their fear in his 1973 book:

> When the women demanded "control over our own bodies," they. . . were in fact invoking one of the most extreme claims of the movement. . . . For, in fact, few males have come to psychological terms with the existing birth-control technology; few recognize the extent to which it shifts the balance of sexual power in favor of women. A man quite simply cannot now father a baby unless his wife is fully and deliberately agreeable. There are few social or cultural pressures on her to conceive. (Gilder, 1973 as cited in Davis, 1991, pp. 453-454)

Forcing women to bear children not only violates women's right to make their own decisions, it also seriously impedes their ability to compete equally with men in the economic realm. Although the bearing and subsequent rearing of children are deeply rewarding, they are also very costly, especially to women. For poor women, the birth of each new child results in their further impoverishment as well as their continued dependence on the highly stigmatizing welfare system (Hayes, 1987). Children can be so detrimental to the career aspirations of more affluent women that one prominent business consultant suggested, in a much-criticized article, that the corporate world needed to develop a "mommy" track (Schwartz, 1989). It is not difficult to see how legislating women's right to make their own decisions keeps women dependent, both on their partners and on the state.

The right to abortion, achieved in *Roe v. Wade* (1973), has been seriously eroded by Congress, the courts, and administrative actions ever since. This has most affected poor women. Funding for abortions has been seriously curtailed since 1976 when the Hyde Amendment prohibited the use of federal funds for abortions except in cases of rape, incest, or when a woman's life is endangered. In 1981, federal funding was further restricted to cases where the woman's life is endangered. This more restrictive wording has been included in the annual Medicaid appropriations bill ever since (Lieberman and Davis, 1992).

Major Supreme Court decisions have so seriously curtailed *Roe v. Wade* that, at the time this is being written, it is unclear whether there will be any federally guaranteed right to abortion after 1992.[1] In *Webster v. Reproductive Health Services* (1989), the Court upheld a Missouri statute prohibiting abortions from being performed in publicly financed facilities, even if paid for privately. In *Rust v. Sullivan* (1991), the Court upheld administrative regulations that bar clinics receiving public funds through Title X of the Public Health Service Act from providing any information about abortion to pregnant women. Although the Bush administration backed off on this extreme infringement on free speech for physicians, the regulations continue to bar social workers and other health care professionals in these clinics from providing such information to their clients. This is especially outrageous given that abortion is still a constitutionally protected right.

This onslaught of government attacks on reproductive freedom combined with an antichoice movement increasingly engaging in direct actions to prevent women access to clinics where abortions are performed has resulted in a decrease in the number of physicians able and willing to perform abortions. This is most visible in rural parts of the country where there has been a 51 percent decline in services since 1977 (Lewin, 1990).

While the battle over the ERA divided the country in the 1970s and 1980s, the battle over reproductive rights divided the country in the 1990s. The depth of passion on both sides of the battles lines (and in some cases there are literal battle lines) suggests that these fights are about more than keeping women out of the military or protecting unborn fetuses. It is about continuing to exclude women from equal participation in society.

REALITY:
A SOCIAL AND POLITICAL CONSTRUCTION

While political activists were fighting to expand women's rights in the public arena, a potentially more seditious political activity was occurring elsewhere at the same time. The very nature of reality was being challenged.

Early feminists had developed an essential political tool: consciousness raising. Women would come together to tell their personal stories, discover the personal and political meaning of their lives, and develop personal and political strategies to transform not only their own lives but society as well. Consciousness raising assumes that reality, or what we have come to think of as reality, "is a political as well as a social construction" (Bricker-Jenkins and Hooyman, 1986, p. 17).

The notion that reality is socially constructed, although adopted by feminists, is not a feminist concept. Berger and Luckmann (1967) deserve credit for introducing the term "the social construction of reality" into the lexicon. Their ideas have been widely accepted by subsequent scholars interested in what is known as epistemology, or the study of knowledge. In their treatise on the sociology of knowledge, Berger and Luckmann observe that it is people who construct and legitimate society and its institutions. Over time, however, people act as if what has been constructed by previous generations has a life independent of its human creators. Two concepts are essential for understanding social constructionism: *reification* and *legitimation*.

> Reification is the apprehension of human phenomena as if they were things, that is, in non-human or possibly supra-human terms. Another way of saying this is that reification is the apprehension of the products of human activity as if they were something else than human products—such as facts of nature, results of cosmic laws, or manifestations of divine will. Reification implies that man [sic] is capable of forgetting his own authorship of the human world, and further, that the dialectic between man, the producer, and his products, is lost to consciousness. . . .
>
> Legitimation is the process of 'explaining' and justifying. . . the institutional order by ascribing cognitive validity to its objectivated meanings. Legitimation justifies the institutional order by giving normative dignity to its practical imperatives. . . . Legitimation not only tells the individual why he should perform one action and not another; it also tells him why things are what they are. In other words, 'knowledge' precedes 'values' in the legitimation of institutions. (Berger and Luckmann, 1967, pp. 89, 93-94)

Although many versions of reality may be constructed, only a few get reified and legitimated. These are the versions of those who wield the power. Until now, those in power have been a small group of privileged white men who have "generalized from themselves to all, established their sex/gender, their race, their class, as norms and ideals for all, while also maintaining their exclusivity" (Minnich, 1990, p. 68). It is these elitist definitions of society and its institutions (which includes its theories, its arts and sciences, its forms of governance and economic structures, the roles it assigns to people and the behaviors it expects of them, as well as its ideologies) that become normative standards against which everything and everyone are judged. What is the effect of one group having exclusive power to define reality?

> Eventually, that one category/kind comes to function almost as if it were the only kind, because it occupies the defining center of power, either casting all others outside the circle of the "real" or holding them on the margins, penned into subcategories. . . There were at the beginning the few, privileged men who generalized from themselves to Man, thus privileging certain of their qualities that, they asserted, distinguished them from 'the horde.' From then on the differences from those few were seen as marks of inferiority. Woman was. . . not the equal opposite of man but a failed version of the supposed defining type, higher than animals but lower than men. (Minnich, 1990, pp. 53-54)

Thus women (and members of other marginalized groups) are first marked as deficient and then their deficiencies are used to justify their exclusion from power. For a long time, women accepted their devalued status, internalizing the belief that they were not good enough to participate in the public arena. Slowly, however, some began to see that it was the normative standards that were deficient, not they.

Some feminists were also coming to understand that it was not only that it was a male-only game, but, more perniciously, it was men who maintained exclusive control over how the game was played. As Belenky and colleagues (1986), in their book on how women learn, write:

> Men move quickly to impose their own conceptual schemes on the experience of women, says French feminist writer Marguerite Duras. These schemes do not help women make sense of their experience; they extinguish the experience. Women must find their own words to make meaning of their experiences, and this will take time. (p. 202)

Transforming How We Think About Reality: Listening to Women's Voices

Some feminists realized they did not want to join the game already in play; they wanted to develop their own games, ones that validated the ways in which women experience life. In the words of writer Grace Paley (1991):

> Most of the Women's Libbers I knew really didn't want a piece of the men's pie. They thought that pie was kind of poisonous, toxic, really full of weapons, poison gases, all kinds of mean junk we didn't even want a slice of.

They wanted instead to transform the way we thought about people and their values, about the arts and the humanities, about politics and philosophy, about science and the professions (Minnich, 1991). Only this time, women (as well as other previously silenced groups) had to become major players in constructing the new realities. Bringing women in as an afterthought meant that women and their work were forever compared to the de facto male model and, through such comparisons, time and again found to be deficient. Bringing women in as an afterthought meant that the models themselves would never be transformed, merely reshaped. Women had to participate in developing versions of reality that more accurately reflected the worlds in which they lived.

One exemplar of a small-scale transformation is Gilligan's (1982) work on moral development. Prior to Gilligan, the most widely accepted model of moral development had been framed around male development and experience (Kohlberg, 1976). At Kohlberg's highest level of moral development, people use abstract universal ethical principles of justice and respect for individual rights to resolve moral dilemmas. Women had been found deficient when judged against this supposedly universal but implicitly male standard. What Gilligan did was listen to women (and men) talk about moral dilemmas. As women struggled with moral dilemmas, they worried about the human consequences of their choices and were loath to apply abstract principles to human problems. Women spoke of the responsibility to care for others; men spoke of the importance of protecting individual rights. As Gilligan listened, she heard different voices. This allowed her to rethink moral development, taking into account both women's concern for connection and men's concern with separation.

> As we have listened for centuries to the voices of men and the theories of development that their experience informs, so we have come more recently to notice not only the silence of women but the difficulty in hearing what they say when they speak. . . . The failure to see the different reality of women's lives and to hear the differences in their voices stems in part from the assumption that there is a single mode of social experience and interpretation. By positing instead two different modes, we arrive at a more complex rendition of human experience. . . . (Gilligan, 1982, pp. 183-184)

No longer are women judged deficient when they fail to adhere to a singular universal standard. Instead their approach to moral dilemmas is seen as equally viable and essential to social well-being.

If this discussion of transforming knowledge sounds very alien to you, step back for a moment and think. If men have been the ones, sitting in Congress and on the Supreme Court, telling everybody—men as well as women—how they could run their lives, haven't men also done the research and written the books that tell everybody—women as well as men—what is truth, what is right behavior, and what is normal? If reality is a political construction, then like other political actions, isn't it those in power who have been the predominant builders?

Feminism Requires a Paradigm Shift

Feminists were not the first to suggest that the ways we think about things need to be transformed. Certainly precedents exist for such transformations. They are what Kuhn has called "scientific revolutions," when the prevailing "paradigm " is discarded in favor of another (1970, p. 10). A paradigm "is what the members of a scientific community share, *and,* conversely a scientific community consists of men who share a paradigm" (Kuhn, 1970, p. 176, emphasis in original; underlining added).

Paradigm shifts begin to occur when facts no longer fit the prevailing paradigm and when another better paradigm is set forth. Even in the more objective world of science, acceptance of a new paradigm takes time. As Kuhn observes, the Copernican revolution was not complete until almost a century after Copernicus' death and Newtonian theory took almost half a century to be accepted.

Kuhn (1970) quotes Max Planck to explain how paradigm shifts occur. "A new scientific truth does not triumph by convincing its opponents and making them see the light, but rather because its opponents eventually die, and a new generation grows up that is familiar with it" (p. 151). It is not that scientists are incapable of admitting their errors; rather, accepting a new paradigm "is a conversion experience that cannot be forced" (Kuhn, 1970, p. 151).

Feminism is just such a conversion experience. Susan Bordo (1990) has called feminism "a cultural moment of revelation and relief" (p. 137). This conversion experience came about for many feminists over the past twenty years as "the category of the 'human'—a standard against which all difference translates to lack, insufficiency—was brought down to earth, given a pair of pants, and reminded that it was not the only player in town" (Bordo, 1990, p. 137).

Conversions are unsettling. The old and familiar world disappears. The taken-for-granted reality is no longer solidly grounded. To turn to Kuhn (1970) once again:

> . . . during revolutions scientists see new and different things when looking with familiar instruments in places they have looked before. It is rather as if the professional community has been suddenly transported to another planet where familiar objects are seen in a different light and are joined by unfamiliar ones as well. (p. 111)

But in the feminist revolution, only some people (and only some feminists) have experienced this conversion, and only some feminists have accepted the need for a new paradigm. If we are really in the process of a revolution, why are so many people acting as if the old paradigm is still adequate?

As Kuhn's study of the history of science has indicated, one paradigm is rejected only when a better one is available that explains something that previously felt amiss. But, for most—or most of those in the community of those we consider scholars—nothing is amiss. Their theories of the world continue to give them comfort. Only those whose stories have been silenced feel that something is seriously amiss. The outsiders are developing competing paradigms, while the insiders remain confident of their social construction of reality. Their ways of thinking about and running the world continue to keep them in power and they have, as yet, no need to think any differently.

At this point in time, only a minority are convinced of the need for an alternative paradigm, one that represents the voices of women and other previously silenced groups. For the majority, an alternative paradigm is not only unnecessary, but absurd. And, at the moment, there is little dialogue between the two. Again turning to Kuhn (1970):

> ... the proponents of competing paradigms practice their trades in different worlds. . . . Practicing in different worlds, the two groups of scientists see different things when they look from the same point in the same direction. . . . That is why a law that cannot even be demonstrated to one group of scientists may occasionally seem intuitively obvious to another. (p. 150)

To understand how people can see such different things when looking at the same phenomenon, one has only to be reminded of the televised confirmation hearings for Supreme Court Justice Clarence Thomas. "They don't get it; they just don't get it" was repeated thousands of times as women throughout the country sat glued to the television set, in wide-eyed amazement as Judge Thomas was confirmed to the highest court in the nation.

Standpoint Feminists: Reality Depends on Where You Stand

For those who do get it, the conversion has been a powerful experience. One group who has participated in this conversion is referred to as feminist standpoint theorists (see Alcoff, 1988; Hartsock, 1990; Stanley and Wise, 1990). The concept of standpoint assumes that all knowledge develops from the objective reality of people's lives. As we look out upon the world or turn inward to understand our inner lives, we are all grounded by our place in society. And our place in society has always been and continues to be firmly grounded by our gender. Most of what society deems worthy of study arises from the standpoint of white men. This ignores, trivializes, and denies vast arenas of life, mostly emanating from the more private realm of family and interpersonal relationships in which women's lives are embedded. It is the "dailiness of women's lives" (Aptheker, 1989, p. 37), cleaning the toilets and nurturing the children and men in private and in public, that leads women to a different understanding of the world than men. And yet it is just these activities and experiences that are made invisible.

Clearly differences exist among women. Women differ on the basis of race, class, sexual orientation, culture, and religion. Not all women share the same standpoint; not all women have the same experiences; not all women have the same view of reality. Nancy Hartsock (1990) expresses this well when she writes of the:

> need to dissolve the false "we" . . . into its real multiplicity and variety and out of this concrete multiplicity build an account of the world as seen from the margins, an account which can expose the falseness of the view from the top and can transform the margins as well as the center. (p. 171)

But at the same time, women, because of their shared gender, are all oppressed and marginalized. Being on the margins gives one a special perspective.

> Because women are treated as strangers, as aliens—some more so than others—by the dominant social institutions, and conceptual schemes, their exclusion alone provides an edge, an advantage. . . . Women's oppression gives them fewer interests in ignorance. . . and fewer reasons to invest in maintaining or justifying the status quo than the dominant groups. . . thus, the perspective from their lives can more easily generate fresh and critical analyses. (Harding, 1991, p. 126)

The oppressed survive only if they understand not only their own world but that of their oppressor. As a result, they have a more complete, although perhaps not more valid, picture of the world. Collins (1989) vividly captures this point in writing about African-American women: "Black women cannot afford to be fools of any type, for their devalued status denies them the protections that white skin, maleness, and wealth confer" (p. 759).

In their eagerness to articulate a way to think about the oppression that *all* women share, some theorists assumed that all women share the same standpoint. But voices even more marginalized and oppressed than white, middle-class women reminded them of their different experiences, their different visions of reality.

As new narratives began to be produced, telling the story of the diversity of women's experiences, the chief imperative was to listen, to become more aware of one's own biases, prejudices, and ignorance, to begin to stretch the borders of what Minnie Bruce Pratt calls the 'narrow circle of the self.' (Bordo, 1990, p. 138)

There was clearly a need to listen to other women's voices, other women's standpoints. But how many different women's standpoints are there? A lesbian women's standpoint, a black women's standpoint, a Chicane standpoint, a Jewish women's standpoint? If there are so many diverse standpoints, is it even useful to articulate women's standpoints? Is gender itself even a useful construct?

POSTMODERNISTS:
IS GENDER STILL A USEFUL CONSTRUCT?

For some feminists, the answer is "no." These are the feminists who have turned to postmodernism, a philosophical perspective that holds that there is no truth; that each individual, situated in her own time, her own place in history, in society, constructs her own reality. Not even oppressed persons can step outside of the social constraints of who they are and the conditions under which they live (Flax, 1987). Postmodernists hold that there can be no universal claims. In their commitment to pluralism, they seek to obliterate all group distinctions, all metanarratives. By privileging all perspectives, no one perspective can become the absolute standard against which to judge truth and fiction. In their commitment to hearing multiple voices, all categories, including that of women, become fictions, needing to be dismantled and deconstructed (see, for example, Nicholson, 1990).

WHY WE STILL NEED A WOMEN'S AGENDA
FOR SOCIAL WORK

These are complex philosophical issues. In this brief discussion, only the contours of the arguments have been drawn. Although they may seem far removed from social work, they are important to setting a future agenda for women. Should we continue to think about women and their issues as separate from a broader social agenda? Or have we entered the postfeminist era, as Betty Friedan has suggested, where we should be focusing on human issues, not women's issues (Friedan, 1986)?

For me, the answer is clear. As I look around me and see male privilege and female oppression, I know it is too soon to move on to a society in which gender is no longer a defining variable. I worry along with Christine Di Stefano (1990), who writes, "In our haste to deconstruct hierarchical distinctions such as gender as harmful illusions we may fail to grasp 'their tenacious rootedness in an objective world created over time and deeply resistant to change'" (p. 78).

As you read through this book, you will be reminded continually of the tenacious rootedness of the gender hierarchy in the objective world and the deep resistance to change in our society and even in our profession.

Women may not have a privileged perspective, but women do have many strengths that have for too long been denied and suppressed. Women need to have these strengths recognized and applauded. Many of what are now being written of as women's values have arisen in response to their oppression. Some may bring harm to them by keeping them oppressed. Although we need to articulate the previously silenced viewpoints of women and rethink "our ideas about what is humanly excellent, worthy of praise. . . we need to be careful not to assert merely the superiority of the opposite" (Flax, 1987, p. 641). Yet Linda Alcoff (1988) observes:

> After a decade of hearing liberal feminists advising us to wear business suits and enter the male world, it is a helpful corrective to have cultural feminists argue instead that women's world is full of superior virtues and values, to be credited and learned from rather than despised. (p. 266)

This brings me to a conclusion that can guide us in our work to construct a more equitable world where women's strengths are validated. Alcoff (1988) goes on to write about "identity politics," a concept originally developed by the Combahee River Collective, a black feminist group. Identity politics acknowledges that one's identity is both a social construction and a point from which to act politically. Although women differ from one another in many important ways, these differences are not sufficient to override our common interests. As women, we have just begun to claim our own power, to speak in our own voice, to use our identity as women as a point from which to act politically. Nancy Hartsock (1990) poses a pointed question:

> Why is it that just at the moment when so many of us who have been silenced begin to demand the right to name ourselves, to act as subjects rather than objects of history, that just then the concept of subjecthood becomes problematic? Just when we are forming our own theories about the world, uncertainty emerges about whether the world can be theorized. Just when we are talking about the changes we want, ideas of process and the possibility of systematically and rationally organizing human society become dubious and suspect. (pp. 164-165)

Jeffner Allen (1989) has asked:

> Does difference enter the scene only to vanish in a time when women perform two-thirds of the world's work, receive five percent of the world income, own less than one percent of the world land; when in the United States every seven minutes a woman is raped, every eighteen seconds a woman is battered; when women and children in female-headed households are estimated to comprise almost all of the population in poverty by the year 2000? (p. 41)

NOTE

1. (Editor's note) As of 2000, the Constitutional right to an abortion remains in place. However, laws that make abortions more difficult to obtain under various state laws have proliferated in the intervening years.

REFERENCES

Abramovitz, M. (1991). Putting an end to doublespeak about race, gender, and poverty: An annotated glossary for social workers. *Social Work, 36:* 380-384.

Alcoff, L. (1988). Cultural feminism versus post-structuralism: The identity crisis in feminist theory. In E. Minnich, J. O'Barr, and R. Rosenfeld (Eds.), *Reconstructing the academy: Women's education and women's studies* (pp. 257-288). Chicago: University of Chicago Press.

Allen, J. (1989). Women who beget women must thwart major sophisms. In A. Garry and M. Pearsall (Eds.), *Women, knowledge, and reality: Explorations in feminist philosophy* (pp. 37-46). Boston: Unwin Hyman.

Aptheker, B. (1989). *Tapestries of life: Women's work, women's consciousness, and the meaning of daily life.* Amherst, MA: University of Massachusetts Press.

Belenky, M. F., Clinchy, B. M., Goldberger, N. R., and Tarule, J. M. (1986). *Women's ways of knowing: The development of self, voice, and mind.* New York: Basic Books.

Berger, P. L. and Luckmann, T. (1967). *The social construction of reality: A treatise in the sociology of knowledge.* New York: Anchor Books.

Boles, J. K. (1979). *The politics of the Equal Rights Amendment: Conflict and decision process.* New York: Longman.

Bordo, S. (1990). Feminism, postmodernism, and gender-scepticism. In L. J. Nicholson (Ed.), *Feminism/postmodernism* (pp. 133-156). New York: Routledge, Chapman, and Hall.

Bricker-Jenkins, M. and Hooyman, N. R. (1986). A feminist world view: Ideological themes from the feminist movement. In M. Bricker-Jenkins and N. R. Hooyman (Eds.), *Not for women only: Social work practice for a feminist future* (pp. 7-22). Silver Spring, MD: National Association of Social Workers.

Collins, P. H. (1989). The social construction of black feminist thought. *Signs, 14:* 745-773.

Conover, P. J., and Gray, V. (1983). *Feminism and the new right: Conflict over the American Family.* New York: Praeger.

Davidson, N. (1988). *The failure of feminism.* Buffalo, NY: Prometheus Books.

Davis, F. (1991). *Moving the mountain: The women's movement in America since 1960.* New York: Simon and Schuster.

Di Stefano, C. (1990). Dilemmas of difference: Feminism, modernity, and postmodernism. In L. J. Nicholson (Ed.), *Feminism/postmodernism* (pp. 63-82). New York: Routledge, Chapman, and Hall, quoting Jay, M. (1984-1985). Hierarchy and the humanities: The radical implications of a conservative idea. *Telos* 62: 140.

Flax, J. (1987). Postmodernism and gender relations in feminist theory. *Signs, 12:* 621-643.

Freeman, J. (1975). *The politics of women's liberation: A case study of an emerging social movement and its relation to the policy process.* New York: David McKay Co.

Friedan, B. (1986). *The second stage,* Revised edition. New York: Summit Books.

Gelb, J. and Palley, M. L. (1987). *Women and public policies.* Princeton, NJ: Princeton University Press.

Gilligan, C. (1982). *In a different voice: Psychological theory and women's development.* Cambridge: Harvard University Press.

Harding, S. (1991). *Whose science? Whose knowledge?: Thinking from women's lives.* Ithaca, NY: Cornell University Press.

Hartsock, N. (1990). Foucault on power: A theory for women? In L. J. Nicholson (Ed.), *Feminism/postmodernism* (pp. 157-175). New York: Routledge, Chapman, and Hall.

Hawkesworth, M. E. (1990). *Beyond oppression: Feminist theory and political strategy.* New York: Continuum.

Hayes, C. (Ed.) (1987). *Risking the future, Volume 1.* Washington, DC: National Academy Press.

Hazou, W. (1990). *The social and legal status of women: A global perspective.* New York: Praeger Publishers.

Jagger, A. and Struhl, P. (1978). *Feminist frameworks: Alternative theoretical accounts of the relation between women and men.* New York: McGraw Hill.

Kohlberg, L. (1976). Moral stages and moralization: The cognitive-developmental approach. In T. Likona (Ed.), *Moral development and behavior: Theory, research, and social issues.* New York: Holt, Rinehart, and Winston.

Kuhn, T. S. (1970). *The structure of scientific revolutions,* Second edition. Chicago: University of Chicago Press.

Lewin, T. (1990). Abortions harder to get in rural areas of nation. *The New York Times,* National, June 28, p. 9.

Lieberman, A. and Davis, L. V. (1992). The role of social work in the defense of reproductive rights. *Social Work, 37:* 365-371.

Minnich, E. K. (1990). *Transforming knowledge.* Philadelphia: Temple University Press.

National Association of Social Workers (NASW) (1990). *Code of ethics of the National Association of Social Workers.* Washington, DC: NASW Press.

Nicholson, L. (1990). Introduction. In L. J. Nicholson (Ed.), *Feminism/postmodernism* (pp. 1-16). New York: Routledge, Chapman, and Hall.

Paley, G. (1991). Conversations. In G. Paley, *Long walks and intimate talks.* New York: The Feminist Press.

Roe v. Wade 410 U.S. 113 (1973).

Rust v. Sullivan, Nos. 89-1391, 89-1392, Slip opinion. U.S. (1991).

Schwartz, F. N. (1989). Management women and the new facts of life. *Harvard Business Review, 67:* 65-76.

Stanley, L. and Wise, S. (1990). Method, methodology, and epistemology in feminist research processes. In L. Stanley (Ed.), *Feminist praxis: Research, theory and epistemology in feminist sociology* (pp. 20-60). New York: Routledge.

Vandiver, S. T. (1980). A herstory of women in social work. In E. Norman and A. Mancuso (Eds.), *Women issues and social work practice* (pp. 21-38). Itasca, IL.: Peacock Publishers.

Webster v. Reproductive Health Services 492, U.S. 109 S.Ct., 3040, 106 L.Ed. 2d 410 (1989).

Chapter 2

Building on the Romance
of Women's Innate Strengths:
Social Feminism and Its Influence
at the Henry Street Settlement, 1893-1993

Barbara Levy Simon

> I believe that women have something to contribute to the gov-
> ernment that men have not, as men have something to contribute
> that women have not; that their traditions and their experiences
> combined will make for a more perfect understanding of com-
> munity needs. (Wald, 1914 [quoted in Coss, 1989, pp. 74-76])

INTRODUCTION

Nineteenth-century women, according to the beliefs of many a
contemporaneous minister, philanthropist, and agent of charity in the
United States, were endowed by their Creator with a unique ability to
soothe, to serve, and to salvage the poor and the vulnerable (Chambers, 1986:4; Hewitt, 1984; Sklar, 1973). Womanly duties were the
sacred duties of mothering, nursing, teaching, and uplifting (Koven
and Michel, 1990; Rendall, 1990). These fundamental functions of
womanhood were carried out at home and in volunteer work in reli-

The author wants to express particular appreciation to Dr. Elinor Polansky, Assistant to
the Henry Street Settlement's Executive Director, Daniel Kronefeld, for her generous
assistance in providing information about current activities at Henry Street and for her
invaluable observations about its present priorities.

gious benevolent societies, two domains unsullied by the contaminating influence of the profane—that is, by wages, competitive market relations, and secular authority.

With consummate artfulness, social feminists in the United States from the 1880s to the onset of World War I fought to expand the sphere of the sacred rather than to transfer women into the realm of the profane. Society, they argued, was in desperate need of good mothering and "civic housekeeping" (Chambers, 1986; Cohen and Hanagan, 1991). Why not encourage women—social feminists such as Jane Addams proposed—to bring the same generosity, empathy, and constancy to urban reform that they had brought historically to their caring for husbands, children, and aging parents? Stepping forward at a historical moment of extreme turbulence, one characterized by massive immigration, migration, industrialization, and urbanization, social feminists claimed that women were suited for two heroic roles at once. Their talents charged them with anchoring and sustaining their families, as they had always done. Now their womanly benevolence was also needed to save a fast-fragmenting society (Cohen and Hanagan, 1991; Koven and Michel, 1990).

Social feminists exploited and extended the metaphor of mothering in an era in which industrial capitalism was orphaning millions, stripping several continents of their resources, and shortening the lives of members of entire occupations and regions. Their message appealed to many inhabitants of a country nostalgic for a slower, kinder, and more comprehensible social order. The ideal of the nurturant mother who gently but firmly brings order to daily chaos was recognizable and compelling to millions of Americans in the tempestuous period between 1880 and 1920.

SOCIAL FEMINISM

Social feminists, according to historians Miriam Cohen and Michael Hanagan, were:

> those women (and sometimes men) who advocated women's rights as part of a broad agenda of social reform. As women's rights advocates, they championed the cause of women's suffrage and the expansion of women's rights in the workplace, but

their highest priorities concerned the poor, both adult and children. (Cohen and Hanagan, 1991, p. 470)

Social feminists viewed the battle for woman's suffrage and for the multiplication of women's occupational, educational, professional, and public roles as a necessary means to the overarching end of improving the lot of endangered and impoverished women, children, and families, both at home and at work (Cott, 1987, 1989).

In mounting their many social reform campaigns, social feminists organized local and state bodies that soon became national leagues and organizations. In 1874, for example, the Woman's Christian Temperance Union, whose motto was "Do Everything," became the first nationally organized social feminist body (Bordin, 1990). Other national organizations soon followed. The General Federation of Women's Clubs (GFWC) was founded in 1890; the National Council of Jewish Women in 1893; the National Association of Colored Women in 1896; the National Congress of Mothers in 1897, known in present-day terms as the National Congress of Parents and Teachers; the National Federation of Day Nurseries in 1898; and the National Federation of Settlements and Neighborhood Centers in 1911 (Koven and Michel, 1990; Leiby 1978). These groups organized a wide variety of projects in the voluntary and public sectors for children, families, and women throughout the country and actively lobbied at local and state levels for expanded services for poor and dependent people. For example, the GFWC, the National Congress of Mothers, and the National Federation of Settlements and Neighborhood Centers were central leaders in state campaigns to win passage of mothers' and widows' pensions, the forerunner of federal Aid to Families with Dependent Children (Abramovitz, 1988; Katz, 1986; Koven and Michel, 1990). They achieved success in forty states by 1920, a remarkable accomplishment given that in 1910 no states had mothers' pension legislation (Katz, 1986; Koven and Michel, 1990).

Most social feminists of the Progressive Era held the view that women were morally superior to men, having been equipped either by nature, God, or cumulative experience with special capacities for helping, teaching, and healing others, especially dependent others. This view, rooted in the much older nineteenth-century ideologies of "the cult of true womanhood" and "republican motherhood" (as historians have characterized them), was held not only by religiously inspired social feminists such as Frances Willard, founder of the Woman's

Christian Temperance Union, but also by irreligious, politically inspired women such as Florence Kelley, the leader of the National Consumers League and a founder of the U.S. Children's Bureau (Kerber, 1980; Welter, 1966). Kelley, the widely known social reformer who represented the left wing of social feminism, argued as late as 1923 that women had special wisdom in matters of social welfare and social justice (Kelley, 1923; Koven and Michel, 1990).

Despite their shared belief in "woman as moral force" and their common commitments to improving the living and working conditions of vulnerable adults and children by means of woman's suffrage and the formal insertion of women into public and professional life, social feminists were a highly divergent group (Cott, 1987). Some were militantly prounion while others were not (Cohen and Hanagan, 1991). Some were propelled into feminism and good works by spiritual impulses. Such was the case of Frances Perkins, a Progressive-Era social feminist who became U.S. Secretary of Labor under Franklin Roosevelt. Others were agnostics or atheists, inspired to action through secular and political identification with the disenfranchised. Florence Kelley and Mary van Kleeck, the influential director of industrial studies for the Russell Sage Foundation, embodied this strain. Some became strong advocates of Margaret Sanger's birth-control movement; others opposed it or were ambivalent about it (Gordon, 1976). For many social feminists, the interests of children came before the rights of women (Gordon, 1990). For others, the interests and rights of children were considered inextricably bound to the political, economic, social, and sexual freedom and power of women—especially poor women.

Notwithstanding these internal differences, social feminists found common justification for their heterogeneous visions and activities in "maternalism," a term crafted by historians Koven and Michel (1990) to characterize a cluster of convictions which:

> exalted women's capacity to mother and extended to society as a whole the values of care, nurturance, and morality. Maternalism always operated on two levels: it extolled the private virtues of domesticity while simultaneously legitimating women's public relationships to politics and the state, to community, workplace, and marketplace. (p. 1079)

The maternalist views of many social feminists led them to concentrate their energies primarily on issues of maternal and child welfare. Toward that end, reformers such as Julia Clifford Lathrop, Lillian Wald, and Grace Abbott, all settlement house activists who became nationally recognized architects of maternal and child health policies, helped secure widows' pensions, outlaw child labor, and shape the U.S. Children's Bureau, which mobilized Congress to pass and fund precedent-setting federal maternal and child health legislation in 1921 (Muncy, 1991). Other social feminists, such as Frances Perkins, Rose Schneiderman of the National Women's Trade Union League, and Alice Hamilton, who was a founder of the field of industrial medicine, poured their talents into reducing the dangers to women and children's welfare that loomed in the workplace.

Maternalist thinking created an indispensable ideological bridge between women's traditional devotion to family and their emergent leadership in the polity. By invoking their belief that women had special motherly insights and strengths upon which the entire society needed to draw in grappling with its multiple escalating crises, social feminists made citizens out of women by capitalizing on the very essentialism—the belief in the innate moral and temperamental distinctions between the genders—that had, until then, so effectively justified their total exclusion from citizenship and most paid work.

THE HENRY STREET SETTLEMENT

Nowhere were female citizens more eager to apply their "special capacities" to the polity than at Henry Street Settlement on the Lower East Side of New York City. Lillian Wald founded Henry Street Settlement in 1893, a year of a severe economic depression. She was a trained nurse who, while pursuing a medical degree, had volunteered to teach a weekly home-nursing class for immigrant women on Manhattan's Lower East Side. Horrified by her first encounters with the misery of tenement life and disillusioned with more traditional forms of nursing which she had encountered in nursing school and in an internship in a juvenile asylum, Wald quit medical school and, with her friend from nursing school, Mary Brewster, decided to "live in the neighborhood as nurses, identify ourselves with it socially, and, in brief, contribute to it our citizenship" (Wald, 1915, pp. 8-9).

What exactly did citizenship mean to Lillian Wald and Mary Brewster and the dozens of nurses, social workers, educators, union organizers, college-student volunteers, social scientists, journalists, and social reformers who were soon drawn into their mushrooming social feminist experiment? How did their devotion to a social feminist version of progressivism manifest itself in everyday life and work?

Social feminist expressions of citizenship at Henry Street and other similar settlements were direct offsprings of those modes of women's service that had been prized in nineteenth-century middle-class family life and Christian and Jewish benevolent associations (Smith-Rosenberg, 1971; Smith-Rosenberg, 1975). The self-sacrificing altruism, the round-the-clock responsiveness, and the total immersion in the daily rounds of caregiving that had characterized women's domestic lives of the midnineteenth century constituted the core characteristics of the role of women "settlers," as they called themselves, at settlement houses like Hull House in Chicago and Henry Street in New York City (Muncy, 1991). Settlement houses, the primary incubators of twentieth-century public health care, community-based social services, and social reform, evolved a highly distinctive ethos of social feminist citizenship (Sklar, 1985).

It is an ethos that merits detailed scrutiny because of its centrality to Progressive-Era social movements and because of its coevality with the beginnings of the social work profession. To understand the guiding beliefs of social-feminist residents of the settlement-house movement in the first two decades of the twentieth century is to comprehend one fundamental portion of the bedrock of both past and present feminism and past and present social work. The Henry Street Settlement, which recently celebrated its centennial year, serves as a microcosmic primer in social feminism's meaning and influence.

Social Feminist Citizenship

Service

Sustained service to others was the reason for being for the Henry Street settler in the early twentieth century, as had been true for her predecessor, the nineteenth-century's "Angel in the House." Yet at Henry Street, the service was public and visible rather than domestic and invisible. Head worker Lillian Wald, for example, established the world's first independent public health nursing service between 1893 and 1895; she then used Henry Street as a base to organize a national and international movement of public health nurses (Coss, 1989; Muncy, 1991).

A long list of other forms of highly visible public service followed. Wald took a leading role in shaping New York City's antituberculosis campaign, serving as a charter member of the first Committee on the Prevention of Tuberculosis of the Charity Organization Society of the City of New York in 1902 (Teller, 1988). Together with her settlement colleagues, she created a milk station in 1903 at Henry Street, which provided free sanitary milk to poor mothers with small children, maternal and child health workshops, and a system of home health visitation (Wald, 1915a). This milk station, and others like it in urban settlement houses, later became the model for the maternal and child health program of the federal Sheppard-Towner Act of 1921 (Combs-Orme, 1988).

Henry Street pilot projects at Public School #1 on the Lower East Side of New York and advocacy on the part of Henry Street staff with school system leaders led to numerous reforms in the public school system. The institutionalization of school playgrounds, school nursing, hot lunches, vocational guidance, after-school recreational programs, classes for children with physical and mental disabilities, and kindergartens throughout New York's school system was a direct outgrowth of Henry Street residents' experimentation and politicking (Coss, 1989; Wald, 1915a).

This ceaseless devotion to public service and social reform in the first era of Henry Street Settlement's life was fueled, in part, by social feminism's late-nineteenth-century essentialist version of womanhood. If one believed that women were endowed from birth with special gifts of charity and compassion and, furthermore, that these inborn gifts carried with them a particular moral charge to serve others, then it followed that one should do all within one's power to make more humane and healthy the housing, neighborhoods, schools, streets, hospitals, and workplaces of the United States.

Social feminism's call to women to save an industrializing society from itself was a message which harmonized gracefully with the teachings of Christian socialism, also known as social gospelism, a movement that spread widely within elite Northeastern colleges and universities and liberal Protestant denominations in the United States between 1870 and 1920. Leaders of Christian socialism, such as Edward Beecher, Washington Gladden, Richard Ely, and Walter Rauschenbusch, preached that the duty of Christians was not to seek a future place in heaven, but, instead, to create heaven on earth by working toward the immediate enactment in the United States of Christ's vision. To accomplish this, they proposed the abolition of poverty and capitalism through the construction of cooperative and collective systems of production and distribution (Cort, 1988; Handy, 1966).

Middle-class female college students in the 1870s and 1880s received a two-pronged charge. Social feminism taught them that, as women, they had a special vocation to serve a deteriorating social order, while Christian socialism directed them to honor the vision of Jesus by helping to eradicate poverty and injustice. These two allied messages received an especially warm reception among female college students educated in the three decades after the Civil War. They were the first generation of females to attend the fledgling women's colleges and the handful of coeducational colleges and universities that existed at the time. As the first generation of American women permitted to earn liberal arts degrees equivalent to those of men, they saw themselves as bearing particular responsibilities to employ constructively the higher education that had been denied to their mothers and grandmothers. However, upon graduating from college, they found that all of the major professions and vocations—the ministry, medicine, law, engineering, government service, diplomacy, architecture, the military, the professoriat, science, and business—were still completely closed to them. Small wonder that these pioneers sought to carve new paths to usefulness, recognition, and citizenship in institutions of their own making, such as Hull House, Henry Street, Andover House, University Settlement, and many other settlements.

Knowledge Building

A second attribute of citizenship at Henry Street was the staff's commitment to discovering social scientific knowledge and making it accessible and understandable to their neighbors and key governmental policymakers. Like numerous counterparts in what historian Robyn Muncy has called the "female dominion in American reform," social feminists at Henry Street Settlement vigorously endorsed the coupling of scientific discovery with popular education and the linking of scholarship with activism (Muncy, 1991, p. 64). "A characteristic service of the settlement to the public grows out of its opportunities for creating and informing public opinion," wrote Lillian Wald (1915a, p. 310).

With its passion for popularizing knowledge and for yoking research to advocacy, female and male social researchers in the female-led settlement-house movement were guided by a markedly different epistemology than was the male-dominated academy. At the very time that Progressive-Era leaders such as Lillian Wald, Grace Abbott, and Paul Kellogg, a reporter who became a leading social researcher and advocate for vulnerable groups, were forging the intimate links among good service, good data, and good government, most university-based social scientists of the Progressive Era, almost all of whom were men, were distancing themselves and their research from social reform movements. They were doing so in consonance with their increasing devotion to positivistic "scientism," Dorothy Ross's (1991) term for an approach to knowledge building that defined science only by its method. Natural scientific method rapidly became the sole standard of excellence in the emergent social sciences. Rather than creating a cluster of research methods that grew out of the particularities of the varied contexts, purposes, and constraints of social scientific discovery, academically based social scientists looked outside their own disciplines to the far older and more prestigious natural sciences (Ross, 1991). The carefully controlled conditions and procedural requirements of the chemist's or biologist's laboratory experiment became the model for investigation in social science.

Meanwhile, the women and the minority of men at Henry Street and other leading settlements, the U.S. Children's Bureau, and the emergent schools of social welfare took a decidedly different route to the construction of knowledge. They gathered quantitative and qualitative data about social problems in situ, that most uncontrolled of states. From home visits, physical examinations, clinical interviews, historical archives, neighborhood surveys, community studies, and the records of public schools, trade unions, municipal and county offices of vital statistics, immigration centers, and charity organization societies, settlers derived information about the everyday conditions and problems of the urban poor. At Henry Street, as at other major settlement houses, data rapidly were put to use in educational groups and courses with parents and adolescents, in discussions with adults and children during home visits and health examinations, in public health pamphlets, and in a cascade of formal testimonies and reports submitted to local, state, and federal officials, governing bodies, and public interest organizations.

The topics of Henry Street's research were as varied as the forms in which the findings were communicated to the public. The conditions of new immigrants, newborns, child laborers, older residents of the Lower East Side, "tuberculars," prostitutes, pregnant women, and juvenile delinquents were subjects of study, testimony, lobbying, and reporting by Henry Street residents. Between 1893 and 1920, Henry Street staff investigated, documented, and publicized the circumstances of mothers who were widows, women workers, the unemployed, workers in the garment trades, unvaccinated and vaccinated children, children with "mental defects," tenements, public schools, recreational sites, street sanitation, night courts, and factories (Chambers, 1986; Chambers, 1973; Coss, 1989; Davis, 1967; Muncy, 1991; Wald, 1915a; Wald, 1934; Woods and Kennedy, 1911; Woods and Kennedy, 1922).

Service provision, data collection, reportage, and advocacy were an interlocking quartet of activities that possessed, for Henry Street staff, an internal integrity that would have been flawed if any of the four functions had been missing. To collect data without providing service or vice versa was unthinkable. Also inconceivable was the prospect of collecting information about pressing social and psychological problems without spreading the word about their findings in the most vigorous manner possible to the public and to relevant governmental and voluntary bodies. It was equally unimaginable for them to testify or advocate without an authoritative database from which to draw generalizations and recommendations.

This settlement-house belief in the indissoluble interdependence of serving, researching, publicizing, and lobbying sprang primarily, in Robyn Muncy's (1991) words, from "a gender-specific need to reconcile their professional goals with Victorian ideals of womanhood" (p. 45). Since altruism had been their justification for moving women's "special virtues" into the public domain, service to others remained their basis for conducting research. As a consequence, a model of inquiry that separated knowledge development from service and politics was incompatible with their conception of womanhood, of female professionalism, of female citizenship, and of social feminism (Furner, 1975; Ross, 1979).

Cultural Diversity

For Henry Street staff, public service entailed far more than attention to the material necessities of life; it also required attentiveness to the cultural and aesthetic longings of their Lower East Side immigrant neighbors. Those longings, thought Wald and her staff, encompassed the entire spectrum of music, the arts, the language, and the crafts of neighbors' own countries of origin and of the heritage of Western Europe and the United States. Lillian Wald embedded in Henry Street's structure and repertoire of activities her double-barreled resistance to two movements which she despised: the Americanization movement of the second and third decade of the twentieth century and the effort to stratify the universe of the arts by removing "high" art from arenas of popular culture and from popular access.

"Great is our loss when a shallow Americanism is accepted by the newly arrived immigrant, more particularly by the children, and their national traditions and heroes are ruthlessly pushed aside," wrote Wald (1915, p. 303). To help prevent that loss of ethnic heritage, Wald consciously borrowed from Japan and Paris the tradition of cultural street fairs, instituting in 1913 a Fourth-of-July street festival and dance to commemorate the twentieth anniversary of Henry Street (Wald, 1915; Wald, 1934). Thousands of costumed people, representing dozens of racial and ethnic groups from New York City, took part in the street fair (Coss, 1989). It became an annual celebration along with other seasonal Henry Street Festivals held in the streets.

Classes for neighborhood children in drama, music, poetry, and dance were introduced in Henry Street's second decade of operation. In 1915, the Neighborhood Playhouse was formed at the Settlement, which became a nationally recognized arena for poetry readings and the production and performance of drama, music, and dance (Wald, 1915). Works created by neighbors of Henry Street; classical and experimental plays by well-known black, Jewish, Irish, Italian, and Hindu writers; and the works of Shakespeare, Whitman, Ibsen, Shaw, and Galsworthy were presented, earning, on many occasions, critical acclaim (Wald, 1915; Wald, 1934).

That Henry Street's mission encompassed "roses" as well as "bread" was partly an artifact of the continuity between Victorian conceptions and enactments of womanhood and those of Progressive-Era social feminism. One of the few areas of human knowledge to which nineteenth-century middle-class women in the United States had been exposed in a sustained way was that of literature, music, the arts, and the French language. Middle-class mothers were expected to educate their children in the fine arts and literature, as well as the Bible. Genteel womanliness in bourgeois families was demonstrated through women's performance of music, writing of poetry, and recitation of classical literature to family friends. A necessary emblem of social respectability for a husband was a home equipped with a piano or harp, a library, servants, and a wife whom he had freed from wage labor and some aspects of household labor so that she had sufficient time to raise cultured children and ornament the household with her own tasteful gentility (Berg, 1978; Sklar, 1973; Stansell, 1987).

The women who founded and shaped Henry Street Settlement had been raised in middle-class households during the decade following the Civil War. In their childhood and adolescence, literature and the arts had been fundamental sources of nourishment, exposure, and inspiration in an era that offered girls few avenues of exploration and expression. Wald and her Victorian-bred female colleagues carried with them into adult life a firsthand appreciation of the liberating force of the arts. In locating drama, dance, music, crafts, and art at the center of Henry Street's priorities, they merged their own personal knowledge of the freeing powers of cultural activity with a lesson learned from the socialism of Florence Kelley and others: that art is not a class-bound privilege, but instead is a universal resource and entitlement (Chambers, 1963; Sklar, 1986).

Serving the public by creating a more humane commonwealth, integrating social scientific research with service and advocacy, and melding cultural commitments with campaigns for social justice were the trinity of ambitions that drove Henry Street social feminists. Their underlying belief in the special capacities and responsibilities of women to salvage society constituted the cementing force of the community of believers at Henry Street for four decades.

Social Feminism's Influence at Henry Street: 1933-1993

In 1933, ill health forced the sixty-seven-year-old Lillian Wald to retire as Henry Street's head worker, a position she had held for forty years. Before resigning, Wald recruited her own successor. She selected Helen Hall, a social worker and social activist who had attended the New York School for Social Work (now the Columbia University School of Social Work); organized a settlement in Westchester

County, New York; performed relief work in France, Alsace, the Philippines, and China during World War I; and served as head worker for eleven years at University House, a settlement in Philadelphia (Hall, 1971; Trolander, 1975).

Wald had managed the nearly impossible—she had found for Henry Street a successor who would quickly prove to be as much of a social reform visionary, community servant, and national leader as she herself had been. Within the first year of her leadership at Henry Street, Helen Hall became a leading national voice for federal relief programs, testifying and lobbying in Washington, DC, for cash relief, federal employment projects and insurance, and for legal protections against evictions for the unemployed (Trolander, 1975). From 1935 through 1940, she served as president of the National Federation of Settlements and Neighborhood Centers, a body whose vigorous and informed advocacy helped accelerate the onset and expand the scope of New Deal employment and Social Security programs.

In 1935, Hall married Paul U. Kellogg, the editor since 1912 of the *Survey*, a widely read publication of the Russell Sage Foundation that explored social welfare and social policy issues, social movements of disenfranchised people, and campaigns for human rights. Hall's predecessor, Lillian Wald, considered Kellogg her "old friend and comrade in numerous adventures" (Wald, 1934, p. x). Kellogg moved into Henry Street where his new wife, Head Worker Hall, already was in residence. There they resided together for a quarter century until Kellogg's death in 1958.

Throughout their marriage and after it, Hall led the Henry Street Settlement through multiple phases of its existence, in which she and her staff pioneered and tested out a variety of community services, social reform strategies, and community arts programs that came to be recognized nationally as prototypical social and cultural experiments. During the years of her leadership, Henry Street conducted numerous studies of housing, unemployment, and gang patterns; created a neighborhood credit union in 1937; a community mental hygiene clinic in 1941; the Predelinquent Gang Project in 1955; the Lower Eastside Neighborhoods Association in 1954; and Mobilization for Youth in 1959, which soon became the model for the next decade's federal antipoverty programs (Hall, 1971). Hall's leadership also ensured the continuation of community-based experimental theater at Henry Street and the creation and licensing of Alwin Nikolais'

Dance School and the Henry Street Settlement Music School, under the direction of Grace Spofford, former dean of the Curtis Institute of Music (Hall, 1971).

In her thirty-four years as head worker, Helen Hall's code of citizenship for herself and her settlement resembled closely that of Lillian Wald. She insisted upon involving the settlement in incessant and multiform public service; in ongoing data collection that served as the basis for the formulation and modification of federal, state, and local legislation and regulations; and in the sustenance and multiplication of the settlement's major cultural projects.

Yet these three forms of citizenship that were concocted originally by turn-of-the-century social feminists endured long after the core beliefs which had inspired their formation died. Notions of the moral superiority and special strengths of women did not survive in the written discourse or recorded speeches of the post-Wald era at Henry Street. Nor did articulation of the desirability of women's "mothering" society. Helen Hall, in her retrospective account of her work at Henry Street, *Unfinished Business in Neighborhood and Nation,* described herself from age ten on as a "passionate adherent of women's suffrage" (Hall, 1971, p. 5). Nonetheless, she made no other reference to social feminism or any other form of feminism in her 354-page book that is otherwise replete with references to important social causes, such as the fight against red-baiting, the formation of unemployed councils in the 1930s, and the importance of working toward racial equity and equality (Hall, 1971).

Maternalism, social feminism, and, more generally, feminism itself vanished as coherent and explicit ideologies at Henry Street after Wald, just as they did in the public at large during the exigencies of the Great Depression and the fragmented and attenuated phase of the U.S. women's movement in the 1940s and 1950s (Cott, 1987; Ferree and Hess, 1985). Belief in women's special ability and responsibility to reform the commonwealth held little appeal to a generation of voting women who were fully engaged, alongside men, in New Deal reforms or socialist or communist activities. Maternalist strains of social feminist thought, especially, had outlived their usefulness and were perceived as relics of a bygone era. Notions of women's particular aptitudes appeared old-fashioned and "unscientific" to reform or revolution-minded women and men of the 1930s, who were busy staffing the burgeoning programs and professions of the expanding welfare state (Koven and Michel, 1990).

By the time of Wald's retirement in 1933, widespread unemployment, homelessness, and hunger preoccupied the settlement house staff at Henry Street. Gender-linked rights, disadvantage, suffering, and injustice disappeared as salient categories of professional concern there until the early 1970s, except for the hard and sustained work that Helen Hall and her staff put into the creation of child-care centers for working mothers during and after World War II (Hall, 1971). Nonetheless, one element of social feminism did endure at Henry Street: the three-tiered version of citizenship that had so passionately consumed the energies of Lillian Wald, Mary Brewster, and Florence Kelley.

Henry Street During the Past Quarter Century

If Lillian Wald could return to evaluate Henry Street today, would she find her code of citizenship still honored in daily practice by its staff? Is, for example, public service still a principle commitment of Henry Street, and are data collected in the course of serving neighbors that are used in campaigns for social reforms? The record suggests clear evidence that these first and second planks of Wald's ethos of citizenship remain intact.

For example, staff members' desire to reduce homelessness and wife battering led them in 1972 to establish Henry Street's Urban Family Center, a model transitional shelter for housing approximately 90 homeless families and battered women in temporary individual apartments in six buildings, each with a live-in social worker who offers vocational, educational, and personal counseling. While at the Center, individuals and families obtain job training, independent-living skills, and basic education. For two decades, Henry Street has succeeded in moving 95 percent of its families in the Urban Family Center into permanent housing (Simpson, 1987).

In working at the Urban Family Center, staff members gather information from residents and from their own experiences about the causes and familial consequences of urban homelessness and the range of economic, psychological, and social supports people need to regain their own homes and jobs. With this information, Henry Street staff devised the Shelter Management Training Program, which educates social workers in homeless shelters from other parts of the country to move people from homelessness into stable independence. Data collected from the Urban Family Center are also used in testimony and official reports submitted to city, state, and federal authorities.

Henry Street also took early action in response to the AIDS epidemic. Its Community Consultation Center, a state-certified mental health clinic, is an official provider of AIDS mental health services for the Lower East Side of Manhattan and has pioneered in developing a counseling and bereavement program for children whose parents have AIDS (Henry Street Settlement, 1990).

As is true in its work with homeless families and battered women, the staff of Henry Street's Community Consultation Center view adult and child clients as important sources of information about the nature, scope, and effects of the AIDS epidemic. In keeping with Wald's earlier efforts against tuberculosis, influenza, and unsanitary milk for infants, Henry Street staff members rely on their experiences as service deliverers and advocates on the Lower East Side to guide their involvement in international, national, and local health campaigns to slow and stop the spread of AIDS.

Public service, research, and advocacy also go on in relation to other key populations. Mobile and homebound older residents of the Lower East Side, pregnant teens, adolescents who have left school, preschool-age children, illiterate adults, children in foster care, and unemployed single mothers are a partial listing of the continuum of groups engaged by Henry Street programs, studies, and lobbying.

Finally, Wald would wonder, does Henry Street sustain its commitment to the arts in the neighborhood? The Gallery at Henry Street's Louis Abrons Arts Center won its fourth national grant from the Institute of Museum Services in 1991. The Gallery has used its four awards to expand its outreach to families, children, and elders (Henry Street Settlement, 1991).

Henry Street's Playhouse, Music Program, and Arts Center continue to sponsor classes, workshops, exhibitions, and productions in opera, theater, dance, visual arts, and music. The Master Arts Series promotes the work of little-known but mature artists through its career retrospectives. In 1991, the Settlement's Folk Art Series sponsored an Asian-American Outreach Program, a five-week festival of Chinese-American arts and crafts. Additionally, Henry Street's Arts-in-Education program exposes 15,000 children each year in surrounding community school districts to arts education in their own classrooms. (Henry Street Settlement, 1990). It would appear that Wald's requirement concerning a settlement house's cultural responsibility to its surrounding community is being honored in full.

CONCLUSION

In a 1915 address at Vassar College, Lillian Wald declared:

> The roots of public social service and responsibility are deeply planted in the nature of woman and what we are witnessing in our generation are the new manifestations of her unchanged and unchanging interests and devotions.
> Her circle of human experience and human feeling has widened. . . . She is capable of doing more, of being more than at any time. (Wald, 1915b [reprinted in Coss 1989, p. 84])

It was woman's nature, Wald believed, to serve more than her family; the whole of humankind required her attentions and talents. The first third of the one-hundred-year history of the Henry Street Settlement serves as detailed testimony to the catalytic force of gender consciousness among Progressive-Era social feminists. Their shared faith in the romance of women's particular inborn worth inspired them to build enduring institutions of service, reform, and culture against significant odds.

Wald's conception of maternalist feminism has long been abandoned by most feminists and most social workers, even as her version of feminist citizenship continues to form the bedrock of many contemporary projects and agencies. Her essentialist premise, that women are innately superior to men in their facility for caring for others, has been discounted in many quarters as an artifact of a Victorian past that was contorted by gender-segregated spheres and roles. Nonetheless, maternalist feminism of the social constructionist variety has grown up in place of essentialist maternalism during the past two decades of resurgent feminism. Not women's genetic makeup, but industrialized cultures' gendered forms of child rearing and women's daily rounds of parenting, caregiving, and befriending have developed in them a greater capacity and sense of responsibility for nurturance than most men have developed, claim Jean Baker Miller (1986), Nancy Chodorow (1978; 1989), Carol Gilligan (1982; 1990), Nel Noddings (1984), and many others. The practice of mothering, with its particular activities, aims, and requirements, has created a way of thinking and knowing that is distinctly "maternal," Sara Ruddick suggests (Ruddick, 1989).

Contemporary feminist social workers have cast a wide net throughout the humanities, the social and behavioral sciences, and the multidisciplinary world of women's studies in their search for knowledge that will help them make sense of the marked and sustained differences between the behavioral proclivities and life chances of men and boys as a group and those of women and girls as a group. Whether working with single teenage mothers on welfare, aged widows, battered women, or incest survivors, social workers who are attempting to assist women and girl clients in restoring and empowering themselves are doing so with the help of multiple "feminist frameworks" of analysis (Bricker-Jenkins, Hooyman, and Gottlieb, 1991; Jaggar and Rothenberg, 1984). These varied paradigms through which to view relations between women and men are products of a turbulent contemporary women's movement and an equally turbulent domain of women's studies in the academy, whose participants have come to understand the salience of the intersections of gender, race, age, class, sexuality, religion, and disability in shaping the meanings, constraints, and choices in women's daily lives.

Yet despite feminist social workers' wide-ranging pursuit of intellectual and political inspirations for their work and despite earnest efforts to draw on the strengths of female clients and colleagues, one major resource is commonly overlooked. Neglected is the rich history of prior social work with women. Neglected is the wealth of example provided by women clients of earlier eras who have sought to overcome abandonment, psychological depression, poverty, sexually transmitted diseases, alcoholism, and myriad other difficulties.

To study the history of women is, in part, to excavate the traditions of surviving, healing, resisting, enduring, and transforming that women clients and women social workers have accrued over time in response to every imaginable kind of internal and external challenge. Some of the dreams, visions, and plans of our predecessors are still accessible to those of us who would look. Also retrievable are some of their strategies, interventive approaches, and methods of framing, assessing, and solving problems. The nature, scope, and causes of their major failures as well as their memorable successes as clients and as workers are still available to us in varying degrees. Some of their assumptions, ideas, and philosophies can be recovered.

However, it is important to ask, why take the trouble to do so? Why, in the midst of the exigencies of responding to clients' escalating crises, stop to look back at the workers and clients of a different era? Why discuss Lillian Wald's perspectives on women, service, knowledge building, and cultural diversity in a historical moment in which the AIDS epidemic, homelessness, the impoverishment of women, violence, and unemployment preoccupy us and the clients to whom we are accountable?

We look back in order to increase the visibility of women's leadership and of women's paid and unpaid labor. We look back in order to decrease clients' sense of isolation and marginalization by making more available to them the accounts of others who have faced and negotiated similar circumstances in the past. Perhaps most importantly, we look back in order to replenish the reservoir of our imagination, courage, and hopefulness, three elements that undoubtedly will prove as indispensable to social work practice in the new century as they have during the nineteenth and twentieth.

REFERENCES

Abramovitz, M. (1988). *Regulating the lives of women.* Boston: South End Press.

Berg, B. J. (1978). *The remembered gate: Origins of American feminism, the woman and the city, 1800-1860.* New York: Oxford University Press.

Bordin, R. (1990). *Women and temperance: The quest for power and liberty,* Second edition. New Brunswick, NJ: Rutgers University Press.

Bricker-Jenkins, M., Hooyman, N., and Gottlieb, N. (Eds.) (1991). *Feminist social work practice in clinical settings.* Newbury Park, CA: Sage.

Chambers, C. A. (1963). *Seedtime of reform: American social service and social action, 1918-1933.* Minneapolis: University of Minnesota Press.

Chambers, C. A. (1973). *Paul U. Kellogg and the survey: Voices for social welfare and social justice.* Minneapolis: University of Minnesota Press.

Chambers, C. A. (1986). Women in the creation of the profession of social work. *Social Service Review, 60: 1-33.*

Chodorow, N. (1978). *The reproduction of mothering.* Berkeley: University of California Press.

Chodorow, N. (1989). *Feminism and psychoanalytic theory.* New Haven: Yale University Press.

Cohen, M. and Hanagan, M. (1991). The politics of gender and the making of the welfare state, 1900-1940: A comparative perspective. *Journal of Social History, 24:* 469-484.

Combs-Orme, T. (1988). Infant mortality and social work: Legacy of success. *Social Service Review, 62:* 83-102.

Cort, J. C. (1988). *Christian socialism: An informal history.* Maryknoll, NY: Orbis.

Coss, C. (Ed.) (1989). *Lillian D. Wald: Progressive activist.* New York: Feminist Press at the City University of New York.

Cott, N. F. (1987). *The grounding of modern feminism.* New Haven: Yale University Press.

Cott, N. F. (1989). What's in a name? The limits of "Social Feminism"; or, Expanding the vocabulary of women's history. *Journal of American History, 76:* 809-929.

Davis, A. F. (1967). *Spearheads for reform: The social settlements and the progressive movement, 1890-1914.* New York: Oxford University Press.

Ferree, M. and Hess, B. (1985). *Controversy and coalition: The new feminist movement.* Boston: Twayne.

Furner, M. O. (1975). *Advocacy and objectivity: A crisis in the professionalization of American social science, 1865-1905.* Lexington, KY: University of Kentucky Press.

Gilligan, C. (1982). *In a different voice: Psychological theory and women's development.* Cambridge, MA: Harvard University Press.

Gilligan, C. (1990). *Mapping the moral domain.* Cambridge, MA: Harvard University Press.

Gordon, L. (1976). *Woman's body, woman's rights.* New York: Penguin.

Gordon, L. (1990). Putting children first: U.S. welfarism in the 20th century. Paper presented at Columbia University Institute for Research on Women and Gender, November 9, Conference on Work and Family Policy.

Hall, H. (1971). *Unfinished business in neighborhood and nation.* New York: Macmillan.

Handy, R. T. (Ed.) (1966). *The social gospel in America, 1870-1920.* New York: Oxford University Press.

Henry Street Settlement (1990). *Biennial report.* New York: Henry Street Settlement.

Henry Street Settlement (1991). *News from Henry Street.* New York: Henry Street Settlement.

Hewitt, N. A. (1984). *Women's activism and social change: Rochester, New York, 1822-1872.* Ithaca, New York: Cornell University Press.

Jaggar, A. and Rothenberg, P. (1984). *Feminist frameworks: Alternative theoretical accounts of the relations between women and men,* Second edition. New York: McGraw-Hill.

Katz, M. B. (1986). *In the shadow of the poorhouse.* New York: Basic Books.

Kelley, F. (1923). Should women be treated identically with men by the law? *American Review, 3:* 277.

Kerber, L. (1980). *Women of the Republic: Intellect and ideology in Revolutionary America.* Chapel Hill, NC: University of North Carolina Press.

Koven, S. and Michel, S. (1990). Womanly duties: Maternalist policies and the origins of welfare states in France, Germany, and the United States, 1880-1920. *American Historical Review, 95:* 1076-1108.

Leiby, J. (1978). *A history of social welfare and social work in the United States.* New York: Columbia University Press.

Miller, J. B. (1986). *Toward a new psychology of women,* Second edition. Boston: Beacon.

Muncy, R. (1991). *Creating a female dominion in American reform, 1890-1935.* New York: Oxford University Press.

Noddings, N. (1984). *Caring.* Berkeley: University of California Press.

Rendall, J. (1990). *The origins of modern feminism: Women in Britain, France, and the United States, 1780-1860,* Second edition. Chicago: Lyceum.

Ross, D. (1979). The development of the social sciences. In A. Loeson and J. Voss, (Eds.), *The organization of knowledge in modern America, 1860-1920* (pp. 107-138). Baltimore: Johns Hopkins University Press.

Ross, D. (1991). *The origins of American social science.* New York: Cambridge University Press.

Ruddick, S. (1989). *Maternal thinking.* New York: Ballantine.

Simpson, J. C. (1987). Enduring service: A 'Settlement House' has new constituency but same old mission. *The Wall Street Journal, 209,* January 23, 16, 1 and 11.

Sklar, K. K. (1973). *Catharine Beecher: A study in American domesticity.* New Haven: Yale University Press.

Sklar, K. K. (1985). Hull House in the 1890's: A community of women reformers. *Signs, 10:* 658-677.

Sklar, K. K. (Ed.) (1986). Introduction. *Notes of sixty years: The autobiography of Florence Kelley* (pp. 25-30). Chicago: University of Chicago Press.

Smith-Rosenberg, C. (1971). *Religion and the rise of the American city.* Ithaca, NY: Cornell University Press.

Smith-Rosenberg, C. (1975). The female world of love and ritual: Relations among women in nineteenth-century America. *Signs, 1:* 1-29.

Stansell, C. (1987). *City of women: Sex and class in New York, 1789-1860.* Urbana, IL: University of Illinois Press.

Teller, M. E. (1988). *The tuberculosis movement.* New York: Greenwood.

Trolander, J. A. (1975). *Settlement houses and the Great Depression.* Detroit: Wayne State University Press.

Wald, L. (1914). Suffrage. (Speech of February 1914.) In Coss, C. (Ed.) (1989), *Lillian Wald* (pp. 74-76). New York: Feminist Press.

Wald, L. (1915a). *The house on Henry Street.* New York: Henry Holt.

Wald, L. (1915b). New aspects of old responsibilities. (Address to Vassar College students of October 12, 1915.) In Coss, C. (Ed.) (1989), *Lillian D. Wald, Progressive activist* (pp. 76-84). New York: The Feminist Press at the City University of New York.

Wald, L. (1934). *Windows on Henry Street.* Boston: Little, Brown.

Welter, B. (1966). The cult of true womanhood, 1820-1860. *American Quarterly, 18:* 151-174.

Woods, R. A. and Kennedy, A. J. (Eds.) (1911). *Handbook of settlements.* New York: Russell Sage.

Woods, R. A. and Kennedy A. J. (1922). *The settlement horizon: A national estimate.* New York: Russell Sage.

Chapter 3

What Is Needed for True Equality: An Overview of Policy Issues for Women

Dorothy C. Miller

What we can't imagine, we can't come to be. (hooks, 1989, p. 176)

INTRODUCTION

Less than ten years ago, when the first volume of this book was published, society seemed closer at least to wanting to know what was needed for "true equality." Today, the word "equality" has entered the realm of passé language, something "retro" that the media, at least, have jettisoned. The media report Mick Jagger, twentieth-century icon personified, as saying, "There's nothing wrong with a bit of sexism. Just as long as it's not overwhelming" (*Wichita Eagle*, 2000). Easy for a multibillionaire to say, adored by women everywhere for reasons other than his personal philosophy. But many women, from all walks of life, agree. The most effective antifeminist weapons used to be ridicule and stonewalling. Now one simply needs to frame feminist aspirations or complaints as unfashionable or tedious. After all, things *have* "gotten better" for women. So, what is the problem?

Modern feminist leaders recognized in the mid-1960s that for true equality between men and women to exist, men had to accept a central role in caring for children and women had to play a central role in providing for their upkeep. In 1966, NOW's Statement of Purpose called for "a true partnership between the sexes," including a "different concept of marriage, an equitable sharing of the responsibilities of home and children and of the economic burdens of their support" (Harrison, 1988, 56). Almost forty years later, we have fallen short of achieving that goal, which is fundamental to true equality.

Today, U.S. women are still expected to do most of the housework and child care while they are *also* bringing home paychecks. Single parents are expected to do likewise and blamed for not having the husbands to help them financially and otherwise. Meanwhile, women are presumed to have limitless choices in the job market and in life. Criticisms of toys with gender labels are simply considered "politically correct," an opprobrium to be feared, and the critics viewed as ignorant of either sociobiological forces and/or a true understanding of what most women want. Barriers to education, job success, marital success, and maternal bliss are hidden in the interstices of bureaucratic behavior and the framing of popular culture. Furthermore, even as women are performing two shifts of work per day while bringing home unfair wages, they must also watch their backs. Violence against women, still culturally pervasive, is either ignored or portrayed as bizarrely and particularly unusual. Underlying all else, the prevailing cultural ideal is the pursuit of wealth; anyone who does not obtain it must be viewed as proportionately inadequate. This resurgence of social Darwinism, strangely bolstered by right-wing religious tenets, prevails, just as it did one hundred years ago. Such is the backdrop to the social policy spectrum at the dawn of the twenty-first century.

Behind the policy scenes, so to speak, one can examine why some social trends have resulted in progress and others have not. Theorists Gelb and Palley (1987) submit that policy proposals that imply role equity are more likely to be politically acceptable than those that are thought to promote "role change." Thus, "equal pay for equal work," a role-equity issue, makes sense to our democratic society's notion of fairness. Affordable and accessible child care, on the other hand, may be seen as promoting unwanted role changes among women (Gelb and Palley, 1987).

From this perspective, feminist social workers and policy analysts face a dilemma as they look to achieve equality-based policy changes. Policies that would ensure true equality for women often suggest changes in women's and men's roles and are consequently threatening to society. Gelb and Palley have described how feminist advocates have downplayed the role-change aspects of policies in order to achieve political acceptance. Indeed, the changes that have been achieved, at least on paper, tend to promote role equity. The more difficult role-change issues, centered on family, have been stalled. As society becomes more sensitive to feminist concerns, it will be increasingly difficult to obscure the role-change implications of needed policies. Instead, feminists will have to bear the burden of proof that role-change policies would in fact be beneficial also to men and children and would build a better society.

In this chapter, I address several fundamental issues that cut across social policy and social work practice initiatives for women and children in the United States. These include family as it intersects with race, class, and gender imperatives; women's economic well-being; and the continuing threat of violence against women. I examine aspects of these issues that are often ignored or denied because they threaten mainstream gender-role ideology or, for advocates, seem so insurmountable that they must be accepted as the "status quo." Yet they produce a climate that makes it hard to move forward. Feminist social workers must include the social and political context of American life in our discourse in order to better understand the opposition to policy proposals that suggest gender-role changes. A vision for the future requires clarity about what constitutes desirable change versus what incremental changes are acceptable for now.

FAMILY, GENDER, AND CLASS

Politicians continue to play to the needs of the wealthy, white, heterosexual nuclear family, ignoring or punishing families who do not fit this structure. With few exceptions, existing public policies and reform proposals continue to use the traditional nuclear family as the basic unit of concern. The need to preserve existing two-parent families and promote their formation is a constant theme among policy analysts and in the popular press. In addition, increasing benefits to the wealthy has become an assumed but unacknowledged prerequisite for Congressional consideration of most proposed family and tax policies.

Social Security is perhaps the social welfare program most heavily invested in the traditional family structure. It continues to favor married couples with one large income over couples with the same total income earned equally by both spouses. This antiquated policy privileges rich families with wives out of the labor market and penalizes lower-class families that require the labors of two people to achieve the same income. The "standard of living" for the latter family may well be less because of the time involved with juggling two careers and the demands of home. Yet even as the system favors one-earner families, women's work at home is not valued or even acknowledged. Homemakers cannot receive disability benefits. Moreover, women who take time out of the labor force to care for children and/or elderly relatives are penalized.

The system is designed to favor workers whose lifetime work patterns, namely forty years of continual full-time midlevel employment, resemble those of white males (Miller, 1990). Aside from the spousal retirement and employment rules, dependents' benefits are restricted to spouses and children. As a consequence, nontraditional families, low-income families, and many people of color, whose adult work lives are likely to be interrupted with layoffs and unemployment, are less well served by the system. Neither does welfare provide a safety net for those falling through the cracks of Social Security.

The Personal Responsibility and Work Opportunity Reconciliation Act (PRWORA) was signed into law in August 1996. This law created our current welfare program, the Temporary Assistance for Needy Families (TANF) program, which replaced Aid to Families with Dependent Children in 1997. The statute, among other things, provides states with money to be used to reduce out-of-wedlock births without increasing the rate of abortion (House of Representatives, *Green Book,* 1998, p. 509). Less money is being spent on economic development and more on "incentives" for behavioral change. Always difficult, humiliating, and inadequate, now the system is even less of a "safety net" but still a mechanism of social control. It attempts to get poor people to conform more to ideal family models without any related attempt to aid these families' ties to the rewards of the middle-class work world.

With the notable exception of the food stamp program, the availability of assistance to a person in need is usually related to the structure of the person's family and the history and current labor force attachment of a family member. For example, children of deceased fathers who were gainfully employed receive Social Security survivor's benefits. (This policy is "gender neutral" in that it applies as well to children of deceased mothers. However, in reality, most beneficiaries are women and children.) These benefits are much more generous than those provided by the means-tested welfare system, TANF, still mostly available to poor children whose fathers are living but absent, unemployed, or who died without having been covered by Social Security. Thus, a needy child's family circumstances, and not need alone, determine the adequacy of the benefit she or he receives.

Shaping social policies with the family as the centerpiece favors the upper classes and places constraints on people's behavior toward and expectations of one another, encoding the primacy of family caregiving in upper-class women's lives while ignoring it among the poor. Underlying these policy perspectives is an effort to maintain traditional gender roles and class privileges. Thus, marriage incentives and divorce disincentives, school vouchers, subsidies for private schools, and tax breaks for stay-at-home mother two-parent families favor the middle and upper classes while doing little for the working class and the poor. Poor women with children are encouraged to look to marriage rather than welfare as the answer to their economic problems. Help in maintaining the families they already have—themselves and their children—is not forthcoming.

The ideal of a good mother has shifted from one who stays at home all the time. However, the new ideal is a woman who arranges for child care, including expenses and transportation, continues to be the more nurturing parent, and does almost all of the housework, in addition to bringing home a paycheck that adds to, but does not replace, her husband's. She has a job with flexible hours and leave policies so that she can pick the children up when they are sick and/or attend school functions when necessary. She also has either occupational mobility or a lack of ambition sufficient enough to allow her to move to another city should her husband be transferred.

Like many ideals, this one does not fit the reality of most people's lives. Almost three in ten children live with only one of their parents. Eighty-five percent of custodial parents are women. About thirty percent of these families are poor (Census Bureau, 1999). These families rely on one income, one adult's labor, and have to deal with the inconvenience, poor city services, and safety risks related to living in a poor neighborhood, all of which make the single parent's job even harder.

Current policy debates regarding one-parent families have recently focused exclusively on the ill effects of single-parent families and the importance of the mother's employment to provide "role models" of industriousness and self-sufficiency for her children. Policymakers give the nurturing care of children a top priority only when those children are in middle-and upper-income families. For the lower classes, employment, regardless of the effect of a parent's employment upon her children, is uppermost. The only benefit to children that is universally applauded is education, which of course is directly tied to their eventual ability to get a job and benefits middle-class children the most.

good point

At best, woman-headed families are tolerated as stemming from an unfortunate happenstance that must be set right. At worst, women are flagrantly defying beneficent social norms to the detriment of their children, who lack the "stabilizing" influence of a husband and father. Although some families may feel this way about themselves, it hardly helps children's self-esteem to see themselves constantly depicted as hopelessly lost without fathers. It can also serve as a self-fulfilling prophecy. Note that in the face of violence and drug abuse among poor teenage boys, one hears literally nothing from professionals or the media about encouraging these boys to listen to their mothers. Social critics lament the existence of so many teen boys without fathers while at the same time sending a strong message that their mothers are incapable of disciplining them adequately. It is no wonder that we observe boys in fatherless homes become unmanageable.

Within families, women and children are often victims, rather than beneficiaries, of fathers and husbands. The Bureau of Justice Statistics (1995) estimates that a woman is assaulted every nine seconds in the United States and is six times more likely to be physically assaulted by her husband than by a stranger. About 4 million women are battered each year by intimate partners and some 2,000 of them die as a result (Busch and Valentine, 2000). Yet a chorus of citizens, media. and policy analysts is saying that boys need fathers to make them law-abiding and nonviolent.

The NOW message of the 1960s, which included role changes for both men and women, has effectively been distorted by antifeminists who claim that the early women's movement was solely concerned with careers for women. In fact, most activists in the women's movement have maintained the position that men's involvement and sincere adoption of responsibility for children's overall welfare, without its patriarchal trimmings, would be of enormous help to children in our culture. (It is possible to take this position without contending that families without fathers or without mothers are hopelessly deficient and abnormal.) We would come a long way toward true equality if men were equally responsible for children. Questions about children's care would have deeper meaning to all those male legislators currently ignorant about how it is that children (even their own) are cared for and raised—namely, the vast amounts of time, money, effort, and attention it requires. Such a change would certainly not eliminate all of the economic class issues plaguing the United States, but, because of the children involved, it might help mediate them.

Social service systems, as well as income maintenance policies, ignore the help that extended families and friends give to one another and discourage those (especially those in white society) who might help but see such help as socially unacceptable. We not only assign caregiving responsibilities to women, but we want them to carry out these responsibilities in conventional family systems. Policies that would encourage all adults in society to participate in child care and child rearing are nonexistent, placing the full responsibility (and burden) on the nuclear family or substitute nuclear families. Permanency planning for foster children, while beneficial to alleviating the uncertainty that foster children experience, is geared to deciding once and for all who the child belongs to rather than, for example, providing for shared caring according to caregiver capacity.

If the adoption system were really devoted to helping the children, surely the children most in need would go to the families considered best equipped to help them—families with resources such as a full-time mother and a comfortable income. Paradoxically, patriarchy is upheld through the reward system of giving infants only to families with acceptable structures, while special needs children are available to single persons. Children's needs are subsumed in the interests of institutionalized family arrangements, precluding more creative conceptualizations.

Day care's impact on children is also a threat to traditional notions of family and motherhood. Meyer suggests that day care introduces to children a more expanded sense of socialization and sharing, acceptance of the "population mix of their society," and a different understanding of care and protection. "It is the feminist perspective that allows for a different kind of understanding of day care through its redefinition of the rigid and stereotyped boundaries of the idea of parenting or mothering" (Meyer 1985, pp. 253-254). It may be this underlying meaning of day care that helps to stifle its comfortable acceptance and support in American life.

In sum, the lack of alternatives to women's care of children within the traditional nuclear family structure forces women to make choices that involve a competition between their own and their children's well-being. Children are hostages to women's achievement of equality. To middle-class women, society is essentially saying, "OK, if you want equality, you will have to destroy your children's lives. Do you really want that?" To the poor, it says, "Everything is up to you. Too bad for your children." Formulating children's policies in the context of family policies perpetuates and exacerbates this dilemma for women because it continues to place on mothers, both poor and well off, primary and almost exclusive responsibility for children's well-being.

New Directions: Policies for Families, Lovers, Friends, and Children

A truly inclusive framework for public policy would both acknowledge and encourage caregiving behavior among all persons regardless of family ties. For example, child and elder care provided by friends could be recognized in the tax system. Tax credits could benefit persons who leave the labor force to care for other people's children, ailing relatives and friends, or people dying of AIDS. Such policies would encourage all adults in society to participate in child rearing and well elderly people to help care for infirm elderly. The new policies would promote community interdependence among persons, groups, and extended families.

Such a framework would help people who are living with AIDS and being cared for by partners and friends. It would also adapt to needs in African-American communities, where extended family as well as "fictive kin"—persons considered family but who are not related by blood—have always been important to family care and household tasks (Amott and Matthaei, 1991; National Research Council, 1990; Joseph and Lewis, 1981; McAdoo, 1980; Stack, 1974). The Social Security caregiver provisions could be expanded to include extended families, gay men and lesbians, nonmarried heterosexual couples, and friends who care for and about each other. There are all sorts of ways to think about how we care for each other and to provide help for caring behavior and policies that serve to enhance the possibilities of care.

An alternative to the construction of foster care as a " 'pretend' natural family home" was conceptualized by Meyer (1985), who suggested that foster parents need not be mothers but can be staff members in placements in neighborhoods where the children live, allowing free visiting with their mothers, family, and friends, avoiding the traumatic separations from home, school, and all things familiar. This would replace the common practice of removing children from their poor urban neighborhoods and placing them in middle-class suburban homes, a classist rescue operation that makes it even harder to return the children to their families. The adoption system could assign the care of children to more than one family or attempt to form caring networks for the care of children with many needs. Children most in need could be attended to by clusters of caring adults who might be seen as extending in a circle outward from "core" parents.

If day care were improved and expanded, children growing up in day care might come to accept as commonplace the notion that a variety of persons can offer love, protection, and educational experiences to children. If one considers that day care might usher in a new conception of what it means to be a mother, it is not surprising that a great deal of the research on day care has focused on whether it causes damage to the mother-child bond. In fact, research has shown that children's bonds with their parents are not disturbed by day care, and day care need not be deleterious to children's growth and development, depending on the quality of the specific care provided (Rutter, 1982).

WOMEN'S EMPLOYMENT AND ECONOMIC WELL-BEING

Women's economic well-being in the United States can best be described as precarious among both the poor and the middle class. Women are at a higher risk of poverty than men because they make less money than men and because they are primarily responsible for the care of their children. Most poor people in the United States are women and children in single-parent families. Almost one in every three black and Hispanic children lives in poverty (House of Representatives, *Green Book,* 1998, p. 1303). Child poverty in the United States is higher than in most industrialized nations, including Canada and most Western European nations (Center on Budget and Policy Priorities, 1999). Eighteen percent of children in the United States live in poverty-level households. More than half of all children under age six in mother-only families are poor (Census Bureau, 1999, p. viii). Yet we are doing little in the United States to alleviate this condition.

As mentioned above, Temporary Assistance to Needy Families (TANF) is the major cash-assistance (welfare) program in the United States for families with children. About 90 percent of TANF recipients are single mothers and their children. Although the average amount of time a family spends on welfare is less than two years, many people who escape welfare do not escape poverty (House of Representatives, *Green Book,* 1998, p. 534). Benefit levels are set by the state legislatures and vary considerably. In July 1997, monthly state payments for a family of three with no other income ranged from $120 a month in Mississippi to $923 in Alaska. The median payment was $379 (House of Representatives, *Green Book,* 1998, p. 524-525). TANF payments nationally are more than 40 percent lower today than they were in 1970, taking inflation into account (House of Representatives, *Green Book,* 1998). TANF provides much less financial help per person than welfare programs for the poor elderly and disabled. Unemployment insurance and Social Security payments are also much higher. These other programs include automatic benefit increases to keep up with the cost of living. TANF is not only insufficient but, as designed, indeed temporary.

The new TANF program increased the requirements for work participation among welfare recipients and established a five-year family lifetime limit of welfare receipt regardless of the parents' job situation or good-faith effort to be employed or find a job. Studies of the initial stages of the program have found that most of those who left the welfare rolls were working in jobs that paid below poverty level. Less than half reported using child-care assistance (Schumacher and Greenberg, 1999). In addition, food stamp use, especially among children, has declined. A study by the General Accounting Office (1999) found that at least some of this decline is due to state and local government negligence with regard to imparting information to clients and/or abrogating eligibility rules. There has been no stir among the general public about this. These families, disproportionately made up of people of color in mother-only families, have, in the public's view, no moral right to their legal benefits.

The previous (and fairly recent) round of "welfare reform," the Family Support Act of 1988, was billed as the expression of a "new consensus" in *The New York Times* (Stevens, 1988). This law added significantly more work-related requirements to the AFDC program. This legislation was the result of several years' debates about welfare reform that commenced with the presidential election of Ronald Reagan. It was based on the view, characterized by Lawrence Mead's (1986) *Beyond Entitlement: The Social Obligations of Citizenship,* that welfare benefits should not simply be a handout but should be given as one side of a "social contract," whereby the government expects work efforts in exchange for benefits. Such sentiment was supposedly behind the Reagan administration's encouragement in the early 1980s of demonstration projects in which women on AFDC were required to participate in job search, training, or education programs in exchange for their welfare checks.

In the first edition of this book (Miller, 1994), I criticized the Family Support Act because it was based on research that represented, in my opinion, little evidence that the program would work. I criticized the built-in assumption that families could live on women's wages, produced through low-paying jobs into which the program was funneling women via vocational education and "job search" activities. I said ". . .feminist policy analysts and social workers must make the connections between women's poverty, their family roles, and labor force discrimination. The JOBS program is entirely focused on the individual, ignoring the fact that the jobs out there for women will not offer them subsistence" (Miller, 1994, p. 47). Little did I know that ten years later I would mourn several components of JOBS.

TANF constitutes a "work first" philosophy that denies women opportunities to obtain education or training, forces them into the labor force regardless of the wages they can expect to make, removes the entitlement feature of public assistance to families with children, and places a five-year family lifetime limit on welfare receipt. What I said then, and can still say, about this newest welfare reform is that a strong case can be made that welfare reform was never about bringing women and their children out of poverty. Instead, it is geared toward welfare savings, maintaining a cheap pool of labor, and the social control of women (Miller, 1990; Abramovitz, 1988). In this booming economy, the present emphasis is the need for cheap labor.

Yet the pay gap between men's and women's wages is still quite real and not narrowing rapidly. In literally all job categories, including occupations in which women dominate, women earn less than men do. In 1999, women working full-time earned 75 percent of what men earned (Women's Bureau, 2000). That appears to be progress, since in the 1970s the proportion was 59 percent. Yet college-educated women employed full-time, year round, still earn only 61 cents for every dollar earned by college-educated men (Costello, Miles, and Stone, 1998). Given the pay gap and women's increasing responsibility for all or part of household income, it is little wonder that the percentage of women who are multiple job holders increased from 16 percent in 1970 to 46 percent in 1996 (Costello, Miles, and Stone, 1998).

Today, 30 percent of women workers are either managers or professionals, representing an increase of 8 percent since the early 1980s (Costello, Miles, and Stone, 1998). Yet progress has been slow. For one thing, Hispanic women are much less likely to be in managerial jobs. Moreover, women's choices of work still tend to be limited. In 1998, the top two occupations of employed women were secretary and cashier, comprising 8 percent of employed women. Seventy percent of working women are employed in the services industry or in wholesale or retail trade (Costello, Miles, and Stone, 1998). In 1997, 46 percent of women working full-time, year round, earned less than $25,000, compared with 29 percent of men. The gendered segregation of labor is very effective in maintaining women's low wages. The low numbers of women in nontraditional jobs is related to the wage gap. Not only are women not receiving equal pay for equal work, the fact that men and women have different jobs exacerbates their difficulties. Traditionally, "women's jobs" pay less, even when they require more education and entail more responsibility.

Although they pay 20 to 30 percent more than traditional jobs, blue-collar jobs that are "nontraditional" for women have been especially difficult for women to obtain. Just 15 percent of all working women in 1999 were employed in nontraditional occupations (Women's Bureau, 2000). On the other end, few women receiving advanced degrees earn them in engineering, math, and science (Costello, Miles, and Stone, 1998, p. 242).

Money Matters

For true reform to be initiated, jobs that will bring all persons into the mainstream of American life should be the first consideration. In this regard, it is important that our confusion and ambivalence about maternal employment be resolved. It is a fact of life that, even in married-couple families, women must be in the labor force for most to attain middle-class status. Moreover, the fulfillment of women's talents and occupational aspirations outside of the home will benefit everyone. We also know that quality child care is not harmful to children nor does it interfere with the parent/child bond. As noted above, quality child care might enhance rather than detract from caring connections among people. It would help enormously if the nation acknowledged these facts and aided in creating a society in which women can work and families can experience a quality family life.

The immediate solutions to women's work issues involve policies such as affirmative action, nondiscrimination, and better laws regarding the rights of part-time workers. Pay equity would ensure that women are provided equal pay for jobs of comparable worth and thus mitigate against the wage differentials between "men's" and "women's" jobs. Job requirements, such as skills, education, experience, degree of responsibility and autonomy, and risk would be compared among jobs to prevent instances in which male-dominated job categories, such as truck drivers, are paid more than those dominated by women, such as nurses. By 1987, twenty states were implementing pay-equity plans. Just one state, Minnesota, had achieved equitable wage scales for its state employees (Mezey, 1992).

The community can work with schools and employers to increase employment, education, and training opportunities for young women and men, especially minority youth. Businesses, faith communities, and community groups can establish and support nonprofit affordable quality child care for low-income parents. Also, paid parental leave for parents of newborn and ill children would help bridge the gap between work and family responsibilities. The unpaid leave allowed by the Family Support Act does not go far enough. All of the European countries have mandated maternity or parental leave with full or partial pay (Stoiber, 1989). It can be done, and states need not wait for the federal government to mandate it. Financial incentives to businesses to provide such leaves can be established locally and state-wide.

Increased opportunities for women to enter nontraditional fields are needed as well. These reforms are more difficult to obtain because they are more likely to bring women equal access to money, power, and status in the work world, thereby effecting gender-role changes. Solutions that make women's work and family roles more compatible—flextime, job sharing, on-site child care, work at home, and part-time work—are less threatening to society because they uphold capitalist and patriarchal norms. These alternative work arrangements institutionalize women's second-class status in society and enshrine their primary roles as both wives and mothers. Yet women are not going to be able to gain equal status in society, not to mention escape poverty, without a change in the gendered division of labor.

In the midst of job-related policies is the urgent need for a decent health care insurance policy. Instead of waiting for the federal government to act, advocates at the state level can promote a health insurance plan funded by business and government to ensure that all persons in the state are covered adequately. Ultimately we need a national health insurance plan that is not tied (or at least not exclusively) to employment.

Eleven years ago, I advocated the federalization of AFDC with higher, uniform payments, indicating that doing so would complete the federalization of welfare that began in 1984 with welfare payments for the poor elderly and the disabled. It would eliminate the need for such a large state welfare bureaucracy, be more equitable to clients from state to state, and free the states to administer needed social services and jobs programs that are best designed at the local level (Miller, 1990). Today, TANF, which is even more decentralized, has taken the country many steps away from any thought of federalization. Yet it remains a reasonable, rational goal. On the other hand, there are alternatives to maintaining such a large welfare system. The United States is the only Western industrialized country that does not have a system of children's allowances, payments to families to help defray the cost of child rearing. Although we have a personal income tax exemption for children, the value of this exemption has eroded considerably since its inception and it is not at all helpful to low-income families with little or no tax liability. The National Commission on Children (1991) recommends that we replace the deduction with a new refundable child tax credit of $1,000 per child. With this credit, indexed for inflation, all families would be better off, and low-income families would be helped considerably.

Achieving women's equality and assuring adequate household and child-care arrangements requires changes in the work world. The struggles concerning work and family will not be solved simply through an equalization of household chores between husbands and wives. Because of the demands of the work world, the stress on family life in the absence of change is inevitable (Pleck, 1977). Alternative solutions to this problem might involve shortening every worker's day, for example. In considering alternatives, policy analysts must consider the relative importance of women's full participation in the workforce (and society), and the implications for changes in men's and women's roles. At the moment, even liberal policy proposals do not change women's roles as much as we would like to think. They just make them a little easier.

SOCIAL CONTROL OF WOMEN THROUGH VIOLENCE

Sheffield has coined the term "sexual terrorism" to mean "a system by which males frighten and, by frightening, control and dominate females" (Sheffield, 1989, p. 3). She compares it to political terrorism in that it is supported by ideology and propaganda, is indiscriminate and unpredictable, and relies on "voluntary compliance," that is, numbers of men who are socialized to maintain the fear and numbers of women who are socialized to be victims (Sheffield, 1989). The societal presence of sexual terrorism, which includes rape, wife battering, sexual harassment, and childhood sexual abuse, informs almost every aspect of women's lives, whether these things happen to us as individuals or not. Sexual terrorism dictates to some extent how women dress, how we walk down the street, how we look at men we see on the street, and how we behave toward men we know casually—the guy in the next office, the workman, the janitor. Young women are cautioned about blind dates—or any date. Sexual terrorism dictates where women go at night and what time to go—where to park and when to get home. Sexual terrorism dictates whether we travel alone and, if so, what precautions we take—what protection to

carry, where to stop to eat or sleep. Even two women traveling together on a camping trip on the Appalachian Trail in 1988 were
stalked and shot (Zia, 1990).

Sexual terrorism makes us restrict our daughters' activities, but not
our sons'. Although we protect our daughters, we also socialize them
into forming identities as victims. The point of sexual terrorism is
that women are always potential victims and never safe. If the "safety
rules" held and women obeyed them, they would be prisoners, but at
least could know they would not be attacked. However, it doesn't
work that way. Attacks are perpetrated against women of all ages, at
all times of day and night, however they behave, and however they are
dressed. Sexual terrorism has the effect of keeping women in their
place and on guard at all times. Sexual terrorism functions, therefore,
as an incredible waste of women's energy and human potential. In addition, sexual terrorism is what Griffin has termed a "protection
racket," because women look to men to protect them from other men
(Griffin, 1989).

All men benefit from sexual terrorism because it gives them dominance and control over the women in their lives in the form of "protection." But of course "protectors" sometimes beat and abuse their
wives and children. These crimes against women are the least prosecuted and, when prosecuted, obtain the fewest convictions (Sheffield,
1989). There were 93,103 forcible rapes reported to law enforcement
agencies in 1998, resulting in 31,000 arrests (Bureau of Justice
Statistics, 1999). People known to the victim, including friends,
acquaintances, and "intimates," accounted for three-quarters of all
rapes and sexual assaults in 1992-1993 (Bureau of Justice Statistics,
1995). Research with convicted rapists indicates that most rapes are
planned (Brownmiller, 1975) and committed by men known to their
victims. Anecdotal evidence gleaned through interviews with rapists
also supports this conclusion (Skipper and McWhorter, 1989).

Sexual harassment on the job, perpetrated by bosses and co-workers, is another form of everyday violence against women. Two types
of sexual harassment occur: quid pro quo, which suggests the exchange of sexual favors as a condition of employment or promotion;
and a hostile work environment, in which a woman is made uncomfortable by comments, actions, pictures, etc. One study indicated that
sexual harassment from co-workers is more likely to happen to women
in nontraditional occupations; the message from their co-workers is,

"You don't belong here." Bosses, on the other hand, use it to keep women in subordinate positions. Most women either tolerate sexual harassment or quit their jobs in the face of it. Those who do complain often feel worse than before (Martin, 1989).

Violence Is Not Inevitable

Surely a social push toward decreasing the tendency toward violence in men's domestic behavior and increasing their nurturing abilities would help families tremendously. But social work/feminist communities have concentrated instead on advocacy and counseling for the victims and prosecution of the offenders. A recent article on "empowerment," for example, focused almost entirely on services for victims and serving victims, with supposedly no notion of changing the masculinist system that perpetuates violence against women in the first place (Busch and Valentine, 2000). Of course, determining places and strategies for intervention is not easy. Most feminists acknowledge the need to help women help themselves rather than waiting for men to change. But it is also easier to avoid the role-changing challenge of addressing masculinist socialization for boys. An essential point of intervention would be to address men's lives, including the way we bring up boys. Otherwise, at best we will simply be filling jail cells and staffing better battered women's shelters. Changing men would make marriage and family more appealing to everyone and might decrease youth violence. But it will not obviate the need for a variety of family structures to be allowed and encouraged to grow and thrive.

Policy issues dealing with everyday terrorism and violence against women should take top priority in the twenty-first century. We must promote public policies that enforce existing laws against violence and move society toward nonviolence. Instead of trying to pick and choose what violent acts are acceptable and which are not, we should oppose them all. Promoting new ways of socializing children, particularly boys, to nonviolence, and socializing girls to be assertive (but *not* violent) would help to reduce and prevent sexual terrorism and wife battering. Instead of keeping our daughters behind closed doors at night, let us teach them how to assert and protect themselves. Fewer men would attempt violent acts against women if they knew that most women had learned self-defense from an early age. Empowered to use their energies proactively, women would not identify as victims. Loving, concerned men would be relieved since they cannot always be there to protect the women they love, however sincere their intentions. The far-reaching implications of these changes, however, are profound changes in women's roles.

Women, not bothered by sexual terrorism, would likely have more time and energy to devote to their lives, would be less likely to identify as victims, and would be more self-confident. I suggest that the role-change nature of effective strategies to end sexual terrorism and violence against women blocks efforts to solve the problem.

CONCLUSION

All social policies have an impact upon women in one way or another. It is important to identify the ways in which they do without apology. One of the frustrations of the fight is that some gains, such as reproductive rights, are threatened. Fighting against regression rather than creating new initiatives to move forward is debilitating and an effective strategy of traditionalists.

Much work is needed to support and improve women's lives in the twenty-first century. True equality involves fundamental gender-role changes. Fighting for policies that would facilitate these role changes is difficult, painful, and disruptive. We are not near to this goal in the United States and even further away at various other places around the globe. At this writing, the United States has just experienced large political demonstrations demanding social responsibility of the World Trade Organization and the International Monetary Fund. One would hope that this is the beginning of a trend toward the continuing and vivid recognition that fair wages and prices in the United States must not be obtained at the expense of unfair wages, prices, famine, hunger, and devastation in other parts of the world. We are all in this together, women, men, and children.

Many proposed policies would be helpful to some women while perpetuating their subordination. It is still true that most well-known proposed changes would make it easier for U.S. white, married women to "juggle home and family" better, offering little significant help to single parents, women of color, and poor people everywhere. Incremental gains are terribly appealing but must not be mistaken for fundamental change.

REFERENCES

Abramovitz, M. (1988). *Regulating the lives of women: Social welfare policy from colonial times to the present.* Boston, MA: South End Press.

Amott, T. L. and Matthaei, J. A. (1991). *Race, gender and work.* Boston, MA: South End Press.

Brownmiller, S. (1975*). Against our will: Men, women, and rape.* New York: Simon and Schuster.

Bureau of Justice Statistics (1995). *Violence against women: Estimates from the redesigned survey.* Washington, DC: U.S. Department of Justice.

Bureau of Justice Statistics (1999). Uniform Crime Reports.

Busch, N. B. and Valentine, D. (2000). Empowerment practice: A focus on battered women. *Affilia: Journal of Women and Social Work, 15*: 82-95.

Census Bureau (1999). *Poverty in the United States: 1998.* Current Population Reports, Series P60-207. Washington, DC: U.S. Government Printing Office.

Center on Budget and Policy Priorities. (1999). *Low unemployment, rising wages fuel poverty decline* (Revised October 4, 1999). Washington, DC: <www.cbpp.org/9-30-99pov.htm> Contact: Robert Greenstein, Jim Jaffee, Toni Katayin.

Costello, C. B., Miles, S., and Stone, A. J. (Eds.) (1998). *The American woman: 1999-2000.* New York: W. W. Norton and Company.

Gelb, J. and Palley, M. L. (1987). *Women and public policies,* Second edition. Princeton, NJ: Princeton University Press.

General Accounting Office (1999). *Food stamp program: Various factors have led to declining participation,* July. GAO/RCED-99-185, p. 2. Washington, DC: General Accounting Office.

Griffin, S. (1989). Rape: The all-American crime. In L. Richardson and V. Taylor (Eds.), *Feminist frontiers: Rethinking sex, gender, and society.* New York: Random House.

Harrison, C. (1988). A richer life: A reflection on the women's movement. In S. E. Rix (Ed.), *The American woman: 1988-89, a status report.* New York: W. W. Norton.

hooks, b. (1989). *Talking back: Thinking feminist, thinking black.* Boston, MA: South End Press.

House of Representatives, Committee on Ways and Means (1998). *1998 Green book: Overview of entitlement programs: Background material and data on programs within the jurisdiction of the Committee on Ways and Means.* Washington, DC: U.S. Government Printing Office.

Joseph, G. I. and Lewis, J. (1981). *Common differences: Conflicts in black and white feminist perspectives.* Boston, MA: South End Press.

Martin, S. E. (1989). Sexual harassment: The link joining gender stratification, sexuality, and women's economic status. In J. Freeman (Ed.), *Women: A feminist perspective* (pp. 57-75). Mountain View, CA: Mayfield Publishing Company.

McAdoo, H. P. (1980). Black mothers and the extended family support network. In L. Rodgers-Rose (Ed.), *The black woman*. Newbury Park, CA: Sage Publications.

Mead, L. (1986). *Beyond entitlement: The social obligations of citizenship*. New York: The Free Press.

Meyer, C. H. (1985). A feminist perspective on foster family care: A redefinition of the categories. *Child Welfare, 64:* 249-258.

Mezey, S. G. (1992). *In pursuit of equality: Women, public policy, and the federal courts*. New York: St. Martin's Press.

Miller, D. C. (1990). *Women and social welfare: A feminist analysis*. New York: Praeger.

Miller, D. C. (1994). What is needed for true equality: An overview of policy issues for women. In L. V. Davis (Ed.), *Building on women's strengths: A social work agenda for the twenty-first century* (pp. 47-64). Binghamton, NY: The Haworth Press.

National Commission on Children (1991). *Beyond rhetoric: A new American agenda for children and families: Final report of the National Commission on Children*. Washington, DC: Author.

National Research Council Committee on the Status of Black Americans (1990). *A common destiny: Blacks and American society*. Washington, DC: National Academy Press.

"People in the News." *Wichita Eagle* (2000). January 4, p. A2.

Pleck, J. (1977). The work-family role system. *Social Problems, 24:* 417-427.

Rutter, M. (1982). Social emotional consequences of day care for preschool children. In E. F. Zigler and E. W. Gordon (Eds.), *Day care: Scientific and social policy issues* (pp. 3-32). Dover, MA: Auburn House Publishing Company.

Schumacher, R. and Greenberg, M. (1999). *Child care after leaving welfare: Early evidence from state studies*. Washington, DC: Center for Law and Social Policy.

Sheffield, C. J. (1989). Sexual terrorism. In J. Freeman (Ed.), *Women: A feminist perspective* (pp. 3-19). Mountain View, CA: Mayfield Publishing Company.

Skipper, J. K. and McWhorter, W. L. (1989). A rapist gets caught in the act. In L. Richardson and V. Taylor (Eds.), *Feminist frontiers: Rethinking sex, gender, and society* (pp. 399-401). New York: Random House.

Stack, C. (1974). *All our kin: Strategies for survival in a black community*. New York: Harper and Row.

Stevens, W. K. (1988). The welfare consensus. *The New York Times,* June 22.

Stoiber, S. A. (1989). *Parental leave and 'woman's place': The implications and impact of three European approaches to family leave policy*. Washington, DC: Women's Research and Education Institute.

Women's Bureau (2000). *Women's earnings as percent of men's, 1979-1999.* Washington, DC: Department of Labor.

Zia, H. (1990). Fighting straight hate. *MS*, September/October: 47.

Chapter 4

Child Welfare As a Woman's Issue: Untangling Gender, Race, and Class

Elizabeth D. Hutchison
Leanne W. Charlesworth

For the past century in the United States, the welfare of children has been considered a legitimate concern of government. This concern for the well-being of children has been problematic for the political institution, however, because of the strong belief among opinion leaders that individual families are responsible for the welfare of their own children. From Colonial times, local, state, and federal governments have struggled with the question of whether and, if so, how to aid families who are not capable of meeting the needs of children without organized assistance (Gordon, 1994; Halpern, 1999; Sidel, 1986, 1998).

Almost from the outset, the child welfare system in the United States has accepted without question the consequences for children of unequal power based on gender, race, and class. Child welfare scholars, policymakers, and practitioners, historical as well as current, have too often studied, planned for, and served children and their families without giving special attention to the needs of female caregivers—as if children's needs could be met whether or not their caregivers had access to the resources for providing sufficient care. Consequently, the child welfare system, currently as well as historically, is built on the oppression of several categories of women.

In the first edition of this book, a gender lens was used to analyze child welfare in the United States. In this second edition, we want to draw more focused attention to the intricate interweaving of multiple systems of domination and their impact on child welfare. A gender analysis alone can obscure racial and class oppression.

As in the first edition, an ecological perspective is used, suggesting connections among several societal systems. Our goal is to provide a more holistic understanding of child welfare and to avoid the partialization of issues that has obscured the complexity of child welfare and led to piecemeal solutions that necessarily fail. By using a broad brush, we hope to stimulate more integrative thinking about child welfare policy. The following sections present historical as well as recent trends of gender, race, and class bias in policy related to child welfare and discuss the oppression of selected categories of women in the child welfare system. Implications and guidelines that flow from this analysis are outlined.

HISTORICAL PERSPECTIVE

After the Revolutionary War, the acceptable method for ensuring the welfare of children was their removal from the family because there was a general feeling that families should not be aided in their own homes and that to do so would destroy parental initiative (Abramovitz, 1988; Halpern, 1999; Sidel, 1986). The most notable example was Charles Loring Brace's (1859) orphan train project in which hundreds of children of poor white ethnic immigrants were transported to the Midwest to be placed with farm families. Beginning in the 1870s, media attention to cruelty to children ushered in the nineteenth-century child-saving movement and Societies for Prevention of Cruelty to Children (SPCCs) were developed.

As the SPCCs matured and began to professionalize, dissatisfaction grew with the method of removal. In 1906, the Massachusetts Society for Prevention of Cruelty to Children (MSPCC) began to integrate the developing social casework method with anticruelty work to serve families with children in their own homes (Anderson, 1989). This new approach to serving children raised an awkward question, however: How can indigent children be maintained in their own families without providing economic resources to caregivers? Support grew for policy initiatives to aid mothers and children, and, by 1923, forty-two states had enacted mothers' aid laws (Hanlan, 1966). Throughout the Progressive Era, government involvement in child and family welfare expanded and the creation of the Children's Bureau in 1912 acknowledged federal responsibility for child and family well-being (Halpern, 1991).

Beginning in the late nineteenth century, two separate discourses existed about the welfare of children. The first discourse was about the need for adequate resources for mothering, especially for single mothers and other poor mothers. Some reformers in this discourse argued that mothers deserve assistance because of the important function they perform for society, arguing in essence that some form of family allowance is warranted as a compensation for services provided. This was not a popular argument, however. The more politically acceptable argument in this discourse was about the innocence of children and the need to aid mothers for the good of the child. A second discourse focused on child saving, the need for social control of parenting to protect children from parental abuse and neglect. This discourse was a continuation of the nineteenth-century child-saving movement.

At the Children' Bureau, it appears that these two discourses were somewhat integrated, and the reformers put great stock in the ability of the newly developed casework method to be an effective tool for assisting poor mothers and protecting children (Gordon, 1994). Over time, however, the issues of assisting caregivers and protecting children became divorced in public discourse and took different paths in the political institution (Halpern, 1999; Lindsey, 1994). For this reason, the historical perspective on each discourse is discussed separately, beginning with the discourse about assistance to mothers.

The Mothers' Aid Discourse

Women dominated the early U.S. Children's Bureau, which became "the heart of white women's welfare thought" (Gordon, 1994, p. 71). More specifically, Children's Bureau reformers were mostly elite, white, Protestant women from the Northeast and Midwest— well-connected women who were among the early college-educated women in the United States, pioneers in the settlement house movement, and activists in the first-wave women's movement. These women were instrumental in envisioning a social welfare system for the country, but their vision was limited by the historical times and political realities in which they lived. These high-status women with prominent careers promoted policies for poor women and children that rested on the patriarchal assumption that women would marry, be supported by their husbands, and devote their lives to the care of children and the home. They endorsed, or at least accepted, the idea of a "family wage" or "living wage" for men so that men could financially support children and a domestic wife. For this social philosophy to hold up, social welfare programs had to fill in for the man economically when he faltered or was absent. And, indeed, the reformers favored social welfare policies that supported the gender-based or "separate spheres" division of labor—policies such as mothers' pensions, Aid to Dependent Children (ADC), protective labor laws, and survivors' benefits. With their acceptance of a gender-based division of labor, the Children's Bureau reformers did not make day care a priority, and, in fact, many opposed it.

Lillian Wald and Florence Kelley, who were the architects of the Children's Bureau, saw women's welfare and children's welfare as one and the same (Costin, 1985; Gordon, 1994). They saw mothers' aid as only a first step in improving the welfare of mothers and children. Their agenda included housing codes, minimum wage laws, protective labor laws for women and children, and maternal and child health programs. Under Julia Lathrop's leadership, the Children's Bureau was instrumental in getting the Sheppard-Towner Act passed in 1921. This act introduced the first federal welfare program, a program of public health nursing for mothers and infants. This was, indeed, a program that benefited both women and children, and the reformers were confident that it was only the beginning of comprehensive federal programming for poor women and children. Unfortunately, however, their ambitions were never realized. Sheppard-Towner was repealed in 1929 and, as the Children's Bureau fought off several waves of conservative attacks, the reformers found that it was easier to build a case for the innocence of children than for the needs of mothers, and their policy development tilted toward the needs of children.

During the Depression, amid an outcry for public relief programs, work began on the several titles of the Social Security Act of 1935, which set the structure of the social welfare system in the United States. The Children's Bureau was asked to draft the ADC title of the Act. Like all legislation, the Social Security Act was enacted out of a process of proposing, negotiating, and compromising. Linda Gordon's (1994) historical analysis demonstrates that gender, race, and class politics all played a role in the final legislation.

All titles of the Social Security Act rested solidly on the patriarchal assumption that women and children will be economically dependent on men. Therefore, the best way to ensure the welfare of women and children is to ensure the economic well-being of men. That leaves, of course, the "single mother problem" to be addressed in some manner. In the midst of the Depression, there was pressure from social movements as well as public opinion for the federal government to develop programs to ensure the "social security" of citizens in a wage-labor economy that appeared destined to cycles of upturn and downturn. At the outset, unemployment insurance, worker's compensation, old age insurance, public works, public medical insurance, and mothers' aid were all considered essentials of "social security" (Gordon, 1994). Opposition from big business and the medical establishment eliminated public works and medical insurance from the reform agenda. The social welfare system that resulted is a two-tier stratified system that reproduces and even exacerbates existing gender, race, and class power structures.

A top tier that includes unemployment insurance, worker's compensation, and old-age insurance (known as Social Security) provides superior payments and enjoys a superior reputation to programs in the lower tier. These programs are federally administered and involve no means testing or intrusion into privacy. Because they are based on prior employment records, and because they exclude some categories of workers, they disproportionately benefit whites, men, and nonpoor families. After 1974, when Old-Age Assistance and Aid to the Blind and Disabled were incorporated into the social insurance system, the lower tier included only one program, ADC. ADC was state and locally based, involved intrusion into family life, and from the outset provided much smaller payments than the social insurance programs. A 1939 amendment made it a means-tested program, serving only poor families. It disproportionately served women and minorities, and association with this program carried increasing stigma over time.

Gender, race, and class played out in complex ways in the story of ADC. The proposed legislation was written by privileged women for poor women, without the voice of poor women. These privileged reformers were genuinely concerned about the lives of poor mothers, but they did not recognize the potential for class oppression with their formula of "financial assistance plus counseling." They saw ADC as only one small program of assistance for mothers and children, a foot in the door for the development of a more comprehensive welfare program for mothers and children. Their vision was short lived. The Ways and Means Committee added a maximum amount of grant to the ADC title, a very meager one that could not possibly provide for the basic needs of mothers and children and was significantly less than the grants for top-tier programs.

The reformers at the Children's Bureau were not attentive to race issues and did not anticipate the strong influence that race politics would have on the various titles of the Social Security Act as they made their way through a legislative process controlled by southern congressmen. The Children's Bureau had proposed that standards of eligibility should be federally determined and were dismayed when eligibility was left to states. They had not been opposed to the "suitable homes" provision in the law, but they did not foresee that it would be used by Southern states to systematically deprive black families of ADC.

Indeed, the Southern congressmen were able to use their power to protect the interests of Southern employers who wanted cheap access to black agricultural and domestic labor. They did this by exempting these two types of labor from the Social Security Act, as well as from other depression-era legislation aimed at protecting workers from insecurities in the labor market (Jones, 1985). Federal government programs in the 1950s, such as veterans' benefits, education subsidies, housing loans, and job training, continued to advance the position of white middle- and working-class men and their families and jeopardize poor, minority, and single-parent families (Sidel, 1998). Gordon (1994) reports that by the 1980s, 80 percent of social welfare monies went to the nonpoor.

The reformers at the Children's Bureau had assumed that they would administer ADC and develop further programs to promote the welfare of children. They had a special interest in maternal and child health. In the end, ADC was not assigned to the Children's Bureau, and the influence of the women's network in and around the Bureau waned as the first wave of feminism came to an end.

We have told the story of white women's discourse about assistance to mothers in securing the welfare of children. There was also a discourse among black women activists who began to organize in the 1890s (Gordon, 1994). It was a separate discourse because, with few exceptions, black women were shunned when they attempted to integrate the white women's reformist movement. In some ways, the black women's discourse was similar to that of white women: both were interested in elevating the status of women; both accepted the gender-based division of labor which made women responsible for the domestic sphere; both gave a special priority to the needs of children; and both believed that poor women needed "education and training as well as material provision" (Gordon, 1994, p. 112).

But there were also differences, born out of the different experiences of the reformers (Gordon, 1994). Although both networks included the elite women of their race, historical and continued discrimination meant that there was less social distance between the black women activists and those they sought to help. The black women focused on racism as well as women's issues. Because they had no political influence, they used their mutual benefit societies, church groups, and women's clubs to build private institutions to care for members of their race and to compensate for their systematic exclusion from existing governmental and private programs. They were particularly interested in education and medical care. These black women were more willing to challenge both racial and gender domination, drawing attention to rape, an issue not bridged by the white women reformers of the era. They favored universal programs instead of the means-tested programs developed by the white women welfare activists, and they were less caught up in moralizing about the situations of single mothers. Although they resented the ways that slavery and Jim Crow policies had undermined their ability to manage domestic life, they were more accepting than the white women reformers of the idea of wage labor for married women. Consequently, in contrast to their white peers, they put a high priority on the development of day care programs. They were interested in ways to help women be successful in simultaneous role performance in both the private and public spheres. In this way, they were far better attuned to the world of the future than the white women welfare activists. It is unfortunate that they had no voice in the political discourse about welfare during the New Deal.

The Child-Saving Discourse

Linda Gordon (1988) has made a significant contribution to the child-welfare literature by using a gender lens to analyze the child protection movement. After reviewing case records of the MSPCC from 1880 to 1960, Gordon identifies five stages (through the 1970s) of the political construction of child maltreatment in the United States. She describes the first stage as the nineteenth-century (or first) child-saving stage (1875-1910). During this stage, family violence was defined as cruelty to children and emphasis was placed on the "depraved immigrant man"—often under influence of alcohol—as perpetrator. Gordon reported that this was the only stage in which child-welfare reforms represented gains for women as well as children. Maternal and child health programs are the best example.

During the second stage, the Progressive Era and its aftermath (1910-1930), child welfare was defined in terms of child neglect. The concern during this stage focused on the weakening of the family, particularly on increases in single-parent families. With the professionalization of social work, the earlier concern about brutal men seemed "moralistic and unscientific" (Gordon, 1988, p. 21) and spousal violence was portrayed as interactive. In general, case records of this era indicate a cover up of wife beating.

During the Depression, the third stage described by Gordon, emphasis was on supporting the cohesiveness of nuclear families. Social service organizations de-emphasized family violence and focused on economic neglect of children. The de-emphasis on family violence continued through the fourth stage, World War II and the 1950s, but now it took another turn. Social work, heavily influenced by psychiatry, viewed interpersonal problems through the lens of individual personality structure. Agency records indicate that during this stage wives were often blamed for their abuse by their husbands. Child neglect continued to be emphasized during this period, but was now constructed as deriving from parental neurosis. Emotional neglect was introduced as a new category of child maltreatment.

During the 1960s and 1970s, the final stage identified by Gordon, a second child-saving movement refocused attention on physical abuse and neglect and brought public attention for the first time to sexual abuse of children. During this era, an active feminist movement garnered recognition that family violence often involves violence to women.

RECENT TRENDS

In recent years, both the mothers' aid discourse and the child-saving discourse have become increasingly hostile to poor single mothers. These mothers have had to withstand a relentless rhetoric that identifies them as the enemy of the state; they have been called "welfare queens," animals, and "rotten mothers" (Dodson, 1998; Halpern, 1999; McLaughlin, 1997; Sidel, 1998). Ruth Sidel (1998) argues that this image of the evil poor single mother is held together by the erroneous stereotype that "most poor people are black" (p. 167), and she questions whether the country would have tolerated recent harsh rhetoric and legislation without this racist imagery. We will look first at recent trends in the mothers' aid discourse, and then at recent trends in the child-saving discourse. Both discourses have led to policies that are heavy on social control and light on material and nonmaterial support.

These harsh policy directions become even more troubling when one considers the social context in which they are implemented. This social context includes changes in family structure leading to a sharp rise in female-headed single-parent households, changes in the labor market with women participating more but increasingly trapped in low-wage jobs in the service sector, and assaults on social welfare programs that serve women and children.

A convergence of these changes in the family system, the labor market, and the social welfare system has intensified the climate of vulnerability for women and their dependent children. In 1997, the poverty rate was 31.6 percent for all female-headed single families with children compared to 5.2 percent of married couple families, 27.7 percent for white female-headed single-parent families with children, 39.8 percent for black female-headed single-parent families with children, and 47.6 percent for Hispanic female-headed single-parent families with children (Dalaker and Naifeh, 1998). These poverty rates become even more jolting when they are analyzed for their impact on children. In 1996, one of every five children under the age of eighteen in the United States was living in poverty. The rates are higher for minority children and children under the age of six (Sidel, 1998).

The Mothers' Aid Discourse

In the early 1990s, tremendous public attention focused on the inadequacies of the social welfare system. Specifically, led by the rhetoric of Charles Murray (1984, 1996) and Lawrence Mead (1992, 1996), the view that Aid to Families with Dependent Children (AFDC, earlier known as ADC and the program typically viewed as equivalent to "welfare") caused a variety of social dysfunctions became increasingly popular. This attention culminated in the 1996 enactment of the Personal Responsibility and Work Opportunity Reconciliation Act (PRWORA) (P.L. 104-193), legislation that eliminated AFDC and replaced it with Temporary Assistance to Needy Families (TANF). Although AFDC had been "reformed" several times during the preceding three decades, PRWORA brought radical changes to the program. For example, under the new TANF block grant system, eligible families are no longer entitled to assistance. Nonexempt adult recipients must work or participate in work-oriented activities in order to receive cash assistance and such assistance is time limited. Most recipients cannot receive aid for more than five years in their lifetime, and in several states this time period is shorter. In addition to these changes, PRWORA awarded states widespread discretion in designing and implementing new welfare-to-work programs. In essence, PRWORA altered the nature of public policy toward impoverished children and their caregivers (see U.S. Department of Health and Human Services, 1998a).

Perhaps most important, the legislation endorses a "work first" philosophy. That is, it accepts the notion that recipients of public aid—typically, impoverished single mothers—should be required to be involved in wage labor. Although certain groups of recipients—for example, those with documented disabilities or children under age one—are exempted from the "work first" requirement, the vast majority are not. As a result, in order to receive financial assistance, impoverished mothers must now work outside the home or engage in a work activity. Moreover, in defining "activity," PRWORA shifted the emphasis away from the human capital development emphasis of its predecessor, the 1988 Family Support Act and toward rapid labor force attachment (for a discussion of these two philosophies, see Gueron and Pauly, 1991).

This "work first" philosophy reverses the "separate spheres" philosophy that undergirded the Social Security Act, a philosophy that children should be cared for at home by their mothers. In reality, however, the new philosophy of "work first" applies only to poor mothers in the public welfare system. The same conservative politicians who demonized poor women as lazy "welfare queens" and demanded that they "go to work" continue to urge middle- and upper-class women to return to the domestic wife role. For more privileged women, domestic work seems to be a legitimate form of work, one that does not carry the label of "lazy." For poor black women, unfortunately, this is not the first historical era in which they have engaged in coerced labor that benefits other families more than it benefits their own (Jones, 1985).

PRWORA has been praised for increasing the flexibility available to states and localities and for encouraging innovation at the local level. Indeed, many states and localities have capitalized on their newfound flexibility, increasing earned income disregards and other supports available to recipients in, or transitioning into, the workforce (Zedlewski, Holcomb, and Duke, 1998). Although these are potentially positive developments, local flexibility also brings additional discretion at both the agency and worker level. Given the historical use of discretion to constrict dispersion of program funds, the net product of local flexibility could be either positive or negative. Unfortunately, we are reminded of another historical era when states rights arguments were used for blatantly racist intents (Gordon, 1994).

There are a number of other areas of concern raised by PRWORA:

1. The "work first," or rapid labor force attachment, emphasis means that many recipients are mandated to take any or the first job available to them. Education and skill development activities are deemphasized if not eliminated, despite the fact that considerable evidence exists to support the need for such investments in order to improve the earning power of public assistance recipients (D'Amico, 1997). The most troubling aspect of this development is that the assumption is not that recipients will be able to earn a living wage through the work-first approach. Instead, public responsibility to ensure an adequate wage for recipients and their children has been abdicated. The accepted view is that although the first job available may not provide a living wage, rapid attachment to the labor force is the best approach to encouraging development of a work ethic which may (or may not) lead to better paying jobs in the future (Mead, 1996). In either case, it is believed that a working family in poverty

free of all government assistance is better off than a family in poverty receiving such assistance. This view has become extremely popular despite the lack of evidence supporting such an assertion.

2. PRWORA brought a dramatic increase in funding for child care, and states were given greater flexibility in administering their child care programs. However, despite this expansion of child care funding and flexibility, many state officials worry about the long-term adequacy of federal and state funding. Specifically, TANF's work requirements and time limits, caps on federal funding, and an absence of funding guarantees in times of economic hardship have made state officials cautious about expanding their child care programs. As was true before PRWORA, very few states have been able to serve all nonwelfare low-income families in need of child care assistance. Thus, although child care for welfare families has dramatically expanded, nonwelfare wage-earning families continue to represent an area of unmet need (Long et al., 1998). And given the low child care subsidies provided to recipients of public aid, the quality of care obtained should be scrutinized. In addition, many mothers obtaining work in traditional low-skill, service-sector jobs will face the ongoing lack of quality care available for very young children and during shift-work hours (weekends, nights, evenings).

3. Recently, as welfare caseloads have continued to fall, growing attention has focused on those public-assistance recipients who face substantial barriers to success in the labor force. This population is believed to comprise approximately one-third of the nation's welfare caseload. Members of this "hard to serve" population, as it has come to be known, are believed to face one or more barriers such as substance abuse, disability, or mental illness (Pavetti et al., 1996). The consequences of PRWORA's work requirements and time limits will be, or may have already been, most severe for individuals facing such barriers. Research has indicated that 40 percent of women who use welfare for extended periods have disabilities (McLaughlin, 1997). Typically, these individuals should, under the law, be exempted from such requirements, but in most cases the response to such individuals is dependent on the local agency or attitude, skill, and knowledge level of the worker.

4. When PRWORA was first enacted, many expressed concern that its work requirements (and the sanctioning that may result from noncompliance) and time limits would force thousands of families

even further into poverty. To date, it appears that most families driving caseload declines are leaving voluntarily. However, despite their minority status, families leaving involuntarily—those sanctioned for noncompliance or whose cases are closed for miscellaneous other reasons—should raise concerns about declines in family well-being. Most evidence indicates that even those with "successful" departures—those leaving due to employment—are obtaining jobs that pay below-poverty-level wages. Though many former recipients may report they are "better off" working, there is, to date, no documented evidence that departure from public assistance, voluntary or otherwise, leads to concrete improvements in family or child well-being. Indeed, in states where families have already reached their time limits, the overwhelming majority is remaining in poverty and a substantial minority is suffering from declines in income (Bloom, Kemple, and Rogers-Dillon, 1997). Research by the Center on Budget and Policy Priorities (Primus et al., 1999) found that the income of the poorest 20 percent of female-headed families with children fell by an average of $580 per family between 1995 and 1997, a period when welfare "reform" was being implemented. And, of course, PRWORA has been implemented to date in good economic times. The real test will be during the next economic downturn.

After a century of government commitment to the welfare of children, PRWORA and the rhetoric that led to its passage demonstrated more concern with mothers' behavior than with family well-being. It is important to note that the preliminary evidence suggests that some families may be benefiting from some features of the new legislation, such as enhanced earned income disregards, and expanded child care subsidies. On the other hand, one researcher (Shook, 1999) found that declines in welfare income were associated with involvement with the child welfare system, but only in the absence of employment. It is likely that the consequences of PRWORA for women and children will be extensive and diverse (see, for example, Child Trends, 1999). Unfortunately, it seems inevitable that some families, perhaps those already quite fragile, will be harmed by the recent changes.

The Child-Saving Discourse

Throughout the 1990s, thirty years into a second child-saving movement in the United States, general support grew for Leroy Pelton's (1990) claim that "public child welfare is in chaos" (p. 19). This

child-saving movement narrowly defines child welfare as child protection (Hutchison, 1993; Kamerman and Kahn, 1990). Current protective policy was legislated on the assumption that child welfare policy could be divorced from general social welfare policy or, more
specifically, from antipoverty policy (Nelson, 1984). The evidence is
clear that this was a faulty assumption—one that has been costly for
poor families in general but particularly costly for women and children,
because economically disadvantaged families are overrepresented in the
child welfare system (National Research Council, 1994; U.S. Department of Health and Human Services, 1996; Vondra, 1993; Zellman,
1992).

The current child-protection movement focuses on policing family
life rather than enhancing the resources for family caregiving. The recent construction of child maltreatment inspired a child welfare system
that relies on mandatory reporting laws as the case-finding method,
emphasizes involuntary rather than voluntary services, and seeks solutions to cope with individual caregiver deficiencies (Hutchison, 1990).
The continuing allegiance to the separate spheres ideology ensures that
it is usually women's deficiencies that are noted in the child welfare
system; even when men are the perpetrators of maltreatment, it is
women who are held accountable for controlling the maltreating behavior.

In recent years, with the skyrocketing rates of reporting, increasing
portions of child welfare budgets have gone toward the process of in-
vestigative disposition and out-of-home placement, with little left for
services to families at risk (Geen, Waters Boots, and Tumlin, 1999;
Kamerman and Kahn, 1990). The Third National Incidence Study of
Child Abuse and Neglect found a sharp increase in the scope of child
maltreatment between 1986 and 1996, but it also found that only a
quarter of severely and moderately injured children were even investigated by CPS in 1996 (U.S. Department of Health and Human Services, 1996). In 1997, only 49.1 percent of child victims with substantiated reports received postinvestigative services, such as in-
home service, family preservation services, counseling, parent training, and foster care (U.S. Department of Health and Human Services,
1999).

Although no standardized data exist on states' total child welfare
spending or how it has changed over time, based on survey data for all
states, the Urban Institute concluded that little funding is being allo-

cated for prevention and family preservation services (Geen, Waters Boots, and Tumlin, 1999). They found that for every one dollar spent on "other services" (including prevention, child protective services, and case management activities), over three dollars was spent on out-of-home placement, adoption, and administrative costs. Between 1986 and 1996, federal payments to states for foster care and adoptive placements increased by 450 percent and the number of children in foster care increased by 79 percent. Has child removal once again become the preferred method for ensuring the welfare of children?

The Urban Institute report points out that PRWORA made few changes to federal child-protection programs, but federal devolution of fiscal authority for other social programs is likely to have an impact on the states' financing of child welfare services. For example, PRWORA eliminated the federal Emergency Assistance Program, rolling these funds into the TANF block grant and reducing the funding for the Social Services Block Grant. It is not known how states will respond fiscally to these changes or what impact this will have on the child protection system.

WOMEN AND THE CHILD WELFARE SYSTEM

Gillian Dalley (1988) describes the role of women under the separate spheres ideology as revolving around "enforced dependency and compulsory altruism" (p. 17). That description, unfortunately, is an apt one for many of the women who play central roles in the current child welfare system. To understand the construction of child welfare as a women's issue, one must look more closely at some of the women involved.

Mothers

When children's needs are not being met, mothers are scrutinized and held accountable. To the many women who already blame themselves for not being able to provide for their children, this comes as a double insult (Dodson, 1998; Sidel, 1986). Although child maltreatment reports often include a mixture of allegations of neglect, physical abuse, and sexual abuse, it is informative to examine the mothers involved in these categories of allegations separately.

Allegations of Neglect

Throughout child welfare history, neglect has been the type of child maltreatment most frequently reported to, and investigated by, child welfare agencies. Neglect is a category that was developed by powerful groups and has been used primarily to describe the parenting of poor women, who are usually single mothers and disproportionately women of color (Gordon, 1988; Swift, 1995; U.S. Department of Health and Human Services, 1999). Gordon (1988) found that approximately 83 percent of single mothers known to child protection agencies in Boston between 1880 and 1960 were known for child neglect. Noncustodial fathers, who are typically far more neglectful than custodial mothers, are seldom labeled as neglecting (U.S. Department of Health and Human Services, 1996). Therefore, the child welfare system supports and reinforces the gendered division of labor.

Neglect is the vaguest of the categories of child maltreatment. Sometimes allegations arise due to differences in definition—especially with allegations of failure to supervise. Most of the mothers who are labeled as neglecting have no access to the resources for adequate care of children. Halpern (1999) suggests that "parental exhaustion or survival-related adaptations" (p. 15) are often mistaken for neglect. To paraphrase Dorothy Miller (1987, p. 290), everyday mothers must make choices about what to neglect. Although sometimes children are neglected, mothers—particularly poor mothers—probably neglect their own basic needs more often. One study of childhood hunger found that in the great majority (97 percent) of hungry households, adults reported that they cut the size of their meals or skip them altogether to allow children to eat (reported in Sidel, 1998). These sacrifices are not usually noted in the child welfare record, however, because the purpose of the protective investigation is to find fault and failure (Swift, 1995).

Allegations of Physical Abuse

Although the second child-saving movement was predicated on the imagery of the "battered child syndrome," now, as in the past, most cases of physical abuse documented by child protection agencies involve excessive corporal punishment (Gordon, 1988; U.S. Department of Health and Human Services, 1998b). Again, issues of definition arise. In contrast with neglect, women and men are considered to be the perpetrators in approximately equal distribution for allegations of physical abuse. Gordon (1988) found that mothers were perpetrators in 46 percent of physical abuse cases and fathers in 54 percent. These data are consistent with more contemporary findings (U.S. Department of Health and Human Services, 1996). Clearly, women are capable of violence within the context of the family, but caution must be exercised in interpreting the finding of similar rates of physical abuse by mothers and fathers, taking into account the far greater amount of time mothers spend with children. It is important to note that even when women are not the perpetrators, they are held accountable for monitoring the man's violence toward children. Protective service workers usually meet only with the mother, and their assessment focuses on the mother's ability to protect the child from the perpetrator (American Humane Association, 1992; Gordon, 1988). Again, this is in keeping with the gender-based division of labor.

Allegations of Sexual Abuse

Although it is only in the past twenty years that child sexual abuse has been recognized as a phenomenon with more than rare occurrence, Gordon (1988) found in the early days of the first child-protection movement that at least 10 percent of case records referred to incest. Men were the perpetrators in 98 percent of the incest cases in this historical analysis. Since the "discovery" of child sexual abuse, the literature has been replete with propositions that mothers collude with fathers in the sexual abuse of their daughters (Fong and Walsh-Bowers, 1998; Wattenberg, 1985). Although Gordon (1988) found that some mothers felt they had no options for protecting their daughters, many others took vigorous measures to provide protection. Gordon also noted a strong correlation between incest and wife beating. This correlation is substantiated by contemporary research (Elbow and Mayfield, 1991; Sirles and Franke, 1989; Truesdell, McNeil, and Deschner, 1986). Across time, many mothers have been advised by a variety of "helpers" that their husbands' abuse of a daughter is a reflection of the mother's sexual inadequacies. There has been a reluctance on the part of the child-protection system and society in general to hold men accountable for their own sexual behaviors.

Foster Mothers

When a birth mother is judged to be not "good enough," children may be removed from her and placed with a foster mother—someone approved as "good enough" by the child welfare system (Smith and Smith, 1990). Children are placed in foster families, but the "adequacy" of the nurturing mother is central in the assessment of foster homes. Carol Meyer (1985) painted this poignant picture of the life of a foster mother:

> To be a woman, to be a mother, to be lower middle class or poor, to be in a minority group, to work for (with? under?) a child welfare agency, to be paid a pittance, to be asked to parent a child whom no one else is able to parent, to try to love that child and to lose him or her when loving has been achieved, to be supervised by a 22-year-old social worker, to have to deal with school teachers, police, courts, medical appointments, angry biological parents, and the impact of all of this upon one's own family— that is the lot and life of a typical foster mother in America. (p. 252)

In the last few years, kinship foster care has become "the new child placement paradigm" (Hegar, 1999, p. 225). Kinship foster care is "out-of-home care provided by relatives to children in the custody of state child welfare agencies" (Scannapieco and Hegar, 1999, p. 2). Of course, it is not a new idea for grandparents or other relatives to care for a child when the parents cannot. What is new is for kinship care to be a formal part of the state foster-care system. This formalizing of kinship care arose largely out of the concerns among minorities of color, particularly Native Americans and African Americans, about the placement of minority children in white foster homes. They noted that the foster child population is disproportionately African American, and the foster parent population is disproportionately white (Brown and Bailey-Etta, 1997; U.S. Department of Health and Human Services, 1999). Minority children are overrepresented in kinship care, and, for the most part, they are placed in the homes of relatives who are single older women who are themselves poor and in need of support. In many places, children are placed in kinship foster care with little or no evaluation of the home (Fennoy, 1997) and, because the social welfare system has yet to adequately respond to this shift, kinship foster parents receive smaller payments and fewer services than nonkinship foster parents (Brown and Bailey-Etta, 1997).

Child Welfare Workers

At the direct service level, child welfare agencies are staffed predominantly by young, white, middle-class women who have no children of their own (Swift, 1995). They receive comparatively low pay, work in highly charged situations, deal with life and death issues, and are under constant public attack for being both overintrusive and underprotective. When harm comes to children, they, as well as the mothers, are blamed. They are mandated to intervene in the lives of families, and, for a variety of reasons, their most intrusive services are directed toward women who are poor, often minority, single parents—women who are already seriously disempowered (Swift, 1995).

Swift (1995) reminds us that "the very beginnings of casework were embedded in both class and gender relations through which members of the middle class rationed services and support to poor and marginalized groups; and women of the middle and upper classes assumed responsibility for providing both inspiration and limited services to mother-led households" (p. 48). In her research with Canadian child-welfare workers, Swift found that they are often anxious about the decisions they make. They are mandated to amass evidence against parents, not to note parental strengths or the lack of resources for the parenting role. They typically encounter underresourced homes, but their case files focus selectively on the types of parental behaviors noted in child protection law, stripping mothers of their social, economic, and political contexts. The only resources they can provide to parents are resources aimed at improving parenting, translated as mothering. They are asked to implement a public mandate that is vague and ripe with inconsistencies and given responsibilities that they do not have the power to carry out.

Day Care Providers

The contradictory views about the desirability of day care based on the race/class status of the mother, cited earlier, prevents sustained focus on and improvement in our nation's child care system. Despite their concerns about the adequacy of child care environments, most mothers transfer their delegated responsibilities for the care of children to day care providers, another exploited group of women. Recently, in order to meet PRWORA work requirements, public-assistance recipients are being encouraged to leave their children in day care or to become day care providers themselves, thereby continuing the trend of child care as a low-skill, low-wage career path. Recent research found that for-profit day care chains are twice as likely as nonprofit centers to hire public-assistance recipients (cited in Sidel, 1998), and these chains seldom put money into training. Sidel (1998, p. 213) cites the following Bureau of Labor Statistics data: "The median hourly wage of child care workers is $6.12, less than that of a parking lot attendant ($6.38) or an animal caretaker ($6.90)." Recent government "reform" therefore contributes to maintenance of a problematic child care system in two ways—forcing more children into care, particularly poor children, and simultaneously taking no action to improve child care as a career option.

Adolescent Females

Historically, gender bias has been evident in programs for pregnant and parenting adolescents. Social service programs that deal with adolescent sexuality, pregnancy, and child rearing have seldom involved young men (Chilman, 1985). It is true that with child support systems, we have developed an interest in determining paternity and requiring financial child support. But we did not hear fathers condemned in the recent demonizing of adolescent mothers in the political arena. And the public discourse about adolescent pregnancy usually does not acknowledge research findings that the males who impregnate teen mothers are themselves often over twenty or research findings that a majority of young women who have sex during adolescence do so involuntarily (Sidel, 1998). The clear message to adolescents of both sexes is that women are responsible for the sexual behavior of men as well as for themselves—and they carry almost sole responsibility for the care of the children.

Evidence exists that mothers who bear their first child at a young age are at greater risk for bearing additional children during their teen years and for becoming involved with the child-welfare system, compared to those who delay child bearing (Jones and Smith, 1997; Sidel, 1998). Rather than demonizing teen mothers after the fact, the focus should be on pregnancy prevention efforts; however, combating teen pregnancy is a complex matter and must include efforts to improve the social and economic opportunities available to economically disadvantaged teens and teens of color. As noted, prevention efforts must address the role that males play in the teen pregnancy problem.

Minority Women

It is ironic, given our country's history, that the public rhetoric about "welfare queens" going to work has been predicated on imagery of black welfare mothers. Black women have always worked in both the public and private spheres. Under slavery, they worked long days, doing heavy labor for the "master" and "missus" and longed to have more time to care for their own families. Later, black domestic laborers incurred the wrath of their white women bosses by refusing to continue to do live-in work, so that they could go home to their own families in the evenings (Jones, 1985). Black women, as well as many poor white women, learned early what many middle-class white women have only recently discovered—that the separate spheres ideology makes them secondary laborers in the labor force while robbing them of their sense of successful role performance in their assigned domestic domain.

Women of color suffer the double jeopardy of race and gender discrimination. Policymakers and direct service practitioners often hold, simultaneously, two opposing stereotypes of women of color (Cropper, 1997), both of them dangerous to women and children of color. On the one hand, they hold the stereotype of the "all-coping indestructible African Caribbean matriarch" (Cropper, 1997, p. 32). This stereotype often leads to policy and practice that withholds resources because they are not considered necessary or fails to protect children in the care of these women. The opposite stereotype is also prevalent, that of the lazy, "rotten," mother; this stereotype leads to punitive, coercive interventions. Research indicates that the child-protection system responds more slowly and less comprehensively to crises in minority families. Once they do respond, however, their assessments and interventions are harsher than those directed toward white families (Ahmed, 1990; Hogan and Siu, 1988; Swift, 1995).

IMPLICATIONS FOR SOCIAL WORK IN THE TWENTY-FIRST CENTURY

In the contemporary era, women have done wage labor more than in previous eras at jobs that pay less than what men receive. They have served more often as the sole support to children while being held increasingly accountable for adequate nurturance of children by a system that has cut social welfare benefits and has been halfhearted about developing alternative methods of child care. They have had to withstand blows to self-esteem caused by a well-orchestrated campaign to demonize them, some for their involvement in wage labor and some for their lack of involvement. The poorest women have been accused of having babies for profit—an accusation that, in the words of one welfare-rights advocate (cited in Jones, 1985, p. 307), "is a lie that only men could make up, and only men could believe." Recent legislation ended the sixty-one-year-old federal guarantee of aid to poor children and gave tax cuts to wealthier Americans, thus clearly illustrating our nation's current priorities.

In the first edition of this book, we suggested that the welfare of children in the United States could not be secured without changes in several social institutions to further three goals: elimination of gender-based division of labor; elimination of child poverty; and greater support for the caregiving functions of society. Changes were recommended for the family, the labor market, the general social welfare system, and the child welfare system. Unfortunately, events of the past few years reveal that we remain a country with deep ambivalence about issues of gender, race, and class, and this ambivalence prevents progress in ensuring the welfare of children, particularly the country's poorest children.

As we enter the twenty-first century, highest priority should be given to influencing the public discourse about the welfare of children. We must be vigilant in tracking economic and political trends and exposing greed, protected privilege, victim blaming, scapegoating, prejudice, and discrimination. We should be particularly forceful about demanding greater democracy in the political process and more authenticity in public discourse. We should work to ensure that poor women's voices are included in the discourse, and we can insist that "child welfare" be used to refer to the quality of life for children, and not for some narrow construction of child protection. We must help educate the public about the serious risks related to early childhood poverty and the inextricable links between child well-being and policies toward women and families.

Practice Guidelines

There is much evidence that in spite of the oppressive context in which child welfare services have been offered, individual mothers have been able to seek and obtain some of what they need from public social welfare programs (see, for example, Dodson, 1998; Gordon, 1988, 1994). Individual social workers have been able to respond to the pain of mothers, as well as children, in the child welfare system (see Fadiman, 1997). These courageous social workers have recognized that there is always some room to move, some degrees of freedom in implementing the mandates of oppressive systems. They have made noble efforts to see, hear, and know their female clients and the contexts of their lives. Several important practice guidelines are suggested by historical and current analysis.

1. Focus on women as people rather than just on women as mothers; know as much about their hopes and their dreams as you know about their parenting skills.
2. Focus on the strengths rather than the inadequacies of mothers—on their efforts to solve problems and their survival skills. Ask yourself often, "Have I encouraged a mother today?"
3. Be sure that case records note parental strengths, efforts to cope, and resource deficiencies.
4. Work in the least hierarchical fashion possible with clients; involve women in decision making even when providing involuntary services.
5. Recognize and validate the emotions expressed by women.
6. Work with women and agencies to recognize when a private woe should be constructed as a public problem.
7. Be sensitive to and challenge "blame the victim" assessments of women clients presented by other professionals.
8. Help women to see their struggles in historical, social, cultural, economic, and political contexts.
9. Share information with clients honestly—even when the news is bad. Coach them on how to successfully negotiate the social welfare system.
10. Develop networks of support for families (in churches, workplaces, neighborhoods, schools, etc.) to enhance their caregiving functions;

use those networks intensively and creatively in times of family crisis.

11. Ensure that all contacts with families support women in their development as persons—and support, to every extent possible, the sharing of the caregiving load. Help women create a space (even a small space) for themselves.

12. Approach foster parents with an honest exploration of the complex demands of their roles. Encourage collaborative relationships between birth parents and foster parents.

13. Evaluate programs for pregnant and parenting adolescents for their gender bias.

14. Do not hold women accountable for acts of maltreatment that they did not perpetrate. Question your own, and others', tendency to expect less from fathers than mothers.

15. Empower yourself by organizing your scarce resource of time to allow the development of some innovative service that you care about.

CONCLUSION

As the United States entered the twentieth century, the mothers' aid discourse (family assistance) and the child-saving discourse were intertwined; with the beginning of the twenty-first century, time is long overdue to bring these two discourses back together. Just as the Social Security discourse of the New Deal reflected the special challenges of the Depression era, the new discourse must reflect the social trends of the current era. These trends include growth in economic inequality, growth in female-headed, single-parent households, increase of mothers in the labor market, and a sharp increase in families reported to the child-protection system. These trends, most of them shared by other late-industrial countries, require structural analysis and structural solutions. At the current time, gender, race, and class politics are producing distributive injustice, with women and children, particularly poor women and children, absorbing the costs of the most recent industrial cycle.

The general welfare of children would be greatly enhanced if economically disadvantaged and/or dependent women were not assigned sole responsibility for their care. Women—particularly poor women— are being asked to do too much with too little and are vilified if they fail at an impossible task. Cross-cultural studies provide convincing evidence that societies in which caregiving is shared have the lowest rates of child maltreatment (Korbin, 1981). Until we move in that direction, the welfare of children will continue to come at considerable cost to the welfare of women—or the welfare of women will come at the expense of the welfare of children.

REFERENCES

Abramovitz, M. (1988). *Regulating the lives of women: Social welfare policy from colonial times to the present.* Boston: South End Press.

Ahmed, B. (1990). *Black perspectives in social work.* London: Ventura.

American Humane Association (1992). *Helping in child protective services: A competency based casework handbook.* Englewood, CO: Author.

Anderson, P. (1989). The origin, emergence, and professional recognition of child protection. *Social Service Review, 63*: 222-244.

Bloom, D., Kemple, J., and Rogers-Dillon, R. (1997). *The Family Transition Program: Early impacts of Florida's initial time-limited welfare program.* New York: Manpower Demonstration and Research Corporation.

Brace, C. (1859). *The best method of disposing of pauper and vagrant children.* New York: Wyncoop and Hallenbeck.

Brown, A. and Bailey-Etta, B. (1997). An out-of-home care system in crisis: Implications for African-American children in the child welfare system. *Child Welfare, 76*(1): 65-83.

Child Trends (1999). *Children and welfare reform: A guide to evaluating the effects of state welfare policies on children.* Washington, DC: Author.

Chilman, C. (1985). Feminist issues in teenage parenting. *Child Welfare, 64:* 225-234.

Costin, L. (1985). Introduction. *Child Welfare, 64:* 197-201.

Cropper, A. (1997). Rethinking practice: Learning from a black feminist perspective. In J. Bates, R. Pugh, and N. Thompson (Eds.), *Protecting children: Challenges and change* (pp. 31-41). Brookfield, VT: Ashgate Publishing Co.

Dalaker, J. and Naifeh, M. (1998). *Poverty in the United States: 1997.* Washington, DC: U.S. Department of Commerce, Economics and Statistics Administration, Bureau of the Census.

Dalley, G. (1988). *Ideologies of caring: Rethinking community and collectivism.* London: Macmillan Education Ltd.

D'Amico, D. (1997). Adult education and welfare to work initiatives: A review of research, practice, and policy. *Literacy Leader Fellowship Program Reports, 3*(1): 1-72.

Dodson, L. (1998). *Don't call us out of name: The untold lives of women and girls in poor America.* Boston: Beacon Press.

Elbow, M. and Mayfield, J. (1991). Mothers of incest victims: Villains, victims, or protectors? *Families in Society: The Journal of Contemporary Human Services, 72:* 78-85.

Fadiman, A. (1997). *The spirit catches you and you fall down: A Hmong child, her American doctors. and the collision of two cultures.* New York: The Noonday Press.

Fennoy, I. (1997). The intersection of child welfare and health services. In A. Carten and J. Dumpson (Eds.), *Removing risks from children: Shifting the paradigm. Strategies for culturally competent child welfare services* (pp. 113-126). Silver Spring, MD: Beckham House.

Fong, J. and Walsh-Bowers, R. (1998). Voices of the blamed: Mothers' responsiveness to father-daughter incest. *Journal of Family Social Work, 3*(l): 25-41.

Geen, R., Waters Boots, S., and Tumlin, K. (1999). The cost of protecting vulnerable children: Understanding federal, state, and local child welfare spending. Assessing the New Federalism, Occasional Paper #20. Washington, DC: The Urban Institute.

Gordon, L. (1988). *Heroes of their own lives: The politics and history of family violence.* New York: Viking.

Gordon, L. (1994). *Pitied but not entitled.* New York: Free Press.

Gueron, J. and Pauly, E. (1991). *From welfare to work.* New York: Russell Sage Foundation.

Halpern, R. (1991). Supportive services to families in poverty: Dilemma of reform. *Social Service Review, 65:* 343-364.

Halpern, R. (1999). *Fragile families: Fragile solutions.* New York: Columbia University Press.

Hanlan, A. (1966). From social reform to social security: The separation of ADC and child welfare. *Child Welfare, 45:* 109-120.

Hegar, R. (1999). Kinship foster care: The new child placement paradigm. In R. Hegar and M. Scannapieco (Eds.), *Kinship foster care: Policy, practice. and research* (pp. 208-240). New York: Oxford University Press.

Hogan, P. and Siu, S. (1988). Minority children and the child welfare system: An historical perspective. *Social Work, 33:* 493-498.

Hutchison, E. (1990). Child maltreatment: Can it be defined? *Social Service Review, 64:* 61-78.

Hutchison, E. (1993). Mandatory reporting laws: Child protective case-finding gone awry? *Social Work, 38:* 56-63.

Jones, B. and Smith, A. (1997). Mental health needs: Underserved and increasing in complexity. In A. Carten and J. Dumpson (Eds.), *Removing risks from children: Shifting the paradigm. Strategies for culturally competent child welfare services* (pp. 127-147). Silver Spring, MD: Beckham House.

Jones, J. (1985). *Labor of love, labor of sorrow: Black women, work and the family, from slavery to the present.* New York: Vintage.

Kamerman, S. and Kahn, A. (1990). If CPS is driving child welfare —where do we go from here? *Public Welfare, 48*(1): 9-13.

Korbin, J. (Ed.) (1981). *Child abuse and neglect: Cross-cultural perspective.* Berkeley and Los Angeles: University of California Press.

Lindsey, D. (1994). *The welfare of children.* New York: Oxford University Press.

Long, S., Kirby, G., Kurka, R., and Waters, S. (1998). Child care assistance under welfare reform: Early responses by the states. Assessing the New Federalism, Occasional Paper #15. Washington, DC: The Urban Institute.

McLaughlin, M. (1997). Toward real welfare reform. In A. Carten and J. Dumpson (Eds.), *Removing risks from children: Shifting the paradigm. Strategies for culturally competent child welfare services* (pp. 83-111). Silver Spring, MD: Beckham House.

Mead, L. (1992). *The new politics of poverty: The nonworking poor in America.* New York: Basic Books.

Mead, L. (1996). Welfare reform at work. *Society, 33*(5): 37-40.

Meyer, C. (1985). A feminist perspective on foster family care: A redefinition of the categories. *Child Welfare, 64:* 249-258.

Miller, D. (1987). Children's policy and women's policy: Congruence or conflict? *Social Work, 32:* 289-292.

Murray, C. (1984). *Losing ground: American social policy 1950-1980.* New York: Basic Books.

Murray, C. (1996). Keeping priorities straight on welfare reform. *Society, 33*(5): 10-12.

National Research Council (1994). *Understanding child abuse and neglect.* Washington, DC: National Academy of Sciences.

Nelson, B. (1984). *Making an issue of child abuse: Political agenda setting for social Problems.* Chicago: University of Chicago Press.

Pavetti, L., Olson, K., Pindus, N., Pernas, M., and Isaacs, J. (1996). *Designing welfare-to-work programs for families facing personal or family challenges. Lessons from the field.* Washington, DC: The Urban Institute and American Institutes for Research.

Pelton, L. (1990). Resolving the crisis in child welfare. *Public Welfare, 48*(1): 19-25.

Primus, W., Rawlings, L., Larin, K., and Porter, K. (1999). *The initial impacts of welfare reform on the incomes of single-mother families.* Washington, DC: Center on Budget and Policy Priorities.

Scannapieco, M. and Hegar, R. (1999). Kinship foster care in context. In R. Hegar and M. Scannapieco (Eds.), *Kinship foster care: Policy, practice, and research* (pp. 1-13). New York: Oxford University Press.

Shook, K. (1999). Does the loss of welfare income increase the risk of involvement with the child welfare system? Joint Center for Poverty Research Working Paper #6.

Sidel, R. (1986). *Women and children last.* New York: Viking.

Sidel, R. (1998). *Keeping women and children last: America's war on the poor,* Revised edition. New York: Penguin Books.

Sirles, E. and Franke, P. (1989). Factors influencing mothers' reactions to intrafamily sexual abuse. *Child Abuse and Neglect, 13:* 131-139.

Smith, B. and Smith, T. (1990). For love and money: Women as foster mothers. *Affilia, 5*(l): 66-80.

Swift, K. (1995). *Manufacturing "bad mothers": A critical perspective on child neglect.* Toronto: University of Toronto Press.

Truesdell, D., McNeil, J., and Deschner, J. (1986). Incidence of wife abuse in incestuous families. *Social Work, 31:* 138-140.

Tweedie, J., Reichert, D., and O'Connor, M. (1999). *Tracking recipients after they leave welfare: Summaries of new state tracking studies.* National Conference of State Legislatures, April.

U.S. Department of Health and Human Services (1996). The third national incidence study of child abuse and neglect. (DHHS Publication, Contract #105-91-1800.) Washington, DC: U.S. Government Printing Office.

U.S. Department of Health and Human Services (1998a). *Comparison of the prior law and the Personal Responsibility and Work Opportunity Reconciliation Act of 1966.* Office of the Assistant Secretary for Planning and Evaluation. Washington, DC: Author.

U.S. Department of Health and Human Services (1998b). *Child maltreatment 1996: Reports from the states to the National Child Abuse and Neglect Data System.* Washington, DC: U.S. Government Printing Office.

U.S. Department of Health and Human Services (1999). *Child maltreatment 1997: Reports from the states to the National Child Abuse and Neglect Data System.* Administration on Children, Youth, and Families. Washington, DC: U.S. Government Printing Office.

Vondra, J. (1993). Childhood poverty and child maltreatment. In J. Chafel (Ed.), *Child poverty and public policy* (pp. 127-166). Washington, DC: Urban Institute Press.

Wattenberg, E. (1985). In a different light: A feminist perspective on the role of mothers in father-daughter incest. *Child Welfare, 64:* 203-211.

Zedlewski, S., Holcomb, P., and Duke, A. (1998). Cash assistance in transition: The story of 13 states. Assessing the New Federalism, Occasional Paper #16. Washington, DC: Urban Institute.

Zellman, G. (1992). The impact of case characteristics on child abuse reporting decisions. *Child Abuse and Neglect. 16:* 57-71.

Chapter 5

Women's Mental Health Issues: Twentieth-Century Realities; Twenty-First Century Challenges

Margaret E. Severson

INTRODUCTION

It is a daunting responsibility to be charged with writing a chapter on women's mental health issues for a book designed to honor the memory and contributions of Liane Davis. There was a time in the not-so-distant past that joining the subjects "women" and "mental health" might have been regarded as oxymoronic; a time when women were solely evaluated through the male-centric lens and subsequently categorized under value-laden headings such as histrionic, schizophrenogenic, codependent, borderline, and neurotic. Thankfully, Liane's contributions and those of her valued colleagues helped to challenge the notion of a singular reality which could be objectified through labels, by revolutionizing our conceptions of reality as being states of minds equally valid; equally worth revealing. Their contributions firmly placed women in the midst of reality making—reminding us that women are not the dependent variables in life's equations, but rather are independent, dynamic, creative, and resilient life forces.

Still, old notions and old habits die hard. Thinking about the kinds of mental health pressures and circumstances affecting women in the twenty-first century, one must be careful not simply to substitute new language for old concepts—*anxious* for *neurotic*; *survivor* for *victim*; *potential* for *problem*; *challenge* for *crisis*. It is tempting to use strategic and powerful language as evidence of real meaningful change in women's conditions, but in the end such rhetoric proves to be as disempowering as the conditions themselves. Early in the past century, Sigmund Freud began building a theory designed around pathologized depictions of women as being anxiety ridden, depressed, conflicted, and dependent—in short, *sick*. The language used, the concepts explored, and the descriptions of his women patients were so seductively powerful that many of the traditional meanings of these concepts have been carried over into contemporary popular verbiage and have developed a referential power of their own. When have the phrases "She is in denial," "She is resistant," "She is dependent" been uttered *with the intention* that they be interpreted in a positive, nonpathological light?

Despite the renewed spirit of the women's movement during the 1960s and 1970s, the illness approach to the assessment and treatment of women's mental health conditions enjoys considerable popularity among clinical professionals as we enter the twenty-first century. What became so pervasive and persuasive at the turn of the past century—the radical and sexistly skewed depictions of women's mental conditions and the language used to describe those conditions—and the perpetuation of these views in this new century should serve as a warning to feminist social work practitioners at the cusp of the new millennium: that reframing women's experiences in the language of strengths, empowerment, and stories must yet address the systemic underpinnings of their struggles. This is social work at its core—working with women in and with their environments.

Chapter Overview

Women may lay claim to a glorious history—one of struggle, heartache, loss, victory, and ongoing challenge—experienced both individually and collectively. Of course, each process and each outcome is worth writing about, and each deserves volumes of contextual exploration. With space limits in mind, the modest goal of this chapter is to provide a way of thinking about women's past, present, and future that honors the elements of herstory and provides a way of thinking about the whole array of mental health struggles women face in the twenty-first century. As defined here, these struggles are not simply or even predominantly those organized around DSM-IV diagnoses, women's interpersonal relationships, and their nondiagnostic but nonetheless suspiciously characterized emotional conditions (see the "V" codes and the myriad other problems proposed in the DSM-IV [American Psychiatric Association, 1994] for further study). Rather, these struggles are explored by focusing on several contemporary social conditions and women's power or lack thereof expressed and experienced within the contexts of those conditions. Social work practitioners and feminist writers have a dual responsibility when working with women and recording their journeys: they must be able to evaluate the institutional and systemic obstacles to mental *health* while simultaneously hearing each woman's account of the impact of those obstacles in her life.

In this chapter, a very brief look at a sample of the historical forces that have impacted women's mental health serves as a backdrop to exploring the sometimes harsh realities of women's mental health conditions in the present day. Although many viable approaches to thinking about the contemporary categorizations and status of women's mental health conditions exist, the discussion here will revolve around a contextualized analysis of women's mental health and power. GlenMaye (1998) suggests that there are three general conditions women share in common "that together produce and enforce" their "subordination and relative powerlessness: (1) profound alienation from the self [analogous to the loss of voice and the loss of self-direction], (2) the double-bind situation of women [the no-win situation that leaves women feeling guilty about their choices], and (3) institutional and structural sexism [the unequal distribution of power]" (p. 31). As an organizational strategy for talking about women's mental health conditions, this chapter's focus on specific mental health issues references these conditions within the context of three structural exemplars: women and poverty; incarcerated women; and women subjected to violence. Accordingly, the social contexts and major mental health repercussions with which all clients and social workers must grapple are highlighted here, along with the power dynamics inherent in the details of the specific mental health contexts, conditions, and challenges that women face.

The final pages of this chapter set out various hypotheses about the structural and emotional issues confronting women in the twenty-first century as well as the responsibilities awaiting social work practitioners working in, with, and for the social systems with which women interface.

TWENTIETH-CENTURY REALITIES—
PAST TO PRESENT

Though both the concept and the state of "madness" have been discussed for centuries, the first major theorist/practitioner to provide a contemplative paradigm of human psychological and sexual development was Sigmund Freud. Theorizing that behavior was primarily determined by the management or lack thereof of the opposing forces of the unconscious, psychoanalytic theory set forth a view of psychological functioning that was both a reflection of the times and a precursor to the future. Consider the era just prior to and during which the early psychoanalytic theories were developed. Women were moving into an awakening of sorts led by early women's rights activists including Matilda Joslyn Gage, Elizabeth Cady Stanton, and Lucretia Mott, all of whom were envisioning equality between the genders and change in the institutional structures that were responsible for their oppression—religion, economics, social life, and government—the "four-fold oppression" of women's lives (Wagner, 1999, p. 62).

Perhaps as a way of understanding and explaining *why* these suffragists and other women were behaving the way they were, ideas were set forth in the psychiatric literature that provided just the type of objectified, seemingly definitive rationalizations that would make men feel more secure in their positions in society. Psychosexual development from birth forward was emphasized as part of Freud's theory and set out particularly in his concept of penis envy. Freud's notion that women's anger at being without a penis and the consequent subordination of those without (women) to those who wielded this powerful physical appendage (men) led to his suggestion that it was this penis envy that constituted the foundation for the development of a woman's madness (Ussher, 1992).

In the context of delivering therapeutic services, originally psychotherapy was something conducted by an emotionally distant and dominant (expert) male who considered himself and was considered by others to be an authority on the female experience, one who could accurately interpret the woman's motivations, reactions (*her narratives*), and behaviors thereby pathologizing her "through disconnecting her struggles from the political realities of poverty, race, class, role, gender oppression, heterosexism, and powerlessness" (Pearlman, 1995, p. 6). Similarly, in the early 1930s, when thousands of women sought the advice of psychiatrist Karl Menninger as they struggled with family of origin, marriage, and gender-role conflicts (Faulkner and Pruitt, 1997), their letters and his responses reflected the impact of Freudian and disease-model thinking on the American woman, the American psychiatrist, and the American press. When Dr. Menninger penned his responses to readers' letters (all of which were from women), he was often "prescriptive and judgmental" (p. 11), blaming wives for their husbands' affairs, encouraging women to make the most of their domestic virtues all the while supporting their men. In describing the process of pulling together a series of these letters for publication, Faulkner and Pruitt relate that at age ninety-six, when Menninger reread the letters, he queried "'Did I do them any good?'" (p. 13), a question which seems to emphasize the work of the therapist—the clinical expert—rather than the work of the writer—who was not only the star, but always the survivor, of the story.

Right or wrong, penis envy or not, historically women have both measured themselves and been measured by others against the male model. Although Freud may have supplied a rationale, he cannot be credited with the actual phenomenon of viewing woman vis-à-vis man. Susan B. Anthony first protested gender-based salary inequities in the 1840s. In the 1850s and 1860s, she, Elizabeth Cady Stanton, and others worked to ensure that women could enter independently into contracts and control their own financial affairs, supported the emancipation of slaves, and of course began efforts that cleared the way for women to vote. At the same time, the forces of men were working against these efforts.

Preceding Freud by several decades, and near the same time that Anthony first registered to vote in the early 1870s, the U.S. Supreme Court (an all male body which would remain so for another 100-plus years) upheld an Illinois court decision denying women the right to practice law (see *Bradwell v. Illinois*, 1872) thus legitimizing male dominance in matters of policy and institutional management. In his concurring opinion, Justice Bradley remarked that "the paramount destiny and mission of women are to fulfill the noble and benign offices of wife and mother" (*Bradwell v. Illinois,* 1872, p. 141). Although the first order meaning of "benign" may have been synonymous with noble, its second order message suggested women's efforts should be seen as supportive, of no direct effect, and innocuous. Women's bodies were the vehicles both to men's power and to women's powerlessness and also to the fulfillment of the woman's proper destiny—that is, one destined to the offices of wife and mother.

Of course, in terms of women's social, civil, and legal rights, much has changed since the mid-1800s in terms of the accumulation of enumerated rights. Women vote, work, pursue educational opportunities, own property, and exercise a political voice. Remarkably for women, these gains have been realized while still fulfilling that destiny—being the "wife"—in whatever way that is defined—and in being the mother. However, the accumulation of rights must be contrasted with the practical realization and yield of the exercise of these rights. It is one thing to have equal access to educational institutions; it is quite another to realize the equalizing resources that make such access feasible on the front end and, on the back end, to reap the benefits such access should afford. It is one thing to fulfill a role physically ascribed, but something quite different when the choice whether to fulfill this role is conditioned on the support of those who biologically cannot do so. In the same vein, it is one thing to suggest that being a wife and mother is "noble"; it is quite another when such singular assignment of nobility means that when the father opts out, it is the noble mother and their children who are cast into poverty. It is one thing to be empowered to compete in the marketplace; it is quite another to realize the fruits of that empowerment in, for example, the supermarket, when earning only 76 cents to the male's dollar (U.S. Department of Labor, 1999).

How does this history relate to women's mental health in the year 2001? These are some of the systemically rooted contradictions that have contributed to the way women's mental health statuses are viewed in current day. Remarkably, the deleterious outcomes of each of these conditions—depression, anxiety, drug and/or alcohol abuse and dependence—are recorded in the social work literature and supported by research (see, for example, the research reviews of Tice and Perkins, 1996; Wilton, 1995; Belle, 1990). Unfortunately, instead of viewing these conditions as symptomatic of "learned helplessness" [and as] normal reaction[s] to disempowering situation[s]" (Manning, 1998, p. 91), these symptoms are interpreted as being evidence of the existence of a mental illness or aberration. Such interpretations are those of mental health professionals who, in that very moment with the woman client, fail to ask and examine for themselves how she has been positioned by the expression of institutionalized power differentials.

From the historical perspective, one does not have to travel back a century to know that the perpetuation of institutional and interpersonal bias and oppression continues and so poses an ongoing danger to women's mental health statuses. Blanch and Levin (1999) point out that two decades of research has resulted in

> scant evidence that "women's issues" are adequately addressed in mental health systems today. . . the role of context and power imbalances in relationships are still infrequently addressed as part of the healing process, and. . . women may not be receiving help in recognizing oppressive conditions and working to overcome them. (p. 7)

If unable to engage with oppression in a way that creates significant systemic change, then mental health professionals and systems are not collaborators in healing and may very well be the unwitting partners of the oppressors.

Twenty years ago, with frightening detail, Broverman and colleagues (1981) reported the relationship between conceptions of health by gender and conceptions of mental health in general. They found that clinicians' conceptions of a healthy and mature man did not significantly differ from their conceptions of a healthy adult. When it came to their conceptions of women, however, these researchers found clinicians to be "significantly less likely to attribute traits that characterize healthy adults to a woman" (p. 94). Other studies investigating the influence of gender on the work of the treatment provider, on the assignment of diagnoses, and on the effectiveness of the treatment itself have reached similar conclusions—that "gender itself is a barrier to effective mental health treatment" (Mowbray et al., 1999, p. 191).

CONTEMPORARY ISSUES IN WOMEN'S MENTAL HEALTH: THE INTERPLAY OF SYSTEMS, STRUCTURES, AND SYMPTOMS

The incidence and types of mental health problems experienced by women are well documented. Women are more likely to have active mental disorders than men are, though the incidence of lifetime disorders is higher for men. Women are more likely than men to be diagnosed with depressive, somatization, and obsessive-compulsive disorders; men are more frequently diagnosed with alcohol abuse/dependence disorders, drug abuse/dependence disorders, and antisocial personality disorder. Women are more likely to have a diagnosed affective disorder and/or an anxiety disorder, and are also more likely than are men to be diagnosed with having three or more disorders (Fellin, 1996).

It is tempting to dispute the pathologizing of women by solely arguing why certain symptoms are not really related to a diagnostic condition but rather are a consequence of the double bind women are in. Although in fact the latter may be true, this type of analysis is susceptible to two pitfalls: it juxtaposes women with men in a way that is not helpful because women experience stress and mental disability independently of men, and it runs short of explaining what can be done to change the symptoms, alleviate the double bind, and ensure that power differentials do not perpetuate the problem(s). Consequently, the focus here on the woman's realization or lack thereof of personal power and the structural contexts in which power or lack of power are revealed and endured helps to move the portrayal of women's mental health needs from a personal and pathological perspective to a contextual analysis: women simply cannot *be* or *be understood* outside of context. Further, while men may be part of the context, they are not in and of themselves the context, so there is no need to view women vis-à-vis men.

Consequently, the exploration of women's mental health issues set out in the following pages is accomplished by viewing them specifically within the context provided by three structural exemplars: women and poverty; incarcerated women; and women and violence. There are no doubt many other contexts in which one could search for a deeper understanding of women's mental health conditions, for example, women and spirituality; women as caregivers; women in employment situations. Poverty, incarceration, and violence were the contexts chosen for exposition here because they are in and of themselves conditions and consequences of institutional structures, making an analysis of their impact on women's mental health conditions rich and complex. It is well documented, for example, that poverty and violence are associated with the existence of mental health problems and that all three are also associated with women (Fellin, 1996).

Exemplar I: Women and Poverty

Although they are indeed families, the terms "child welfare," "family assistance," and "aid to families with dependent children" are all terms used to describe the impoverished condition of women and their children. Fathers may be incarcerated, unknown, or otherwise absent; they all too frequently are not part of the family denoted by the family service label.

There are countless ways that women (and their children) end up living in impoverished situations and at or below the official poverty level. Pearce (1979) coined this outcome the "feminization of poverty," the phenomenon inextricably related to an "inequality of opportunity" (Reitmeir and Christensen, 1994) in family, social, economic and/or political settings. The relationship between poverty and women's mental health is clear; many years of social science research has established the correlation between poverty and "psychological distress and diagnosable mental disorder" (Belle, 1990, p. 385).

Surely one of the most prominent ways this slide into poverty occurs is through fathers abandoning their responsibilities to provide economic and physical support to women and children after the termination of their relationships. A divorce rate of nearly 50 percent in the United States leaves between 85 and 90 percent of children of divorce in the custody of their mothers (Mulloy, 1997). There are an unknown number of nonmarital relationship terminations that also result in children being solely physically as well as economically assigned to the responsibility of their mothers. Irving and Benjamin's (1995) review of the divorce research yielded two conclusions in this regard: (1) while men enjoy stable or enhanced incomes after divorce, during the same period, women "experience a sharp decline in income" and (2) the stress which results from this decrease in income "may be the single most important source of postdivorce adjustment difficulty among women" (p. 56).

And the picture has worsened. In 1996, the welfare income maintenance system, of which Aid to Families with Dependent Children was a part, was replaced by the Personal Responsibility and Work Opportunity Reconciliation Act (1996), which set both lifetime limits and demands for work on the part of recipients and gave to the separate states the power to design how income support would look in each particular jurisdiction. The overall design of the new welfare system "reflects social values that center on the desirability of work, marriage, and positive parenting" (Berrick, 1999, p. 176), a design which, for several reasons, inherently works to the disadvantage of women. Several very restrictive components are included in these reform measures, designed to penalize states if they fail to meet certain mandates set out by the federal government. For example, one cannot receive welfare for more than two consecutive years without being subjected to a work requirement; one cannot have more than a five-year lifetime tenure on welfare; and food stamp eligibility is drastically reduced for nonparent single adults. Further, the separate states are mandated to reduce unwanted pregnancy without increasing the rate of abortion and, while under previous law child care was an entitlement, under this new law, it is no longer so. Now, single, minor parents may not receive aid unless they live with an adult, they abide by procedures intended to establish paternity, they refrain from having additional children while receiving aid, and they ensure that their children have received proper immunizations and, if applicable, attend school (Berrick, 1999).

In the context of poverty, the realities of women's lives were not taken into account by the architects of welfare reform. The time limits imposed are harmful to women who suffer from domestic violence, particularly given that states may now impose residency requirements that work to penalize victims who flee one state because they fear for their safety. Regulations in the child support and enforcement program that require welfare recipients to identify their children's fathers place women in even greater danger. Many women who should be getting financial support from the father of their children do not wish to seek it because of the history of abuse in the relationship. This abuse in and of itself can be a barrier to subsequent employment. Who can blame an employer for not wanting to hire or retain a woman who is chronically late, looks like she has been in a brawl, or whose former abusive partner continues to issue threats against her (see Sable et al. 1999)?

To make matters worse, under the Temporary Assistance to Needy Families (TANF) mandates, states are no longer required to give TANF recipients any child support money collected through the state, bringing to fruition economic consequences for the nearly one million children who have been "expected to be affected by growing impoverishment" (Briar-Lawson and Drews, 1999, p. 167). Further, this policy may contribute another risk factor toward the creation of the next generation of poor, incarcerated, and mentally impaired women.

Growing evidence suggests that disproportionately large numbers of women on welfare were physically and/or sexually abused as children. Goodman (1991) found that 57 percent of her sample of low-income mothers reported having been physically abused and 46 percent reported having been sexually abused as children. Additional research (Banyard, 1999) is confirming these results and revealing the link between "childhood maltreatment and mental health problems in the lives of survivors" (p. 161) and between poverty and psychological distress and poverty and adult victimization as well. Banyard (1999) found that, after controlling for other risk factors, the experiences of physical and sexual abuse as a child resulted in high risk levels, traumatic stress, and negative consequences experienced across the woman's life span.

In essence, the condition of poverty is akin to the crumbling of one essential pillar of support needed for good mental health. The failure to place gender at the center of any analysis of dependency on government services *and* the failure to put the woman's experience of poverty at the center of any analysis of women's mental health issues is untenable. Doing so merely provides a method for ignoring the deleterious effect poverty wreaks on women. First, it perpetuates the economic disadvantage of many single-parent—read mothered—families. When welfare policy is written to promote the ideals of work, marriage, and good parenting but gender biases have the effect of creating social and economic obstacles for women to attain these ideals, women experience the full thrust of an institutionalized power imbalance. Second, in part or perhaps primarily as a product of living in poverty, women experience mental health challenges that result in their being overrepresented in certain diagnostic categories, particularly in categories where symptoms of depression and/or dependence are prominent. This places women in a double bind: poor women have less viable access to mental health services and, as they are released from welfare and the minimal benefits of medical assistance programs, their ability to purchase more effective though also more expensive antidepressant medications is further impeded. Treatment with less efficacious drugs results in side effects that may in turn interfere with their ability to give 100 percent at work and/or with their children. The result is that, once again, the woman is relegated to the position of not having lived up to the ideals set by a body of lawmakers who did not place her in the center of their policy analysis to begin with—*before* changing the law. Further, if in fact the depression is caused or exaggerated by the woman's poor economic status, then treating the depression in isolation is tantamount to treating only the symptom. Empowerment must entail more than access to traditional mental health services because without more, the message to the depressed, poor woman is disempowering: "Take this pill, take this treatment, and live with your plight." This *Stepford Wives* type of intervention changes nothing; meaningful change starts only with the realization that the pill merely alters the experience of the problem, not the problem itself. The problem is poverty. The problem is the impact of poverty on women's mental health.

Exemplar II: Incarcerated Women

Women represent the fastest-growing segment of the incarcerated population in the United States (Beck, 1999), and yet are largely underserved by mental health programming both because of their status as incarcerated women and because of the perception of them, by clinical professionals, as being difficult or resistant clients. In general, incarcerated women, those in jails and prisons, present complex problem sets, including co-occurring health, psychiatric, and substance abuse disorders, life predicaments, and treatment needs. Nearly half of the women confined in state prisons during 1998 had been using drugs and/or alcohol at the time of their offense. Further, women in jail and prison present with important and unique health needs, including pregnancy and HIV-positive statuses, stressful conditions that serve to further aggravate impaired mental health conditions.

At the time of their incarcerations, women are more likely than men to have children and to be their caregivers. In 1998, mothers of 1.3 million minor children were living under correctional supervision; one-quarter of these children had mothers incarcerated in a jail or prison (Greenfeld and Snell, 1999). Probably not unrelated to their status as mothers, incarcerated women are also likely to be poor—almost 30 percent of women incarcerated in 1998 reported that they were receiving welfare assistance prior to their arrest; 37 percent reported having an income of less than $600.00 per month (Greenfeld and Snell, 1999). Not surprisingly, many poor, incarcerated women are also members of minority populations. Veysey (1998) points out that the changes in national welfare and health-care policies are likely to have a particularly negative impact on women who are incarcerated. Generally, these "women have less access to public subsidies, including housing, health care, and financial entitlements" and "face increasing discrimination due to their multiple statuses as offenders, mental health service users, substance abusers, and being predominantly people of color in poverty" (p. 370). White women are already more likely to be on probation status and thus employed than are minority women, who instead are serving time in jail or prison (Greenfeld and Snell, 1999).

Over the past decade, women have consistently reported having personal histories of physical and/or sexual abuse (Greenfeld and Snell, 1999; Veysey, 1998; Bureau of Justice Statistics, 1994; American Correctional Association, 1990). In sum, they are more than three times as likely as men to report having experienced physical or sexual abuse sometime prior to incarceration. In 1996, 48 percent of jailed women reported that they were victims of sexual or physical abuse sometime prior to admission; 27 percent reported that they had been raped (Bureau of Justice Statistics, 1998). Most indicated having been abused before age eighteen. Further, much of the reported abuse was allegedly delivered at the hands of an intimate or family member (Bureau of Justice Statistics, 1997).

Women prisoners are often viewed as being more demanding and more difficult to manage than male prisoners are. In fact, there may be some truth to this, not because they are women, but because of their histories and unique experiences as women—histories that have not been taken fully into account in designing women-centered, jail/prison health/mental health based services. Behaviors that have in the past led to formal diagnoses such as depression, anxiety disorders, or personality disorders, may in fact be symptoms of posttraumatic stress. Even, as Teplin, Abram, and McClelland (1996) found, where symptoms consistent with the formal diagnoses of drug and/or alcohol abuse or dependence, major depressive episodes, dysthymia, and antisocial personality disorders are seen, they may accompany a diagnosis of PTSD. In a prison population, Jordan and colleagues (1996) noted similar findings and also found a significant occurrence rate of the diagnosis of borderline personality disorder, a diagnosis they specifically linked to the woman's experience of sexual abuse at or prior to the age of ten.

Despite these substantiated differences in mental health problems and their etiologies, in the past ten to fifteen years, when mental health services have been offered to incarcerated women, they have resembled the same service programs that are offered to men. Of course, institutions have managed to avoid providing specifically developed, woman-centered services on the basis that there are many fewer women than men being served and so only provision of the same or similar services would be fiscally efficient (Collins and Collins, 1996). More recently, researchers have suggested that women's particular needs—again, largely rooted in histories of violence and abuse—make it necessary to think about equality in services but not sameness—i.e., that women should have services made available that are particularly designed for women and in so doing manage to avoid the formula approach to corrections-based mental health programming.

This idea of offering strategically and specifically designed mental health services to women offenders seems particularly important given the rapid rise in the number of incarcerated females. In fact, it may well be easier to design a package of services for women after their incarceration, given the captive nature of the audience, the potential for additional funding sources to support the services, and the coercive nature of certain judicial interventions.

But there are major problems with holding back services until poor, single-parent, physically unhealthy women with histories of sexual and/or physical abuse become incarcerated—not the least of which is that waiting until incarceration results in many more costs, particularly those social, economic, and personal emotional costs incurred by placing their children in foster care. Differing estimates of 7 to 13 percent (Bloom and Steinhart, 1993) up to 33 percent (Veysey, 1998) of children whose mothers are incarcerated are living in foster care or are otherwise entangled in the child protective services system, causing additional stress for these incarcerated women. Although some women are able to place their children with family members, the opportunity to do so and ensure their financial support through access to welfare programs is diminishing under the TANF regulations. One critical question is why affordable day care that could support mothers in realizing educational and occupational success before they turn to crime is unavailable in this country, yet costly foster care after incarceration is something deemed affordable. That and other questions raised in the same vein, however, are rarely heard when they originate from the mouths of the prisoner—whether she is the prisoner of the jail or the prisoner of the policy system—because the words of her narrative are muffled by the walls of disempowerment.

The criminal justice system is made up of and managed by the law and by the rules that spring from the law—rules that are Eurocentric, male made, and male oriented. This is not to suggest that there is something inherently wrong with this orientation as it applies to males; it suggests only that the mark is missed where women are concerned. This issue is this: when looking at the incarcerated woman, do the rules that guide the treatment of that woman reflect an understanding of her experience, her needs, and her history? Anything less is, by its very nature, disempowering.

In essence, every woman is susceptible to the economic, social, and political circumstances that precede and follow incarceration. Poor women, particularly those of minority status, women raising children as single parents, women who have been victims of domestic violence, and women who have been abandoned by policies that support family values but penalize only one segment of the family are most at risk. These factors must be viewed as contributors to the mental health disabilities and challenges that many incarcerated women and their children face. When assessing the full impact of incarceration, gender must be placed at the center of the analysis. The failure to do so, to put the woman's unique experiences that led to and followed her incarceration at the center of any analysis of women's mental health issues, is negligent.

Exemplar III: Violence and Women

Consider these facts disseminated by the U.S. Department of Justice (Bachman, 1994). Women are ten times more likely than men to be victims of violence at the hands of intimates. During an eighteen-year period, more than two-thirds of the violent encounters against women were committed by persons known to them. Younger, single, less educated, and less economically well off women who were African American or Hispanic and living in central areas of a city were most vulnerable to becoming violent crime victims during this same period of time. Significantly more women who were victimized by intimates rather than strangers did not report the victimization to police out of fear of further offender violence. The economically poorest women in this country experience the highest rates of all forms of violence.

When women leave abusive relationships the lack of affordable housing and long waiting lists for housing assistance mean that women and children are forced to choose between abuse at home or living on the streets. The National Coalition for the Homeless (1999) cites several findings from a series of studies investigating the relationship between violent victimization and homelessness. One finding revealed that 50 percent of the homeless women and children studied reported fleeing abuse; a 1998 study of 777 homeless parents (mostly women) in ten cities found that 22 percent left their last residence because of domestic abuse; and 46 percent of cities recently surveyed by the U.S. Conference of Mayors identified domestic violence as a primary cause of homelessness.

Many of those receiving welfare or who earn low wages experience domestic violence at some point during their lives. Some studies have found that up to 60 percent of recipients in welfare-to-work programs have been victims of physical abuse and more have been victims of verbal or emotional abuse (Sable et al. 1999). Without cash assistance and housing support, many victims are at risk for homelessness and, consequently, more violence.

And the women victims themselves are not the only people at risk for victimization. Recent research into risk and protective factors for youth violence sheds light on both the broader impact of violence and, more significantly, the systemic and inseparable repercussions of poverty, inadequate health and mental health care, and parental criminality. Hawkins and colleagues (2000) reviewed data from long-term studies with the goal of identifying these risk and protective factors. They point to evidence of a predictive association between prenatal and delivery trauma, childhood maltreatment, and parental criminality and violent crimes committed later in life; and between "poor family management practices" and "later delinquency and substance abuse" (p. 3). Further, disruptions in parent-child relationships appear to be related to later violence, as does parent-child separation, particularly at younger ages. With regard to these findings, however, the authors caution that other identified risk factors, for example parental incarceration, necessarily constitute a "disruption" in the parent-child relationship, and, to date, the negative contributions of each risk factor to later violence has not been—though remains to be—determined. Finally, victimization of the adult woman cannot be separated from the victimization of her children—with some research showing the common coexistence of child abuse and partner abuse, and a child abuse rate between 12 and 45 percent in homes where their mothers are battered (Sable et al., 1999).

It is well established that victimization of women is a significant contributor to the onset of major depression, alcohol and drug abuse and dependence, certain types of anxiety disorders, eating disorders, and other major mental health problems (Fellin, 1996). Although violence against women is often accomplished at the hands of an intimate, it is critical to remember that stranger violence wreaks similar consequences. Researchers suggest that 20 percent of adult women have been raped and 25 to 50 percent of women have been subjected to sexual harassment (Mowbray, et al., 1999). What is experienced in the aftermath of all these episodes of violence—whether physical, emotional, or some combination of the two—are ongoing emotional challenges including chronic depression and anxiety, potentially incapacitating fear that interferes with social and occupational functioning, and, for some, the loss of their voices, having been *"beaten into silence, through physical and sexual violence, through poverty and deprivation, through the legal, moral and psychological denial of rights and personhood"* (Smyth, 1995, p. 201).

In addition, poverty is implicated as both a precursor to and a product of domestic violence. Sable and colleagues (1999) express fear that moving women off of public assistance and into jobs without recognition of and intervention into the underlying problem of abuse may prove disastrous, leaving women and their children without employment, without income, and, once again, powerless within a social system which, through its economic and social policies, places women in a double bind. This system demands behaviors consistent with the American work ethic and does little to ensure that women have a fair playing field on which to fulfill their multiple roles and perform their ascribed and assumed functions.

TWENTY-FIRST CENTURY CHALLENGES—
PRESENT TO FUTURE

The year 2000 and the hearkening of the new millennium brought with them both myriad answers to twentieth-century concerns and new worries which form the basis of critical questions for the twenty-first century. In the twentieth century, women earned both the right to vote and to be voted for. In the twentieth century, women realized some success in regulating their own bodies, particularly in areas involving sexual behavior, contraception, and abortion. In the twentieth century, women made strides in the employment arena, attaining positions of power and control in the business world.

As we began the year 2000, concerns about massive, crippling computer failures at the stroke of midnight proved unfounded. Ironically, during the final decade of the past century, much time and energy and resources were expended preventing drastic microchip malfunctions while only minimal efforts were made to prevent or alter the core conditions that have for so long contributed to women's disempowerment, particularly those conditions of poverty, incarceration, and violence, and the drastic human malfunctions that occur in the application of systemic biases. In the early years of the twenty-first century, women are still fighting for control over their bodies; that control having been only tenuously held in the past century. At the same time that there was preoccupation with deciding who would be the new leader at the helm of the nation, a leader for whom women would vote, the populace— men and women alike—seemed uncomfortable with the idea that someday that leader will be a woman. Some suggest the presidency is the ultimate glass ceiling. In reality, a glass ceiling hangs over every woman's head—the ceiling hit when, by virtue of disempowering norms, customs, and laws, women are victimized by violence, by an unresponsive criminal justice system, and by a welfare system that places women (and their children) one divorce, one economic downturn, one aging parent, one abusive partner, and/or one special-needs child away from poverty.

In the twenty-first century, old concerns may be replaced or renewed with more questions. Will the new century usher in a change in the economic progress of the previous decade? Closely related, will women continue to earn less on the dollar compared to men, as they did in the 1900s? Will the new century find powerful women more demonstratively expressing their power on behalf of women who have not yet found the strength of their voices? Will a new DSM-V continue to detail and propose diagnostic criteria that pathologize women? Will hard-fought victories in exercising control over one's body and mind remain secure?

All of these questions culminate in the realm of women's mental health and raise the query whether, in the twenty-first century, mental health professionals will universally embrace approaches to women's issues that demand analysis of the forces of power and oppression in women's lives. For decades, the emotional repercussions of women's confrontation with oppressive forces have shaped the telling of their experiences. Women's mental health struggles have been viewed through the employment of diagnostic labels and therapeutic interventions. Their challenges have been defined as illnesses: women suffer from depression more than men; women have more anxiety-related disorders than men; women are more likely to be identified with "unhealthy" characteristics than are men. Truthful substitutions for this verbiage lend a whole new perspective: women suffer from more intimate violence than men; women more commonly carry the burdens of being the sole parent and economic support for families; in most settings, women do not have the same access to preventive mental health resources as do men. In other words, from a mental health viewpoint, speaking of women only in diagnostic terms is fundamentally an abuse of therapeutic power because it mischaracterizes the woman as being sick and suggests the cure be found in individual work. As Ussher (1992) remarked, "Therapy may now be widely available and practiced by a range of professionals far from the leading edge of science, but its roots are firmly in this arena. Much of the therapeutic discourse is still tied to science, and thus to power, to prestige and to patriarchy" (p. 109).

In the process of writing this chapter, several public events occurred that shored up the ideas being presented here and that surely would have caught Liane Davis's attention. One such event found young women, independently pursuing their own interests in a public setting in one of the great cosmopolitan cities of the world, attacked and emotionally and sexually molested by spontaneously formed mobs of males, while literally hundreds of police officers were in the immediate vicinity. What shall we say about one (or more) of these women when she seeks mental health services? Shall we call her "depressed"? Shall we label her with an "anxiety disorder"? Shall we write "rule out histrionic personality disorder"? When talking about women's mental health issues in the twenty-first century, we must think about the language we use and how it works to reinforce the one-down positioning of women by allowing the problem to be over-looked in the problem definition. If a label must be assigned to this woman, would it not make more sense to say that she is "oppressed," "a victim of objectification," "a person rendered powerless by the misuse of physical power and absence of human respect and dig-nity"?

One viable twenty-first century social work approach to women's mental health issues is an empowerment approach. In part, it incorpo-rates the "careful examination of the power differences that exist be-tween the person receiving services and others, including providers and the community. . . and question[s] traditional therapeutic con-cepts or approaches" (Kalinowski and Penny, 1999, p. 150). Beyond the individual-based intervention, empowerment of and progress for women in the twenty-first century means an unrelenting pursuit of fundamental changes in the social systems that disadvantage women who react appropriately to disempowering situations. This includes viewing "the symptoms of learned helplessness—apathy, submis-siveness, anger, depression, and withdrawal"—as normal reactions to disempowering situations rather than as negative signs of a mental disorder (Manning, 1998, p. 91) and writing and talking about and educating others about the systemic contributors to women's mental health challenges. These normal reactions can be viewed as side effects of the products of a variety of social, economic, and bureau-cratic systemic forces. They are akin to the itch for which an antihis-tamine is prescribed. This itch requires treatment, but only the alleviation of the irritant provides the guarantee of true, real, and last-ing relief.

EMPOWERED PRACTICE
IN THE TWENTY-FIRST CENTURY:
IDEAS FOR SOCIAL WORKERS

The irritants discussed in this chapter are those of poverty, an unresponsive social and criminal justice system that ends in the meaningless abyss of incarceration, and violence against women by strangers and intimates. There are others as well, all perpetuated by the language and the attitudes of the people working in and for these systems. Social workers contribute to the problem and can and should lead the way to change.

As a start, we should begin to talk about the "states" of women's mental health. Nothing in this chapter denies the existence of biological factors in certain types of mental illnesses. How and to what extent the onset of these illnesses is aggravated by environmental and systemic conditions remains unknown, but for women, treatment must always consist of helping them have the opportunity to make choices about and manage their health, while supporting them in succeeding at their assigned or chosen endeavors. This may mean advocating, on their behalf, for child care, income, and housing support. It means steadfastly refusing to buy the still dominant discourse that characterizes women as weak and sickly, and it means incorporating into one's practice a determination to always view the woman in the power context in which she lives. If she has a mental illness or an emotional disturbance, she will not resolve it alone, she will not cure it with a pill, and she lives in the presence of constant risk; of poverty, violence, homelessness, and incarceration. She needs and deserves more than to be described by the sterile language of some diagnostic manual.

In the twenty-first century, empowered practice means asking every woman key questions about her life: her history of victimization and of survival; the demands she faces to take care of others; the stories of her personal fight for basic survival; and her dreams and aspirations as well. It means working with her to find a way out of the oppression and on toward those dreams.

In the twenty-first century, empowered practice means talking about the systems that perpetuate women's oppression. It means taking a flight—be it real, economic, or spiritual—to that cosmopolitan city and challenging the power on any and all levels, until reparations are made to all the women who have been victimized by mobs and victimized again by those other mobs—the systems that allow the objectification of women, sometimes expressed in the form of violence, to happen. It means refusing to report to any insurance company, for whatever reason, that this victimized woman is "depressed" or that she suffers from "borderline personality disorder." In the end, it means instead that we join with her to write the narrative for the insurance company, for the lawmaker and the judge, for the public, and for the record, powerfully asserting two central ideas: first, that this woman's symptoms are the side effects of an irritant for which a cure is being sought, and second, that this woman has an incurably normal condition so long as we are there for her.

REFERENCES

American Correctional Association (1990). *What does the future hold? Task force on the female offender.* Alexandria, VA: Author.

American Psychiatric Association (1994). *Diagnostic and statistical manual of mental disorders,* Fourth edition. Washington, DC: Author.

Bachman, R. (1994). *Violence against women. A national crime victimization survey report.* NCJ-45325. Washington, DC: Office of Justice Programs, Bureau of Justice Statistics, U.S. Department of Justice.

Banyard, V. (1999). Childhood maltreatment and the mental health of low-income women. *American Journal of Orthopsychiatry, 69*(2): 161-171.

Beck, A. J. (1999). Prisoners in 1998. *Bulletin. Bureau of Justice Statistics.* Washington, DC: U.S. Department of Justice.

Belle, D. (1990). Poverty and women's mental health. *American Psychologist, 45*(3): 385-389.

Berrick, J. D. (1999). Income maintenance and support: The changing face of welfare. In J. Midgley, M. B. Tracy, and M. Livermore (Eds.), *The handbook of social policy* (pp. 175-185). Thousand Oaks, CA: Sage.

Blanch, A. K. and Levin, B.L. (1999). Organization and service delivery. In B. L. Levin, A. K. Blanch, and A. Jennings (1999) (Eds.), *Women's mental health services: A public health perspective* (pp. 5-18). Thousand Oaks: Sage.

Bloom, B. and Steinhart, D. (1993). *Why punish the children? A reappraisal of the children of incarcerated mothers in America.* San Francisco: Center on Juvenile and Criminal Justice.

Bradwell v. Illinois, 83 U.S. 130 (1872).

Briar-Lawson, K. and Drews, J. (1999). Child and family welfare policies and services: Current issues and historical antecedents. In J. Midgley, M. B. Tracy, and M. Livermore (Eds.), *The handbook of social policy* (pp. 157-174). Thousand Oaks, CA: Sage.

Broverman, I. K., Broverman, D. M., Clarkson, F. E., Rosenkrantz, P. S., and Vogel, S. R. (1981). Sex-role stereotypes and clinical judgments of mental health. In E. Howell and M. Bayes (Eds.), *Women and mental health.* New York: Basic Books.

Bureau of Justice Statistics (1994). *Special report: Women in prison.* Washington, DC: U.S. Department of Justice.

Bureau of Justice Statistics (1997). *Sourcebook of criminal justice statistics—1996.* Washington, DC: U.S. Department of Justice.

Bureau of Justice Statistics (1998). *Profile of jail inmates, 1996.* Washington, DC: U.S. Department of Justice.

Collins, W. C. and Collins, A. W. (1996). *Women in jail: Legal issues.* Washington, DC: National Institute of Corrections. U.S. Department of Justice.

Faulkner, H. J. and Pruitt, V. D. (1997). *Dear Dr. Menninger: Women's voices from the thirties.* Columbia: University of Missouri Press.

Fellin, P. (1996). *Mental health and mental illness: Policies, programs, and services.* Itasca, IL: F.E. Peacock Publishers.

GlenMaye, L. (1998). Empowerment of women. In L. Gutierrez, R. Parsons, and E. Cox (Eds.), *Empowerment in social work practice: A sourcebook* (pp. 29-51). Pacific Grove, CA: Brooks/Cole Publishing Company.

Goodman, L. A. (1991). The prevalence of abuse among homeless and housed poor mothers: A comparison study. *American Journal of Orthopsychiatry, 61*: 489-500.

Greenfeld, L. A. and Snell, T. L. (1999). *Special report. Women offenders.* Bureau of Justice Statistics. Washington, DC: U.S. Department of Justice.

Hawkins, J. D., Herrenkohl, T. I., Farrington, D. P., Brewer, D., Catalano, R. F., Harachi, T. W., and Cothern, L. (2000). *Juvenile Justice Bulletin. Predictors of youth violence.* Washington, DC: Office of Juvenile Justice and Delinquency Prevention.

Irving, H. H. and Benjamin, M. (1995). *Family mediation: Contemporary issues.* Thousand Oaks, CA: Sage.

Jordan, B. K., Schlenger, W. E., Fairbank, J. A., and Caddell, J. M. (1996). Prevalence of psychiatric disorders among incarcerated women. II. Convicted felons entering prison. *Archives of General Psychiatry, 53:* 513-519.

Kalinowski, C. and Penny, D. (1999). Empowerment and women's mental health services. In B. L. Levin, A. K. Blanch, and A. Jennings (Eds.), *Women's mental health services: A public health perspective* (pp. 127-154). Thousand Oaks: Sage.

Manning, S. S. (1998). Empowerment in mental health programs: Listening to the voices. In L. Gutierrez, R. Parsons, and E. Cox (Eds.), *Empowerment in social work practice: A sourcebook* (pp. 89-109). Pacific Grove, CA: Brooks/Cole Publishing Company.

Mowbray, C. T., Oyserman, D., Saunders, D., and Rueda-Riedle, A. (1999). Women with severe mental disorders: Issues and Service Needs. In B. L. Levin, A. K. Blanch, and A. Jennings (Eds.), *Women's mental health service: A public health perspective* (pp. 175-200). Thousand Oaks, CA: Sage.

Mulloy, T. B. (1997). Women as mental health service recipients and providers. In T. R. Watkins and J. W. Callicutt (Eds.), *Mental health policy and practice today* (pp. 258-273). Thousand Oaks: Sage.

National Coalition for the Homeless (1999). *Domestic violence and homelessness.* NCH Fact Sheet #8, April. <http://nch.ar.net/domestic.html>.

Pearce, D. (1979). Women, work and welfare: The feminization of poverty. In K. W. Feinstein (Ed.), *Working women and families*. Newbury Park, CA: Sage.

Pearlman, S. F. (1995). The radical edge: Feminist therapy as political activism. In E. F. Williams (Ed.), *Voices of Feminist Therapy* (pp. 3-10). Luxembourg: Harwood Academic Publishers,

Personal Responsibility and Work Opportunity Reconciliation Act, P.L. 104-193 (1996).

Reitmeir, M. A. and Christensen, K. R. (1994). Is there a feminization of poverty? In H. J. Karger and J. Midgley (Eds.), *Controversial issues in social policy* (pp. 214-225). Boston: Allyn & Bacon.

Russo, N. F. (1990). Overview: Forging research priorities for women's mental health. *American Psychologist, 45*(3): 368-373.

Sable, M. R., Libbus, M. K., Huneke, D., and Anger, K. (1999). Domestic violence among AFDC recipients: Implications for welfare-to-work programs. *Affilia, 14*(2): 199-216.

Smyth, A. (1995). Haystacks in my mind or how to stay SAFE (sane, angry and feminist) in the 1990s. In G. Griffin (Ed.), *Feminist activism in the 1990s* (pp. 192-206). London: Taylor and Francis.

Teplin, L. A., Abram, K. M., and McClelland, G. M. (1996). Prevalence of psychiatric disorders among incarcerated women. I. Pretrial jail detainees. *Archives of General Psychiatry, 53:* 505-512.

Tice, C. J. and Perkins, K. (1996). *Mental health issues and aging: Building on the strengths of older persons* (p. 206). Pacific Grove, CA: Brooks/Cole Publishing Company.

United States Department of Labor (1999). *What women earned in 1988. Issues in Labor Statistics*. Washington, DC: Bureau of Labor Statistics. U.S. Department of Labor.

Ussher, J. M. (1992). *Women's madness: Misogyny or mental illness?* Amherst: The University of Massachusetts Press.

Veysey, B. M. (1998). Specific needs of women diagnosed with mental illnesses in U.S. jails. In B. L. Levin, A. K. Blanch, and A. Jennings (Eds.), *Women's mental health service. A public health perspective* (pp. 368-389). Thousand Oaks, CA: Sage.

Wagner, S. R. (1999). Is equality indigenous? The untold Iroquois influence on early radical feminists. *Winds of Change, 1* (summer): 62-65.

Wilton, T. (1995). Madness and feminism: Bristol Crisis Service for Women. In G. Griffin (Ed.), *Feminist activism in the 1990s* (pp. 28-39). London: Taylor and Francis.

Chapter 6

Women, Welfare, and Violence: A Look at the Family Violence Option

Jan L. Hagen

Violence against women in the United States is of staggering proportions—one out of two women has experienced physical assault within her lifetime and one out of six has experienced an attempted or completed rape. Each year, an estimated 1.9 million women are physically assaulted and 302,000 are raped (Tjaden and Thoennes, 1998). One major component of this violence is the battering experienced by adult women at the hands of their spouses or male partners. Drawing on the National Violence Against Women Survey, Tjaden and Thoennes (1998) note that women in the United States "are primarily raped and/or physically assaulted by intimate partners: 76 percent of the women who were raped and/or physically assaulted since the age of 18 were assaulted by a current or former husband, cohabiting partner, or date" (p. 8). Tjaden and Thoennes (1998) report that one out of four women in their nationally representative sample experienced rape or some form of physical assault by an intimate partner at some point in their lives. Rape or physical assault was experienced during the past year by 1.5 percent of the sample.

Although estimates on the prevalence and incidence of severe aggression or wife battering vary, a commonly cited figure is that women experience *severe* violence from their cohabiting male partner in 3.4 percent of all households (Straus and Gelles, 1986). Tjaden and Thoennes (1998) report percentages by types of physical assault. For severe forms of physical assault, 6.1 percent of women report an intimate partner choked or tried to drown them; 5 percent report being hit with an object; 8.5 percent being beaten; and 3.5 percent being threatened with a gun.

Although of significant magnitude, wife abuse was considered a "private trouble" rather than a "public issue" until the 1970s. As Davis (1987) stated: "Wife abuse has been endemic for centuries; the women's movement made it a social problem" (p. 311). The recognition of domestic violence as a social problem demanding a public response prompted the development of both state and federal legislation beginning in the 1980s (Davis and Hagen, 1988). Although states initially took the lead in developing policies responsive to the needs of battered women, the federal government finally took action during the Reagan years with the passage of the Family Violence Prevention and Services Act. This was followed by the Violence Against Women Act of 1994, which enhanced the criminal justice response and provided additional support for services to victims, including domestic violence victims.

The general strategy for responding to victims of domestic violence may be characterized as emphasizing women's risks of experiencing battering without regard to distinctions by socioeconomic class or other categorical characteristics. However, the debates surrounding "welfare reform," specifically the revision of Aid to Families with Dependent Children (AFDC), the nation's program for providing income support to poor women and their children, brought to the fore the particular vulnerability of poor women relying on public support who are also victims of battering by their spouses or male partners. For many battered women, welfare provided a safety net when trying to leave abusive relationships. However, new conditions attached to welfare receipt, such as lifetime limits on federal welfare benefits and increased emphasis on quick labor-force attachment, threatened to further the vulnerability of battered women relying on public assistance.

As a result, when AFDC was abolished in 1996 and replaced by Temporary Assistance for Needy Families (TANF), the legislation included an amendment offered by Senators Murray and Wellstone known as the Family Violence Option. This amendment offers states the option of including flexibility in their welfare programs in order to safeguard the well-being of poor women and their children who were also dealing with domestic violence. The purpose of this article is to analyze the federal legislation and regulations governing the

Family Violence Option within the context of TANF, review the research linking welfare and domestic violence, assess the state responses to the Family Violence Option, and delineate the implications of this review for next steps in serving battered women.

TANF AND THE FAMILY VIOLENCE OPTION

TANF is a fundamental transformation of the nation's welfare programs for poor women and their children. In passing the legislation, the primary intent of Congress was to further devolve control of welfare to the states by increasing their flexibility in operating welfare programs (42 USC 601 [a]). To achieve this goal, the federal entitlement to cash assistance for needy families and their children was explicitly ended. Further, financial support for welfare was converted from open-ended categorical funding to block grants, thereby limiting the federal obligation for income support to poor women and their children. Some control over welfare was retained by the federal government; however, by making full block grant funding contingent on several conditions—conditions which have significant implications for welfare recipients.

The first condition is the imposition of new work requirements that apply to almost all welfare recipients, requiring them to work or engage in work-related activities within two years of receiving welfare. What "counts" as work or work-related activities was significantly narrowed under TANF to give emphasis to "work first" approaches to welfare employment programs. These approaches rely on labor-force attachment strategies such as employment, job search, and work experience rather than education and training activities to prepare recipients for employment. The hours of work required each week are twenty for a single mother with children under age six and thirty hours for others. Unlike prior welfare employment provisions, child care is not guaranteed under TANF, but federal funding has been authorized and liberalized. If recipients fail to comply with work requirements, as well as other program requirements, states are required to impose sanctions reducing the level of benefits and may terminate benefits for the entire family. (See Hagen, 1998, for a review of work requirements under TANF.)

A second condition in essence creates a welfare cliff (Hagen, 1999) by imposing a five-year lifetime limit on receiving benefits from federal funds. The majority of states (twenty-seven) have elected to impose five-year time limits but states are free to establish shorter limits and some have done so. Other states such as Michigan and New York have imposed no time limits on benefits, opting to use their own funds to provide support beyond the five-year federal limit (U.S. Department of Health and Human Services, 1998).

In addition to these federal requirements, states are free to impose various other conditions on the receipt of welfare, including making benefit level conditional on children's school attendance ("Learnfare") and imposing family "caps" which preclude increasing benefit levels for any child born after the receipt of welfare begins.

These provisions and others—mandatory work requirements, lifetime limits on welfare, and paternity and child support enforcement procedures—all have the potential of increasing the risks of violence for some victims of domestic violence by increasing or prolonging their economic dependence on abusive partners or by exposing them to abusive behaviors from partners who may resent and therefore interfere with their efforts at economic self-sufficiency (Howell, 1997). Congress recognized that some TANF provisions might prove unrealistic or impose severe difficulties on some adult recipients and addressed this possibility through two provisions.

First, states are allowed to exempt up to 20 percent of the caseload from the five-year time limit for TANF benefits because "of hardship or if the family includes an individual who has been battered or subjected to extreme cruelty" (402 U.S.C. 608 [a][7][C][i]). "Hardship" is not defined in the legislation, leaving that as well as the procedures by which families are deemed to be experiencing "hardship" to state interpretation. Battering and extreme cruelty are defined and include actual or threatened physical injury, sexual abuse, threatened or attempted physical or sexual abuse, and mental abuse.

Second, Congress responded specifically to the potential vulnerability and needs of battered women by including the Family Violence Option (42 U.S.C. 602[a][7]) as part of the TANF legislation, a step that, for the first time, recognizes in federal policy the link between domestic violence and welfare for some welfare recipients (Brandwein, 1999). Imperial (1997) characterizes the Family Violence Option as representing a three-pronged strategy for addressing domestic violence under TANF. First, if selected by states, the Family Violence Option provides flexibility in applying TANF rules to victims of domestic violence. Under this option, states may waive such program requirements as time limits, family caps, work requirements, and child support enforcement requirements for domestic violence victims if complying with them places clients at risk or unfairly penalizes them. Second, the Family Violence Option allows states to offer confidential screening and identification of battered women and third, it allows states to provide referrals for supportive and counseling services.

The relationship between these two provisions, one for "hardship" and the other for domestic violence victims, was unclear and controversial for a period of time. The issue was whether domestic violence victims who were waived from the federal time limits were to be included in the 20 percent states are allowed to exempt from the time limits due to hardship or if time limit exemptions for domestic violence victims were in addition to that 20 percent. Senators Murray and Wellstone's intent under the Family Violence Option was to provide exemptions for domestic violence victims separate from the 20 percent hardship exemption (Raphael, 1999), but others argued that the 20 percent exemption should apply to the entire caseload. This issue was finally resolved in April 1999 with the promulgation of the federal regulations which clarified that states could exceed the 20 percent hardship exemption without penalty if they had adopted the Family Violence Option and they exceeded the 20 percent because of granting "federally recognized" good cause waivers for domestic violence. Additionally, states may also have lower work participation rates than federally required if that lower rate is a result of granting domestic violence waivers (45 C.F.R. 260.58). In essence, the federal regulations provide an incentive for states "to take the maximum advantage offered by the FVO to protect the safety of recipients" (Greenberg and Savner, 1999, p. 38).

In addition, and significantly, the federal regulations encourage states to provide recipients with appropriate services "to help the individual prepare for work and self-sufficiency consistent with ensuring her and her children's safety" (U.S. Department of Health and Human Services, 1999, p. 3). For states to qualify for federally recognized good cause domestic violence waivers, states must base the waiver on an individualized assessment conducted by someone with domestic violence training, have a person with training in domestic violence design an individualized service plan based on the assessment, design that service plan to lead to work if the individual is protected, and make waiver redeterminations every six months (45 C.F.R. 260.55). The inclusion of a service plan leading to work, provided the woman and her children are safe, addresses the concern raised by domestic violence advocates that the Family Violence Option would be used to exclude battered women from employment-related services rather than as a vehicle to address their needs (Imperial, 1997).

States remain free to waive any program requirements for domestic violence victims, but only federally recognized good cause domestic violence waivers qualify for state exceptions to the 20 percent hardship exemption or the federal mandated work participation rates. Waivers for cooperation with child support enforcement may be granted under either the Family Violence Option or child support good cause provisions (Greenberg and Savner, 1999).

The Family Violence Option has been adopted by the majority of states. As of May 1999, thirty-four states, Puerto Rico, and the District of Columbia had adopted the Family Violence Option, five states were in the process of adopting it, and two states offered it as a county option. Six states had not adopted the Family Violence Option but had developed state policies allowing battered women to receive temporary deferrals from work-related activities (Raphael and Haennicke, 1999). With the Family Violence Option in place, states have the opportunity to respond constructively and flexibly to the needs of battered women and their children while maintaining their eligibility for full federal funding under TANF (Pollack and Davis, 1997).

THE LINK BETWEEN DOMESTIC VIOLENCE AND WELFARE

For women who are abused, the Family Violence Option is crucial in light of research findings that suggest economic resources are often a determining factor in women being able to leave their batterers and provide an alternative for themselves and their children. Gondolf and Fisher (1988), in a study of more than 6,000 women receiving shelter services, found that that the best predictors of a woman leaving her abusive partner were related to her having the necessary resources to live independently, such as transportation, child care, and a source of income after leaving the shelter. Maintaining economic control is an important component of a batterer's strategy for maintaining power over his partner. As Davis (1999) notes:

> [A]dequate financial assistance—whether from family members, friends, or public assistance—often is the key factor that enables battered women and their children to leave and remain separated from their abusers. If such assistance were not available as a last resort, many battered women would be forced to remain in, or return to, dangerous or life-threatening situations. (p. 18)

Although research on domestic violence has been extensive, relatively few studies have taken an in-depth look at the extent of violence in the lives of women who are poor, even though findings from representative national studies indicate that poor and low-income women and children face higher risks for violence—particularly severe violence (Browne and Bassuk, 1997). In addition, the link between welfare and domestic violence and the extent to which domestic violence interferes with welfare-to-work programs as well as employment have been investigated only recently, emerging in the mid-1990s concurrently with the political initiatives to reform the nation's welfare programs for poor women and their children.

One of the first investigators to bring this connection between welfare and domestic violence to light was Raphael (1995, 1996). These early works were based primarily on reports from welfare-to-work programs documenting the extent to which their program participants were victims of domestic violence. Also, the reports illustrate the multiple ways in which abusive partners undermine women's efforts to participate in job training or employment. Examples include inflicting violence the night before job interviews or exams, undermining child-care arrangements, hiding or destroying books and homework, and stalking women at training programs or work sites.

Raphael's report (1996) combined with that of Raphael and Tolman (1997) also gave visibility to several studies examining the prevalence of domestic violence among welfare and low-income women, with the incidence of current abuse ranging from 14.6 to 32 percent. Curcio (1997) in a survey of 846 AFDC women in New Jersey found 14.6 percent of the respondents reporting current physical abuse and one-fourth currently experiencing verbal or emotional abuse. Using a random sample of AFDC recipients in Massachusetts, Allard and colleagues (1997) found current physical abuse among 19.5 percent of the respondents. Lloyd (1996), using a random sample drawn from a low-income Chicago neighborhood, found that within the past twelve months, 31.1 percent of the AFDC respondents had experienced physical abuse and 19.5 percent, severe physical abuse. Lifetime rates for physical abuse were higher: Curcio (1997) found 57.3 percent reporting physical abuse and Allard and colleagues (1997), 64.9 percent. Lloyd (1996) reported 33.8 percent of the AFDC recipients in her sample experienced severe aggression as adults.

A major study that begins to address the gap in the literature regarding the link between welfare and domestic violence is an epidemiological, community-based study conducted in Worcester, Massachusetts, the Worcester Family Research Project. Salomon, Bassuk, and Brooks (1996) and Browne and Bassuk (1997), measuring physical violence by male partners and childhood violence among a sample of AFDC mothers, found extremely high rates of violence against the women as both children and adults, and even higher rates for those who received welfare for five years or longer. Overall, more than 60 percent of the AFDC mothers had been victims of severe physical violence by male partners, and almost one-third reported severe physical violence by their current or most recent partner. Physical or sexual abuse as children was reported by 72 percent of the sample. Some form of violence over their life span was reported by 85 percent of the sample.

Salomon, Bassuk, and Brooks (1996) also point out that abused women often live with severe emotional and mental health consequences, including post-traumatic stress disorder (PTSD), which is "highly associated with increased risk of depression and substance abuse" (p. 522). The women in their sample had rates of PTSD that were three times greater than those found in the general population of women. The researchers concluded that "the pervasiveness of violence in the lives of women living in poverty interferes with the capacity of these women to remain economically independent for long periods" (p. 523) and that work-based initiatives will not be sufficient to prevent the need for long-term income support for some women who have been physically or sexually abused. However, in an analysis of individual-level factors that were predictive of the employability of the same sample, Brooks and Buckner (1996) did not find lifetime experiences of family violence or mental health issues to be barriers to employment, but they were not able to consider the impact of current episodes of family violence or mental illness on employment.

Using a random sample of single mothers with children who were receiving welfare in an urban Michigan county in 1997, Danziger and colleagues (1999), in the Women's Employment Study, measured the extent of severe physical abuse using the Conflict Tactics Scale. Almost 15 percent of their sample reported severe physical abuse from a husband or partner within the past year, a finding similar to earlier studies (Raphael and Tolman, 1997). Within the sample, 14.6 percent had PTSD and 26.7 percent had major depression, a rate twice that of women nationally (12.9 percent). The percentage of respondents classified as being drug dependent was higher than the national percentage, 3.3 percent compared to 1.9 percent; alcohol dependence was somewhat lower in the sample, 2.7 percent compared to 3.7 percent for women nationally.

Based on the studies to date, it is reasonable to estimate that between 20 to 30 percent of the women on welfare will have experienced domestic violence recently (within the past year) and that for most of these women, the physical abuse they experienced will be severe. Also, rates of PTSD and major depression will be significantly higher among women on welfare and rates of substance abuse will be somewhat higher. All three mental health consequences may be associated with current or prior experiences with violence, including physical and sexual assault by intimate partners.

DOMESTIC VIOLENCE AND ECONOMIC SELF-SUFFICIENCY

To maintain their victims' economic dependence, batterers may interfere with women's efforts to become economically self-sufficient through job training and employment. Raphael and Tolman (1997), based on early anecdotal reports from welfare-to-work programs, concluded that "many women on welfare who do not comply with work or training requirements while receiving assistance may be prevented from doing so by the direct behavior of an abusive partner, or by the indirect effects of the abuse on their health and well-being" (p. iii). A number of empirical investigations are emerging to support this observation. Shepard and Pence (1988) conducted one of the earliest studies examining batterers' interference with training and employment. Based on a survey of battered women, Shepard and Pence (1988) found that the women's work performance was negatively affected by their abusive partners, including absences, lateness, and job loss. The women also reported that their partners actively attempted to prevent their employment or education.

More recent research supports Shepard and Pence's (1988) initial findings on the effects of battering on women's job training and employment. Based on interviews with service providers in welfare-to-work programs in New York City, Kenney and Brown (1996) found service providers estimating anywhere from 30 to 75 percent of the women in their programs were abused, including physical and emotional abuse as well as stalking and harassment. The domestic violence experienced by these women significantly undermined their efforts to participate in training programs, increasing the likelihood that they will drop out of employment and training programs. If they do secure employment, the ongoing abuse impedes their ability to retain their jobs. As Kenney and Brown (1996) note: "The sabotage takes many forms, from failing to provide promised child care or making harassing visits to a woman's job site to inflicting serious injuries that prevent her from attending classes or going to work" (p. 10).

Cross-sectional studies using representative samples, however, do not find a statistically significant link between recent physical abuse and women's employment. In the Women's Employment Study, Danziger and colleagues (1999) considered the impact of severe physical abuse within the past year on women's employment. Of those with the domestic violence barrier, 55.4 percent were working twenty or more hours a week compared to 57.1 percent of those without the barrier—a difference that was not statistically significant. Neither domestic violence nor PTSD significantly predicted employment. However, the study measured severe physical abuse within the past year and did not attempt to measure the impact of *current* domestic violence on employment. If domestic violence is directly or indirectly linked to other barriers to employment, such as major depression, lack of transportation, or limited employment experience, the likelihood of employment will decrease, as these factors are significant in predicting employment of twenty hours or more each week. As Danziger and colleagues (1999) note: "One or two barriers [to employment] may have little effect on employment, but multiple barriers might seriously impede employment" (p. 17). Finally, the data are cross-sectional at this point and the job retention and consistency of employment have yet to be examined in this study.

Another cross-sectional analysis of the impact of male violence on female employment has been conducted by Lloyd and Taluc (1999), extending Lloyd's (1996) analysis of data gathered from 824 women in a randomly selected sample drawn from a low-income neighborhood in Chicago. Their findings suggest that male violence, whether within the past twelve months or during adulthood, does not significantly affect women's current employment status nor does it significantly affect days absent from work, work-related impairments, or occupational status (Lloyd and Taluc, 1999, p. 375). However, women who have expecienced male violence are more likely to report having been unemployed and to report a range of physical and mental health problems that could affect employability.

Although Lloyd and Taluc (1999) found male violence had a negative impact on labor-force participation, it was not at a statistically significant level. Specific forms of male violence, however, were found to be related to employment status. Women were less likely to be employed if they confront male violence in such behaviors as threatening to harm children, threatening to kill the victims, and being directly prevented from going to school or work. Lloyd and Taluc (1999) suggest that the impact of male violence on women's employment may be complex and that "aggregated measures may obscure the different, possibly offsetting, effects of different kinds of aggressive behaviors. They may also fail to distinguish among women who may react very differently from each other when confronted with similar circumstances" (pp. 384-385).

To more fully track this link between current domestic violence and women's employment, longitudinal studies capable of measuring the impact of different forms of male violence are needed. The only longitudinal study identified that considers the link between current partner violence and the ability of poor women to maintain work over a period of time was conducted by Browne, Salomon, and Bassuk (1999), again using the sample from the Worchester Family Research Project. In this sample of low-income women followed over two years, 30 percent had experienced at least one incident of severe physical attack or threat during that time period. Using a multivariate analysis, Browne, Salomon, and Bassuk (1999) found that recent (within the past twelve months) partner violence served as a predictor of the women's capacity to maintain their work efforts in the year following the violence. Specifically, Browne, Salomon, and Bassuk (1999) report that those with recent experiences of intimate partner violence were less than half as likely to work at least thirty hours per week and one-fifth as likely to work full-time for six months or more during the following year when compared to women who had not experienced physical violence or aggression within the past twelve months.

Given this impact on women's capacity to maintain work over a period of time following recent incidents of domestic violence, Browne, Salomon, and Bassuk (1999) suggest that the expectation for women to engage in work or work-related activities within two years of receiving public assistance may be problematic for those who have recently experienced domestic violence. Women with recent experiences of violence also reported higher levels of psychological distress and were more likely to report substance abuse problems. This suggests a need to provide supportive and supplemental services and resources to address the consequences of recent violence. As Browne, Salomon, and Bassuk (1999) note, "simply exempting women from welfare-to-work requirements without stabilizing interventions may produce little progress in their readiness or capacity to sustain work" (p. 421).

IMPLEMENTING THE FAMILY VIOLENCE OPTION

In their analysis of the Family Violence Option, Pollack and Davis (1997) suggest that the intent was "to extend to domestic violence survivors the flexibility, protections and services necessary to begin or continue on the path away from abuse and toward safety, physical, mental, and financial recovery, and self-sustaining employment" (p. 1079). At this juncture, relatively little is known about the impact of the Family Violence Option on battered women or the capacity of local welfare agencies to implement its provisions. In part, this information is limited because the final federal rules for the Option became effective only recently, in October 1999. Information may also be limited because states have focused their efforts on other components of the new welfare law, particularly the new work requirements for adult recipients and the increased emphasis on "work first" strategies. In this larger implementation context, the Family Violence Option may not be viewed as a significant policy demanding attention. The studies available on the Family Violence Option or its implications predate either the states' enactment of the Option or the promulgation of the final federal regulations. Nonetheless, the studies provide a beginning foundation from which to view the implementation of the Family Violence Option.

The Taylor Institute has conducted two studies on state implementation of the Family Violence Option; one in 1998 (Raphael, 1999) and the other in early 1999 (Raphael and Haennicke, 1999). In both studies, telephone interviews were conducted with state TANF and child support administrators, and state and local domestic violence coalitions to assess policies and procedures in all fifty states, Puerto Rico, and the District of Columbia. Because this is the only information available at this time on how states are proceeding with implementation, the studies will be presented in depth. At the time of the 1999 study, thirty-eight states had adopted the Family Violence Option, five were in the process of adopting the Option, and six had not adopted the Family Violence Option but had state policies covering battered women.

Raphael and Haennicke (1999) found that procedures for notifying welfare recipients of the Family Violence Option and screening for domestic violence vary widely across the states. Some states provide notice and rely on client self-disclosure, others screen for domestic violence but do not universally inform clients about the Family Violence Option, and still others both give notice and screen. In twenty states, the notice and screening procedures were inadequate and characterized as "FVO Lite" (Raphael and Haennicke, 1999, p. 9). Even if screening tools were developed by states, these might not be used or used consistently by workers on the front line. Further, the types of questions in some instances tended to be intrusive in that they asked about a range of abusive behaviors rather than more generally inquiring about violence interfering with work participation or securing child support. In most state materials, child support enforcement and good cause exemptions are not mentioned. The interface between child support enforcement and the Family Violence Option was also problematic in that the processes have remained separate, using different definitions of eligibility for exemptions and different criteria for verification of eligibility for waivers or exemptions.

In granting temporary waivers from work requirements, most states rely on the woman's word or her sworn statement about the domestic violence in determining her eligibility for a waiver. In using the waivers or exemptions, about one-half of the states provide up-front waivers of work requirements that stop the work clock; one-third also offer waivers that stop the clock on the five-year, lifetime limit for benefits; and one-fifth of the states do not give exemptions from the work requirements but count participation in battered women's services as work activity. The length of the waivers also varies widely across the states and may or may not be renewable. In most states, a welfare caseworker is authorized to make the determination about the temporary waiver from work requirements.

If a waiver is granted, most states require the women to cooperate with domestic violence services and to work toward eliminating domestic violence as a barrier to work. To implement this requirement, states are taking varied—and sometimes innovative—approaches, including special appropriations to domestic violence services, the development of specialized domestic violence staff in welfare offices, colocation of domestic violence services in welfare offices, and intensive case management services for families with domestic violence issues. Raphael and Haennicke (1999) suggest that locating domestic violence providers at welfare offices increases the comfort of frontline workers, making them more willing to implement domestic violence policies and increasing the number of women who self-disclose domestic violence.

One study (Angelari, 1998) has tracked the implementation of the Family Violence Option at the county level. Based on telephone interviews with welfare administrators in nineteen of Maryland's twenty-four counties, Angelari (1998) found significant implementation issues in many counties, including the lack of written materials related to the Family Violence Option, lack of tracking or analyzing the implementation of the Family Violence Option, failure to designate a domestic violence expert as required by the state, and discomfort on the part of frontline staff in screening for domestic violence. Angelari also noted that the frequency and timing of screening for domestic violence might be problematic, particularly if not done during the child support interviews and during hearings on women's lack of compliance with work requirements.

In addition to the reports on state and county implementation of the Family Violence Option, several studies have considered the policy from the perspective of domestic violence victims and frontline workers. An early study conducted by Imperial (1997) used focus groups and individual interviewers to provide the perspective of a small number of domestic violence victims ($N = 22$) on issues related to the Family Violence Option and, indirectly, on its implementation. Although none of the women had made use of the Family Violence Option at that early date, as victims of domestic violence and recipients of welfare, their perspective is an important one to consider. Without knowing the specific benefits to be gained from disclosing abuse, participants expressed serious reservations about identifying themselves as domestic violence victims to welfare workers because of possible lack of confidentiality and sensitivity from the workers, including not being believed without physical proof. The women identified several possible consequences of disclosure, including being found by batterers and being reported to child protective services for suspected abuse and neglect of their children. The focus group participants also had reservations about being referred for domestic violence services because this might be perceived by welfare applicants as yet another barrier to establishing eligibility, further discouraging welfare applications.

In Imperial's study (1997), the participants believed that welfare regulations must be flexible for victims of domestic violence and that victims of domestic violence should not be penalized if their efforts at self-sufficiency are undermined by their batterers' intervening behaviors. The women viewed complying with child support enforcement as particularly problematic. Given their need to leave unsafe situations quickly, women may not have their children's birth certificates or social security numbers, which are required by child support enforcement. These women were also fearful that their locations might be disclosed to the batterers, or that in pursuing child support, their batterers might insist on greater involvement with children or sole physical custody of the children. Their recommendations for assisting domestic violence victims included explaining through multiple media both the advantages and disadvantages of disclosing domestic violence to welfare workers; the need for coordinating services between the welfare agency and domestic violence providers; and increased information available to recipients regarding the good cause exemptions for child support enforcement.

The good cause exemption for child support for victims of domestic violence has been considered by Pearson, Thoennes, and Griswold (1999) in a four-county study in Colorado. Using both written notice and follow-up interview questions, welfare workers screened public assistance applicants for domestic violence during a nine-month period. The women who disclosed domestic violence received further information from child support workers regarding the good cause exemptions for child support enforcement. Current or past domestic violence was revealed by 40 percent of the applicants. However, of these, only 6.7 percent were interested in applying for a good cause exemption from child support enforcement. The vast majority of the women were interested in obtaining child support and did not believe pursuing it would initiate or escalate domestic violence.

The women who were interested in the good cause exemption reported threats of harm to themselves or their children, had been prevented from working by the abuser, had been abused within the past six months, and had called the police. For these women, pursuing child support was viewed as dangerous to themselves or their children. Despite the seriousness of these issues, only one-third of the women interested in a good cause exemption were granted one, primarily because they were able to support their abuse claims with official records. Pearson, Thoennes, and Griswold (1999) suggest that the low-income and often poorly educated women will be unable to obtain official records to support their claims, particularly given severely restricted time frames. Given the low level of requests for good cause exemptions, Pearson, Thoennes, and Griswold (1999) suggest agencies relax some of the documentation requirements and accept sworn statements from victims. (The linkage between domestic violence and child support, although an important one, has not been examined extensively. For further information, see Pearson and Griswold, 1997, and Roberts, 1997.)

Only one study to date has considered implementation issues related to the Family Violence Option from the perspective of frontline workers in welfare agencies (Hagen and Owens-Manley, in press). This study, too, was conducted prior to the full implementation of the Family Violence Option, but it provides preliminary information on the views of, and issues confronting, welfare workers. Using focus groups with workers responsible for eligibility determinations in two local welfare offices, Hagen and Owens-Manley (in press) found relatively little agreement among frontline workers regarding waiving TANF requirements for domestic violence victims. However, using hypothetical case illustrations, the workers did prioritize clients for exemptions based on the safety and stability in living circumstances for mothers and children as well as on the extent to which women had already demonstrated independent action to address the domestic violence situation through seeking emergency shelter or orders of protection. This latter criterion was used as a proxy by the workers for measuring the seriousness of the client's claim. Because of the additional resources and waivers available to domestic violence victims, frontline workers were concerned that clients would falsely report domestic violence in order to "scam" the system. As Hagen and Owens-Manley (in press) note, a criterion of independent action to secure an exemption from TANF rules "may result in a system that is unresponsive to domestic violence victims who are not familiar with these alternatives" of orders of protection and emergency shelters.

The findings from Hagen and Owens-Manley (in press) also suggest that "women who follow the cyclical pattern of leaving and returning to abusive partners may be less likely to receive exemptions or waivers from requirements" because workers were frustrated by this pattern and found it difficult to understand. In implementing the Family Violence Option, special consideration needs to be given to how to most effectively serve women and children in these circumstances:

> The women's attempts to leave abusive situations must not be undermined, but costs of serving these women and their children over time combined with worker resistance to these clients may limit their access to welfare services. This, in turn, may further compromise their ability to leave abusive partners due to a lack of alternative resources. (Hagen and Owens-Manley, in press)

NEXT STEPS

The prevalence of domestic violence among women on welfare is now fairly well established, and initial studies have documented a link between abuse and both physical and mental health problems, including PTSD, depression, and substance abuse. The impact of domestic violence on education, training, and employment for battered women is less clear, however, indicating the need to move beyond cross-sectional studies to longitudinal ones such as Browne, Salomon, and Bassuk's (1999), which considers employment patterns and disruptions in relation to the timing of violence as well as its type.

In responding to the needs of battered women on welfare, the Family Violence Option and the accompanying regulations provide a solid foundation upon which state and local welfare agencies can build flexible programs under TANF capable of responding to the individualized needs of battered women. States which have not yet adopted the Family Violence Option should be encouraged by advocates to do so now that the regulations are final. Adopting the Family Violence Option not only serves battered women on welfare but also serve the states' interests by allowing them to serve domestic violence victims without compromising their ability to meet the federal standards for work participation and for the hardship exemption.

The challenge of the Family Violence Option rests in its implementation—on the choices state and local welfare agencies make and their commitment to responsibly serve battered women in their programs. States are now in the early stages of implementing the Family Violence Option. At these stages of early implementation, building on the implementation studies conducted by the Taylor Institute (Raphael, 1999; Raphael and Haennicke, 1999) is paramount. Because states have been granted wide-ranging autonomy and discretion in implementing both TANF and the Family Violence Option, it will be necessary to examine policies and programs within each state. Attention must be directed to the local implementation of the policies—where the client meets the policy. Emerging issues include staffing, service delivery, and service capacity (Johnson and Meckstroth, 1998).

Staffing

Universal notification, screening, and service referral for domestic violence all place new demands on frontline workers in welfare agencies. To fulfill these functions, extensive training of welfare workers, both eligibility workers and child support workers, will be required. The training must go beyond informing workers about the new rules; it must include education and knowledge building about domestic violence and its impact on women on welfare. It may also benefit welfare agencies to invest in extensive education and training for selected workers who specialize in working with battered women or to contract for these services from a domestic violence service provider. For service providers who regularly work with victims of domestic violence in other settings, it is equally important to become knowledgeable about the state's welfare rules and regulations regarding domestic violence. To facilitate collaborative working relationships as well as appreciation for the nature of the work in public welfare settings and in community-based organizations serving battered women, cross training of these frontline workers in both settings may be an appropriate model (Stuart, 1999).

Service Delivery

The most crucial points in addressing the needs of battered women are the notification and screening processes. As Raphael and Haennicke (1999) state:

> The linchpin of any state's FVO effort is thus the method by which the state informs the TANF participant about the FVO or domestic violence policies, and provides the opportunity to self-disclose at all stages of the case processing and throughout the welfare-to-work process. (p. 9)

A wide range of procedures is used by the states to inform clients about the Family Violence Option and to screen for domestic violence among women on welfare. Preliminary data suggest, however, that women may not be receiving information about the Family Violence Option nor the advantages and disadvantages of disclosing domestic violence. Concerns also have been raised about the intrusiveness of screening questions and the lack of multiple opportunities in which to voluntarily disclose domestic violence (Raphael and Haennicke, 1999). The assessment process probably varies as well but little information is available about the purpose of assessments, their scope, or their format. All of these issues must be addressed by local welfare agencies and merit monitoring on both the state and local levels to ensure that women on welfare are being notified about the Family Violence Option and given the opportunity to voluntarily disclose domestic violence in a private and confidential setting.

The nature of the issues presented by some victims of domestic violence also requires that referrals be made from the welfare agencies to supportive and supplemental services, either within the welfare agencies or community-based agencies, particularly domestic violence services and, for some, mental health and substance abuse services. Within the welfare agency, coordination of procedures and requirements under the Family Violence Option and under child support enforcement is required. Ideally, establishing eligibility for a waiver or an exemption under either child support or the Family Violence Option will be sufficient for the other.

To effectively serve battered women needing other supportive services, effective interagency partnerships must be developed on both the state and local levels. Services for battered women continue to be organized around community-based shelters (Hamby, 1998), many of which have expanded their functions to include not only emergency shelter but also other services, including counseling, legal advocacy, employment services, and support groups. Well-developed linkages between the welfare agency and the shelter network are essential if battered women on welfare are to have access to this array of community-based services. Developing a coordinated delivery system for women confronting multiple challenges has the potential for effectively serving victims of domestic violence and their children. Highly coordinated community-based programs have been found to be effective in serving victims of sexual assault (Campbell, 1998; Campbell and Ahrens, 1998). The effectiveness of these models should be developed and evaluated for battered women as well.

Service Capacity

In order to provide effective referrals and to develop effective coordinated community services, "the particular service that is needed must exist, be accessible, and respond in culturally sensitive ways" (Davies, 1997, p. 28). Relatively little is known about the general capacity of local services for battered women. Nationwide, approximately 1,250 shelters serve battered women, with budgets ranging from under $50,000 to over $1 million annually (Roberts, 1998).

Funding for shelters and their related services has expanded from charitable community contributions to include federal and state funding streams. However, the lack of adequate shelter capacities to meet the demand and lack of accessible shelters to all state residents continue to be issues in most states (Davis, Hagen, and Early, 1994).

As welfare agencies move to serve victims of domestic violence under the Family Violence Option, identifying the gaps in services and mobilizing federal, state, and local support for services will be required. As well as insuring the availability and accessibility of supportive services for battered women as they make the transition from welfare to work, attention must be directed to providing ongoing, supportive services once employment is obtained to address the job retention issues confronting victims of domestic violence. For all of these services, monitoring is needed to ensure that women are getting to needed services and that these services are effective in helping them address barriers to employment or stability in employment.

In looking at all three of these issues, obtaining the perspectives of the women themselves—the intended beneficiaries of the Family Violence Option—will help states to design policies responsive to their needs (Imperial, 1997) and the complex ways those needs interact with welfare regulations. As Imperial (1997) notes:

> Because domestic violence victims have differing strengths and needs, the welfare system must be flexible. The complexity of the lives of domestic violence victims . . . calls for individualized responses rather than blanket exemptions from program requirements. (p. 34)

CONCLUSION

The Family Violence Option affords the opportunity to develop flexible and responsive programs for battered women on welfare by taking a strengths-based perspective on the women, the welfare agencies, and the larger community context (Postmus, in press). Part of doing so, however, requires the recognition that "although wife abuse occurs in the interpersonal arena, it is a social problem that requires social solutions" (Davis, 1987, p. 311). Among those solutions must be welfare policies that adequately serve the needs of battered women and their children, including their need for economic support in escaping abusive relationships. But the implications of domestic violence are not restricted to welfare policies alone. The pervasiveness of violence against women and the particular vulnerability of low-income and poor women and their children should alert us to incorporating flexibility and sensitivity to these issues in other social programs as well. As Browne and Bassuk (1997) suggest:

> No programs or interventions designed for very low-income mothers and children—whether they be welfare-to-work policies, health policies, or educational programs for children—can be fully effective if they do not take into account the reality that violence is omnipresent in their lives. (p. 276)

REFERENCES

Allard, M. A., Corten, M. E., Albelda, R., and Cosenza, C. (1997). *In harm's way? Domestic violence, AFDC receipt, and welfare reform in Massachusetts.* Boston: University of Massachusetts, McCormack Institute, Center for Survey Research.

Angelari, M. (1998). *The family violence option in Maryland: A preliminary report.* Towson, MD: The Women's Law Center of Maryland.

Brandwein, R. A. (1999). Family violence and social policy: Welfare "reform" and beyond. In R. A. Brandwein (Ed.), *Battered women, children, and welfare reform: The ties that bind* (pp. 147-172). Thousand Oaks, CA: Sage.

Brooks, M. G. and Buckner, J. C. (1996). Work and welfare: Job histories, barriers to employment, and predictors of work among low-income single women. *American Journal of Orthopsychiatry, 66*(4): 526-537.

Browne, A. and Bassuk, S. (1997). Intimate violence in the lives of homeless and poor housed women: Prevalence and patterns in an ethnically diverse sample. *American Journal of Orthopsychiatry, 67*(2): 261-278.

Browne, A., Salomon, A., and Bassuk, S. S. (1999). The impact of recent partner violence on poor women's capacity to maintain work. *Violence Against Women, 5*(4): 393-426.

Campbell, R. (1998). The community response to rape: Victims' experiences with the legal, medical, and mental health systems. *American Journal of Community Psychology, 26*(3): 355-379.

Campbell, R. and Ahrens, C. E. (1998). Innovative community services for rape victims: An application of multiple case study methodology. *American Journal of Community Psychology, 26*(4): 537-571.

Curcio, W. (1997). *The Passaic County study of recipients in a welfare-to-work program: A preliminary analysis.* Paterson, NJ: Passaic County Board of Social Services.

Danziger, S., Corcoran, M., Danziger, S., Heflin, C., Kalil, A., Levine, J., Rosen, D., Seefeldt, K., Siefert, K., and Tolman, R. (1999). *Barriers to the employment of welfare recipients.* Poverty Research and Training Center, University of Michigan. Retrieved March 25, 1999, from the World Wide Web: <http://www.ssw.umich.edu/poverty/pubs.html>.

Davies, J. (1997). The new welfare law: State implementation and use of the family violence option (Paper #2). Harrisburg, PA: National Resource Center on Domestic Violence.

Davis, L. V. (1987). Battered women: The transformation of a social problem. *Social Work, 32*(4): 306-311.

Davis, L. V. and Hagen, J. L. (1988). Services for battered women: The public policy response. *Social Service Review, 62*(4): 649-667.

Davis, L. V. Hagen, J. L., and Early, T. J. (1994). Social services for battered women: Are they adequate, accessible, and appropriate? *Social Work, 39*(6): 695-704.

Davis, M. F. (1999). The economics of abuse: How violence perpetuates women's poverty. In R. A. Brandwein (Ed.), *Battered women, children, and welfare reform: The ties that bind* (pp. 17-30). Thousand Oaks, CA: Sage.

Gondolf, E. W. and Fisher, E. R. (1988). *Battered women as survivors: An alternative to treating learned helplessness.* Lexington, MA: Lexington Press.

Greenberg, M. and Savner, S. (1999). *The final TANF regulations: A preliminary analysis.* Center for Law and Social Policy. May. Retrieved January 26, 2000, from the World Wide Web: <http://www.clasp.org/pubs/TANF/finalregs.PDF>.

Hagen, J. L. (1998). The new welfare law: "Tough on work." *Families in Society. 79*(6): 596-605.

Hagen, J. L. (1999). Time limits under Temporary Assistance to Needy Families: A look at the welfare cliff. *Affilia, 14*(3): 294-314.

Hagen, J. L. and Owens-Manley, J. (in press). Issues in implementing TANF in New York: The perspective of front-line workers. *Social Work.*

Hamby, S. L. (1998). Partner violence: Prevention and intervention. In J. L. Jasinski and L. M. Williams (Eds.), *Partner violence: A comprehensive review of 20 years of research* (pp. 210-258). Thousand Oaks, CA: Sage.

Howell, S. L. (1997). How will battered women fare under the new welfare reform? *Berkeley Women's Law Journal, 12:* 140-150.

Imperial, M. L. (1997). Self-sufficiency and safety: Welfare reform for victims of domestic violence. *Georgetown Journal on Fighting Poverty, 5*(Winter): 3-37.

Johnson, A. and Meckstroth, A. (1998). *Ancillary services to support welfare to work* (PR98-21). Princeton, NJ: Mathematica Policy Research, Inc.

Kenney, C. T., and Brown, K. R. (1996). *Report from the front lines: The impact of violence on poor women.* New York: NOW Legal Defense and Education Fund.

Lloyd, S. (1996). *The effects of violence on women's employment.* Evanston, IL: Northwestern University, Joint Center for Poverty Research, and Institute for Policy Research.

Lloyd, S. and Taluc, N. (1999). The effects of male violence on female employment. *Violence Against Women, 5*(4): 370-392.

Pearson, J. and Griswold, E. A. (1997). Child support policies and domestic violence. *Public Welfare, 55*(Winter): 26-32.

Pearson, J. Thoennes, N., and Griswold, E. A. (1999). Child support and domestic violence: The victims speak out. *Violence Against Women, 5*(4): 427-448.

Pollack, W. and Davis, M. F. (1997). The family violence option of the personal responsibility and work opportunity reconciliation act of 1996: Interpretation and implementation. *Clearinghouse Review, 30*(11-12): 1079-1098.

Postmus, J. L. (2000). Analysis of the family violence option: A strengths perspective. *Affilia,* 15: 244-258.

Raphael, J. (1995). *Domestic violence: Telling the untold welfare-to-work story.* Chicago: Taylor Institute.

Raphael, J. (1996). *Prisoners of abuse: Domestic violence and welfare receipt.* Chicago: Taylor Institute.

Raphael, J. (1999). The family violence option: An early assessment. *Violence Against Women, 5*(4): 449-466.

Raphael, J. and Haennicke, S. (1999). *Keeping battered women safe through the welfare-to-work journey: How are we doing?* Chicago: Taylor Institute.

Raphael, J. and Tolman, R. M. (1997). *Trapped by poverty/trapped by abuse: New evidence documenting the relationship between domestic violence and welfare.* Chicago: Taylor Institute and University of Michigan Research Development Center on Poverty, Risk, and Mental Health.

Roberts, A. R. (1998). The organizational structure and function of shelters for battered women and their children: A national survey. In A. R. Roberts (Ed.), *Battered women and their families,* Second edition (pp. 58-75). New York: Springer.

Roberts, P. (1997). *Pursuing child support: More violence?* Center for Law and Social Policy. Retrieved December 3, 1997, from the World Wide Web: <http://www.clasp.org/pubs/childenforce/child_support_enforcement.htm>.

Salomon, A., Bassuk, S. S., and Brooks, M. G. (1996). Patterns of welfare use among poor and homeless women. *American Journal of Orthopsychiatry, 66*(4): 510-525.

Shepard, M. and Pence, E. (1988). The effect of battering on employment status of women. *Affilia, 3*(2): 55-61.

Straus, M. A. and Gelles, R. J. (1986). Societal change and change in family violence from 1975 to 1985 as revealed by two national surveys. *Journal of Marriage and the Family, 3:* 465-479.

Stuart, D. M. (1999). Domestic violence victims and welfare services: A practitioner's view. In R. A. Brandwein (Ed.), *Battered women, children, and welfare reform: The ties that bind* (pp. 79-93). Thousand Oaks, CA: Sage.

Tjaden, P. and Thoennes, N. (1998). *Prevalence, incidence, and consequences of violence against women: Findings from the national violence against women survey.* Washington, DC: National Institute of Justice.

U.S. Department of Health and Human Services (1999). *Clinton administration finalizes welfare regulations* [HHS Fact Sheet]. U.S. Department of Health and Human Services. Retrieved January 28, 2000, from the World Wide Web: <http://www.acf.dhhs.gov/news/3tanfreg.htm>.

U.S. Department of Health and Human Services, Administration for Children and Families (1998). *Temporary Assistance for Needy Families (TANF): First annual report to Congress.* U.S. Department of Health and Human Services. Retrieved January 26, 2000, from the World Wide Web: <http://www.acf.dhhs.gov/news/Welfare/congress/tanfp9.htm>.

Chapter 7

Promoting Reentry for Formerly Incarcerated Women: Individual and Community Practice Challenges

Patricia O'Brien

INTRODUCTION

Corrections, especially for women, continues to be a boom industry (Severson, 1994). By mid-year 2000, nearly 93,000 women were incarcerated in state and federal prisons in the United States, accounting for approximately 6.5 percent of all prison inmates (Beck and Karberg, 2001). Relative to their number in the U.S. population, the incarceration rate is about sixteen times higher for men than for women (885 to 57 per 100,000, respectively). However, analysis of imprisonment rates from 1990 to 1997 reveals a 71 percent increase among females as compared to a 49 percent increase among males in the number of sentenced prisoners per 100,000 residents (Beck and Mumola, 1999).

As a profession, social work has historically been concerned with populations who are vulnerable to our greatest social ills. A cursory look at incarcerated female offenders produces a typical portrait of an impoverished, disproportionately African-American, drug-affected, and undereducated woman. Many of the women were or are victims

An earlier version of this chapter was presented at the Council on Social Work Education Annual Program Meeting, San Francisco, March 11, 1999. It received the Barbara Solomon Feminist Scholarship Award from the Women's Commission.

of current abuse, homelessness, substance addiction, mental disorders, and/or poverty (Brownell, 1997).

About 70 percent of incarcerated women are parents of minor children (Greenfeld and Snell, 1999). More than half of the female inmates in a national survey of women inmates reported their children were living with grandparents, with only a quarter living with the child's father, as compared to 89.7 percent of the incarcerated men's children living with the children's mother (Snell, 1994). It is estimated there are more than 1.3 million minor children of women under correctional sanction (Greenfeld and Snell, 1999). Whether contact with the children occurs during incarceration often depends on the caregivers' willingness and ability to transport the child to the prison facility.

A national survey of prison inmates found white females had the highest rate of mental illness (29 percent) of any other group (Ditton, 1999). Nationally, the proportion of female inmates who are HIV positive is higher than that of men (Maruschak, 1999). Young (1996) found that women enter prison in poor physical health due to a combination of personal and societal conditions including poverty, race, and drug use.

Many accounts since the mid-1970s have attempted to describe women's pathways into criminal behavior and their experiences while in prison (see, for example, Adler, 1975; Belknap, 1996; Burke, 1992; Chesney-Lind and Rodriguez, 1983; Fletcher, Shaver, and Moon, 1993; Watterson, 1996). Research describing the aftermath of incarceration for women is scarce and tends to overgeneralize men's experiences to include women. Although men also face barriers when exiting prison, additional barriers for women may derive from sexism (Carlen and Worrall, 1987; Chapman, 1980; Erez, 1992; Visher, 1983; Wilson and Anderson, 1997), racism coupled with sexism (Arnold, 1990; Daly, 1994; Phillips and Votey, 1984; Richie, 1996), challenges in the resumption of the primary parenting role (Fesseler, 1991; McCarthy, 1980), and prior experiences of abuse (Gilfus, 1992; Harlow, 1999).

Consistent with an increasing rate of incarceration and the well-documented lack of adequate resources for women's rehabilitation in prison, women's rate of recidivism is increasing. A three-year follow-up of a sample of women discharged from prisons in eleven states in 1983 found that 33 percent were returned to prison (Beck and Shipley,

1989). A 1991 national survey indicated that 71 percent of all female prisoners had served a prior sentence to probation or incarceration (including 20 percent who had served a sentence as a juvenile) (Snell, 1994). In 1996, about 45 percent of women for whom parole supervision was ended were returned to prison or had absconded (Greenfeld and Snell, 1999). We see an increasing number of women serving short bursts of prison time separated from family and children but without gender-specific treatment, skills development, or necessary community support to successfully return to the community after incarceration.

Today's correctional environment and the trend of women more often to serve sentences of incarceration than probation is being driven by the "get tough on crime" and "war on drugs" policies that emerged in the late 1970s and became codified in the 1980s in mandatory minimum sentencing policies that removed discretion from judges (Chesney-Lind, 1991; Dressel, 1994). The purpose of this chapter is to review briefly the factors and elements that contribute to recidivism for women and describe the findings from a qualitative study of women who identified themselves as successful after incarceration. I then consider the role for social work practitioners to address women's needs during reentry and advance policies to create a more just and responsible response to female offenders.

FACTORS CONTRIBUTING TO POSTINCARCERATION RECIDIVISM OR SUCCESSFUL REENTRY

Recidivism is the consequence of becoming reinvolved in a criminal activity that is reported and acted upon by law enforcement. It can also be the consequence of a failure to meet probation or parole conditions. Although remaining free from crime is an achievement, it is only one of several criteria for successful reintegration into the community.

The overwhelming majority of studies of the process of reentry have focused on male offenders. Additionally, they have been primarily concerned with the risk factors for recidivism—those demographic characteristics that predict which exprisoners will fail after release. Literature describing success after incarceration is scarce. Most studies of adult offenders have focused only on the predictors and the outcome of recidivism rather than on the processes of reentry.

Beck and Shipley's (1989) study of adult releases in 1983 shows that men are more likely to be rearrested, reconvicted, and reincarcerated after their release from prison. The study also showed that recidivism is higher in the first year; older prisoners have lower rates of recidivism; females with more than six prior arrests were just as likely to be rearrested within three years of release as were men; those who served five years or more had lower rates of rearrest; and those released for property offenses were most likely to be rearrested.

Other studies have identified differences in variables associated with recidivism for men and women, such as spouse abuse (Bonta, Pang, and Wallace-Capretta 1995; Danner et al., 1995), higher rates of recidivism for women who come from broken homes (Danner et al., 1995), similar rates of recidivism for older and younger women (Jurik, 1983), and lower rates for black women compared to white women (Robinson, 1971).

Another element affecting reentry is the lack of programs available to women in prisons and in the community. Many women's state prisons are located in rural areas, which removes women from access to schools, training programs, and work release opportunities found in urban areas (Pollock-Byrne, 1990). Additionally, vocational training programs for prisoners continue to be more limited for women (American Correctional Association, 1990; Pollock-Byrne, 1990; Sobel, 1982). Prerelease programs designed to prepare women for the transition from prison to the community variably exist in state correctional systems. Field (1998) describes various studies that demonstrate the importance of continuity of care in reducing recidivism and relapse—a frequent problem related to reincarceration.

Factors that have been identified as indicators of postincarceration success for women include economic support (Jurik, 1983), employment (Lambert and Madden, 1976; Schulke, 1993), family stability (Bloom, 1987; Flanagan, 1995; Hairston, 1991; Lambert and Madden, 1976), positive relationships (Schulke, 1993), substance abuse treatment, and self-efficacy (Fletcher, Shaver, and Moon; 1993).

Zamble and Quinsey (1997) have developed a model that represents recidivism as an ongoing psychological process that examines the interaction between internal dispositions and external events. Thinking about reintegration as a dynamic process can be helpful to programs designed to assist in the reentry process, to the women and families in that process, and to community members involved with these women.

Following is an interview study that attempts to illustrate this dynamic process.

METHODOLOGY

The goals of this exploratory study were to (1) discover the women who, despite the odds, had "made it" after experiences of incarceration and (2) develop a more complete picture of how they had managed their reintegration to home and community (O'Brien, 2001). This study uses data from in-depth interviews with eighteen formerly incarcerated women residing in two Midwestern states in early 1996 to describe the elements that contributed to their successful transition from prison. "Success," for this voluntary sample of exincarcerated women, was not defined beyond the criteria that they must have been at least three months postrelease and self-identify as "successful."

Description of Participants

The women had been incarcerated in four state facilities and five federal facilities and released from 1983 to late 1995. They ranged in age from twenty to sixty-seven years old, with a mean age of 34.6. Of the eighteen, four are African American, two are Hispanic, one is Korean/African American, one is Native American, and the remainder are white (ten). At the time of the interviews, only two of the participants had no children, while thirteen were parents of minor children, and three were parents of adult children. Seven of the women were married or living with an intimate partner, and one of the women identified as a lesbian. Thirteen were employed either part- or full-time.

As compared to state and national samples of incarcerated women, this group of released women had a higher degree of white participants, an older mix of participants, more married women, and a more highly educated selection (ten reported "some college education," some of which they obtained while incarcerated). This group of study participants may represent a more stable group of exoffenders than is typical.

The range of crimes and variation in criminal history is more characteristic of the national profile. For example, seven of the women had been incarcerated for property crimes, an equal number had been incarcerated for drug offenses, and four had served time for crimes of violence against persons. Seven (39 percent) of the participants had been incarcerated two or more times. Two had been incarcerated ten times previously. Participants in the study had served sentences that ranged from six months to eight years and had been released from prison anywhere from three months to twelve years. Ten of the participants were still either on parole with the state department of corrections or on supervised release under jurisdiction of the federal office of probation and parole.

Procedures

In an effort to maximize discovery and description, I employed open-ended questions as a qualitative data-gathering technique (Reinharz, 1992). The questions focused on how family, friends, intimate partners, parole officers, and experiences during incarceration promoted or hindered the women's progress after prison. The design incorporated a semistructured interview guide that attempted to capture similarities as well as identify differences among the participants with a variety of incarceration and exit experiences. Although there were some limitations to this intensive but broad-brush approach, the interviews, which ranged from one-and-a-half hours to six hours in length, elicited information, stories, and recommendations from a highly diverse group of women. In the case of one participant who had been out of prison for twelve years, a second interview was scheduled due to the complexity of her experiences. In addition, a focus group was conducted with about half of the participants both to review initial findings and to build on some of the individual themes that had emerged over the course of the interviews. The women's participation in the study was consistent with both feminist and social work values, both in giving voice to those who have been socially or culturally disempowered and in recognizing the women's many strengths in the process of sharing their stories (Laird, 1989).

Analysis

The primary method of data analysis was an adaptation of the constant-comparative method (Glaser and Strauss, 1967; Lincoln and Guba, 1985). The constant-comparative method is a process of developing categories, concepts, and broader themes inductively from the interview data and testing them out at each step by returning to the data to evaluate their fit. This method, in which there is continuous and simultaneous data collection and processing of data, provides the basis for the integration of similarities and differences to produce the findings.

Coding and comparative analysis of data were accomplished by the use of manual techniques and a data analysis software program *QSR NUD IST* (Qualitative Solutions and Research Ltd., 1995). By applying the constant-comparative method that included both within and between case comparison into categories, the major themes emerged. Dependability and credibility of the findings were enhanced by a limited member check procedure in the focus group held at the conclusion of the interviews.

Findings

Analysis of the interviews and focus group suggested two overarching themes: the women's need to address basic survival issues after leaving prison and the importance of their intrapersonal and interpersonal attitudes about their identity and functioning as exinmates. The women provided many examples of these two interwoven and overlapping themes. For example, all of the participants discussed the necessity of finding shelter or having "someplace to go" as a crucial start of their transition. It was also evident that the women had to address the impact of incarceration upon their relationships, their everyday behavioral choices, and how they thought and felt about themselves as a consequence. Often women expressed insights about their experiences that they had not been aware of up to the point of their articulation in the interviews. They also identified internal strengths that had nourished their sense of survival and hope. These themes were not sequential or hierarchical but rather unique to each woman and her particular psychosocial context. As a heuristic device for conceptualizing what the women defined as markers of success, I constructed the "Empowerment Framework for Assessing Women's Transition from Prison" (see Figure 7.1).

As this graphic representation indicates, the narratives produced five key categories of successful reintegration. The critical elements include: (1) living arrangements, (2) supportive relationships, (3) gainful employment, (4) community attitudes and resources, and (5) self in transition.

FIGURE 7.1. Empowerment Framework for Assessing Women's Transition from Prison

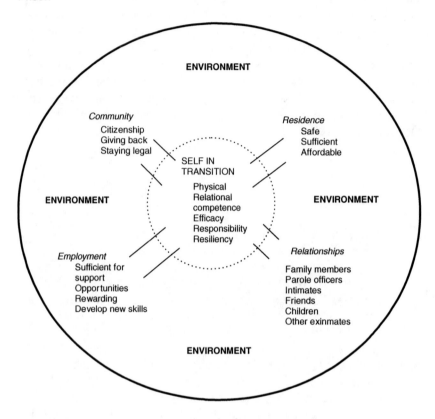

Living Arrangements—Safe and Sufficient Housing

The women in the study had two distinct ways of dealing with housing depending on whether they were federal or state inmates. If they were federal inmates, they were released from the prison to a community placement facility. The facility provided room, board, and supportive services for the remainder of the woman's sentence, in most cases 90 to 120 days. Residents at the facility were expected to obtain employment within their first month and thereafter pay a percentage of their income for "subsistence" while residing at the facility. They were also expected to save the bulk of their earnings to enable them to manage initial living expenses.

Other women came directly out from the state prison to the community with little more than hope in their pockets. These women were much more dependent upon family members or friends for a temporary residence. Therefore, their housing tended to be much less stable. For example, Bernie* called a friend she had known while incarcerated who put her up for a few nights while she completed the paperwork that enabled her to get a subsidized apartment due to her age and health disabilities. Mandi initially stayed on the couch at her brother's home but then moved in with friends from work; eventually, after she was working two jobs, she rented her own home. Ashley stayed with her parents. When that situation became conflictual, she moved in with a boyfriend, before finally moving into her own residence. Two of the women were still living with a family member and trying to save enough money so they could move into independent housing.

Participants who entered the community via the community placement facility moved an average of 1.3 times, while women who entered the community directly from the prison facility moved an average of 2.25 times. Thus, the halfway house concept ameliorated at least one aspect of reentry: the ability to secure housing.

Supportive Relationships

Only two participants had no concrete or emotional family support during incarceration or after release from prison. However, a surprising finding reflected the necessity of repairing fractured relationships with family members, especially inmates' mothers, who had often served as caregivers for participants' minor children during incarceration. Ten of the eighteen study participants described their relationships with their mothers as historically problematic and sometimes abusive. Working out the difficulties in their relationships with their mothers contributed to the women's sense of growth following incarceration, even if their mothers were no longer living, as was true for Bernie. For some women, regaining the ability to parent their children also depended on their mending these relationships.

Despite the triggers for relapse or conflict, the difference was that women described skills of relational competence learned while incar-

---

*All reported names are pseudonyms chosen by the student participants.

cerated or in the context of their transition. Several women in the group discussed the concept of drawing boundaries in their relationships. They no longer tolerated certain behaviors from others, including abusive or criminal conduct. For Ashley, finally asserting herself to her mother opened the door to having a more bounded relationship. She explained,

> My mom and I were never really close . . . because she did abuse me. I would never open up to her and talk to her. So, about a year ago, I just sat her down one day, and I said, "Look, Mom, this is me, and this is the way I am. You either deal with it or you don't because you don't have another daughter. But I'm not gonna let you downgrade me and talk bad about me. You have to accept me the way I am.

Susan took responsibility for the behaviors that resulted in her two incarcerations, but said she also gained insight by examining abuse in her family history that may have contributed to her criminal behavior. For Susan, the examination began during her last incarceration and continued when she was referred for mental health sessions during her parole. Meanwhile, her mother also obtained counseling and began to address some of the damage she had inflicted upon her daughter as a child.

Sixteen of the eighteen participants had children. At the time of the interviews, thirteen of the participants had minor children, including four who had been born since their release. Eight of these thirteen participants had alternative physical or legal custody arrangements for their children. Most resided in the care of their mothers or other family members. These parents chose a more graduated process of regaining custody of their children. They recognized that they were not yet financially able to support their children.

All the parents discussed the pain of being separated from their children while incarcerated. Those who chose not yet to resume their residential parenting role described relationships with their children that were both supportive and challenging. These women felt they were given a chance to address some of the trauma their children had experienced before and during their incarceration. Challenges further existed due to the ambivalence the women felt when they were unable to resume their parenting role and identity.

The reawakened capacity to care for their children made some of the women feel rewarded. Nan, a single mother of five children, including one that was born while she was incarcerated in a federal prison facility, actively continued her parenting role while in prison only because her younger sister moved to the town where she was incarcerated with her children to ensure that she had regular visits with them. She explained how creating a home for her children enabled her to overcome her compulsion for a materialistic lifestyle that had previously resulted in criminal behaviors:

> Havin' to go to prison, livin' in a matchbox room and only havin' X-amount of dollars and havin' nowhere to go and nobody to turn to—I don't ever want that again. All them fine fancy clothes and good livin' . . . I wasn't even happy. Now, I'm so happy bein' right here with my kids. With little money and nothin' because it's real, true love right here in the home with me and my kids.

Women also described receiving assistance from intimate partners, friends, and former inmates. Several of the women had the experience of reconstructing their lives after prison with a new partner. Rene described the process of building the walls of support for her and her two children with the help that her new fiancé provided:

> I started while I was there in prison. It's just like doin' a diagram of a house, and you're gonna have this—what's gonna hold it up, and you're gonna do all these things to keep it standin'. And it's like keeping all the bricks in place. That's what I did, because my boyfriend was there. We was friends before I got locked up. He came to see me. He stuck in there with the kids.

Most of the women discussed the importance of their relationships with their parole or supervision officers in facilitating their transition: "I am so grateful for her today," says Mandi, a former crack addict, about her parole officer. For this group of women, facilitative relationships with correctional staff provided another element to their successful reentry. Some of the women described how they gained a sense of self-efficacy by earning respect from correctional officers for how they did their time. Demi recalled that a correctional officer told her, "You don't belong here," which reinforced her motivation to use the opportunity to enter a drug treatment program while she was incarcerated.

At the time of the study, ten of the eighteen women were still accountable to the system under some form of supervision by state or federal officers. Many of the women described the parole or postrelease supervision process as "doing what I have to do." However, the ways women negotiated meeting their conditions of supervision and their relationship with their supervisory officer were instrumental for success in their reentry. Four of the participants in the study shared the same parole officer who was cited for her willingness to extend herself to meet a parolee's needs and her flexibility in modifying parole conditions when appropriate.

Other officers were recognized for the respect they showed the women. As Suzy said, one officer "treated me like a person instead of a number." Parole officers can assist women exiting prison by providing information about what the women can expect in the parole process, by teaching women how to manage disclosure of their status, and by making referrals for counseling and support. Common to these women's experiences was the development and reconstruction of growth-enhancing relationships and the termination of abusive relationships.

Gainful Employment

The women described how their incarceration was a barrier not only to their obtaining employment due to the associated stigma but also to having a realistic notion for how they would manage day-to-day responsibilities. Suzy compared the new responsibilities she faced relative to the unchanging routine of prison life with some nostalgia:

> I knew what to expect [in prison]. I knew where I was and what my responsibility was. You had a routine and knew what you had to do and how you had to do it, and it didn't change. And here in a normal life, it changes every day. All these different responsibilities and stress factors. I didn't have 'em then there.

Anita discussed how the controlling prison culture reinforced the lack of planning for future responsibilities women face when they exit the institution: "They know when they was in there, they can eat for free. They don't gotta pay no bills. They don't worry about no kids. They don't do nothin' but be there and do what they want ya to do, and that's the same daily routine."

The women who were most successful at managing the unpredictability of the job search, the disclosure of felony status, and the everyday work world were those who had been consistently employed while in prison. Women reported they had to self-advocate to obtain productive prison work, which later helped them qualify for postrelease work opportunities.

The federal women who came out via release to the community placement center had more support and referrals for job placement. These women were already identified as exinmates by virtue of their residence and so did not report as much concern with stigma related to finding a job as did those women who came out to the community directly from a prison facility.

The state-released women managed the disclosure challenge in a variety of ways. Elizabeth did not reveal her exinmate status; but when it was discovered, she was fired from two different jobs. Mandi used the data-entry job training and experience she had gained in prison and personal contacts at a company to secure her first job. Later, she "sold herself" by her friendly demeanor and became a manager at the McDonald's she frequented. Sadie's first job was at the domestic violence shelter that had sponsored the support group she attended while in prison, so she was already known by the agency. Thirteen of the eighteen women reported they were discriminated against on the basis of their criminal record, which prevented them from getting the jobs they wanted.

Most of the women struggled with finances. While one woman received SSI due to a disability, another received a limited amount of public assistance for her newborn child. The overwhelming concern among all the working women was that their income was insufficient to support themselves and their children. They were scraping by, often working more than one job, and drawing upon other family and social resources to supplement their wages.

Community Attitudes and Resources

Study participants reported a number of professionals from various private and public agencies provided concrete assistance to them, especially during the early stage of their transition. Some women praised the charismatic drug counselor at the federal community placement facility as he had "been there" both as an exaddict and exinmate. Elena bragged that he encouraged her to "prove 'em all wrong":

> When I came out of prison, I had the same attitude that I was gonna do everything like before. I wasn't gonna change. I just thought, "They made me wiser." I got caught one time. I was just gonna be slicker, and that was my attitude when I first came out. I had a terrible attitude. I think my drug counselor was the one that really helped me decide on what I really want out of life— he was like my inspiration. If he could do it, I can do it.

Aftercare for drug addiction was more of a challenge for the women released directly to the community from the state prison. Mandi acknowledged relapsing with crack cocaine but, with the help of her work supervisor, was able to get the treatment she needed. Some women worried about using community resources because they had to disclose their record of incarceration. Nan likened the intrusion to an extension of control she already felt in her postrelease supervision. She exploded,

> The federal government was all in my business and turned it upside down and told me what to do, when to do, not 365 days a year, but four times 365 days a year. And I live with my officer that does the same thing. I don't want to go nowhere else and nobody ask me nothin' about my business. Can I have some privacy? Can I be a citizen? Can I have rights? Can I be human?

Nan's questions reflect what many of the women said about how the community contributed to their success, not so much for the resources it provided them, but for the sense that they were able to contribute to others. Bernie shared her experiences with churches and civic organizations, raising funds and collecting clothing for other exinmates. Elena discussed her urge to work with adolescents so they wouldn't get involved in drugs. This notion of "giving back" enabled the women to feel they belonged to their community. As Sadie articulated, and other participants in the study confirmed, it is crucial that people in the "free world" recognize that former inmates are often living and working in the same community as them:

> Almost everybody who goes to prison gets out [and] they are teaching in your school or shopping in the same stores. . . . They are helping you out and doing this and that and the other and in many ways are part of the community. I fix your kids' bicycles now. That's who excons are, you know.

Self in Transition

The women described a phenomenon of growing from the "inside out" that often began when they learned how to manage their incarceration. Many claimed that prison saved them from death or worse. What is certain is that prison allows time away from outside pressures or easy access to drugs. It provides some inmates with resources they might not otherwise have, including some programming, drug treatment, and vocational training. Numerous prisoners take the opportunities offered in prison and other correctional facilities and make positive changes despite soul-deadening limitations imposed on them by the prison structure. Many women in this study have survived circumstances far more perilous than a prison term, and most will continue to survive and even thrive in the new beginnings they are constructing.

Although these women described major struggles in gaining housing and employment, they reflected an ability to bounce back from adversity. Some of the internal strengths they identified included tenacity, stubbornness, problem-solving skills, a willingness to take responsibility for one's behavior and choices, and a sense of competence for handling challenges.

In addition to having some insight about the elements that contributed to their successful reentry, these women expressed aspirations that reflected their sense of hope for transforming their lives. These aspirations included returning to college, better-paying employment, and doing meaningful work.

DISCUSSION AND IMPLICATIONS

Running through these narratives is a sense of both dormancy and growth. The women project a wisdom sharpened by experience for how they must function in order to free themselves from correctional involvement. The process of successful reintegration is dependent upon the woman's development of a sense of self-efficacy and resiliency and the use of family, community, and social resources. These findings are consistent with what others have identified, particularly in the area of receiving drug treatment while in prison (Fletcher, Shaver, and Moon, 1993), developing economic self-sufficiency (Jurik, 1983), and the support of relationships (Schulke, 1993). The central organizing theme for an understanding of women's emancipatory process is how they are able to resurrect their lives and reclaim their identity and power.

Empowerment has at its foundation a dual focus on person and environment. It evolves from a historical understanding of a concomitant need simultaneously to aid people in need and attack social ills (Pinderhughes, 1994; Rose and Black, 1985). In this paradigm, the welfare of individuals and their families is linked inextricably to the life-promoting qualities of their social contexts. Similarly, feminist theorists have pointed to the intertwined nature of the personal and the political realities of women's lives.

The key point is that each woman found a starting point for her transition—sometimes in the way she coped with the incarceration, or in the ways she was able to renegotiate family roles and relationships, or in the ways she managed her obligations of parole or supervision, or in the way she was able to reparent her children. From these starting points, as several of the women described, there was a synergistic effect of other "good things" that followed.

If there is a sequential or temporal order to the process of transition, this study suggests that it begins with the woman herself as an active participant in the social world rather than a passive object, acted upon by the forces in and around her. Most of the women described how they took responsibility for the decisions they had made and used their incarceration experiences both to bolster their internal strengths and to amass other external resources they could use after their release. The reasons some women chose more efficacious behavior at the time of their most recent incarceration remains elusive. For some, it may have been a cumulative effect; as one woman related, she just got "sick and tired" of being "sick and tired." For others, especially those for whom the incarceration was the first and last of their lives, the unexpected seriousness and pain of the consequence, especially as indicated by those women incarcerated for federal drug convictions, may have had a lasting effect.

How the exinmate makes daily choices, the types of relationships she brings into her life, and, finally, the management of the multiple expectations she faces, determine her capacity to begin a cycle of efficacy (Bandura, 1992) that is self-perpetuating and reinforcing of her desire to assert a noncriminal identity. The ways in which the woman creates and maintains supportive relationships, as well as her identification with her community have profound effects on successful reentry. Women recognized the restorative power of the human bond and sought to attach with people with whom they could have shared goals and a healthy interdependence. In addition, they attempted to address some of the disconnections in previous relationships.

The interaction between the women in this study and their environments demonstrates a need for effective coping strategies and a sense of empowerment, but also a need for accessible resources. A lack of financial assistance, drug treatment and aftercare, transportation, or child care and support for parenting are obstacles in this process. Better coping skills and the availability of resources were both necessary to prevent reincarceration. As Denni so eloquently stated, "It has to be a combination. It's just like bakin' a cake. You can't leave out the flour. You need all the ingredients to make it come out right."

PRACTICE AND POLICY LESSONS FOR THE FUTURE

Study participants made the following recommendations that they believed would facilitate women's efforts to make the transition from prison. These include:

- To begin identifying sources of postincarceration support while in prison
- To facilitate women addressing former experiences of childhood or partner abuse and addictions that prevent them from recognizing their ability to manage the transition

- To treat women with respect and believe in their potential to transform themselves
- To provide incarcerated women with "real world" training for employment at a livable wage after incarceration
- To recognize that association with exinmates can be an important source of mentoring and support
- To create awareness about the challenges that women coming out of prison have to face and to be willing to work with women to define strategies for addressing those challenges

Study findings (and these recommendations) have important implications for social work practice and education. They suggest that practice interventions must address both the psychological and the social aspects of women's lives upon release from incarceration.

The study also suggests important policy implications, particularly given the financial and social costs of incarceration (Dressel, 1994). Contemporary sociologists and criminologists have argued that it is time to look at alternatives to incarceration, especially considering the mix of social and environmental factors that are producing female inmates at an increasing rate. Examining the efficacy of community-based programs for female (and male) offenders is also a crucial area of needed research. For example, a nonrandom survey of community-based programs for women and their children demonstrated a 0 to 17 percent rate of recidivism for their graduates (Devine, 1997), much lower than the norm.

Consistent with social work values of self-determination and belief in the individual capacity for growth and change, "Restorative justice" concepts may hold promise for doing justice better. Described as both "an umbrella concept and social movement" (Daly and Immargeon, 1998, p. 38) and based on an idealistic conception of justice, restorative justice is a reparative approach as compared to the current punitive approach. The focus of many of its practices is on the offender repairing ruptured social bonds and being restored to her relationships, her communities, and herself. Traditionally, values associated with feminism have stressed human beings' mutuality and commitment to one another. Restorative justice proposes similar values as the basis for responding to inappropriate or criminal behavior in the public sphere.

A justice process that addresses women's need for healing and promotes reintegration while holding women accountable for harm done to self, victims, and the larger community makes sense. We can begin using this approach immediately with nonviolent offenders through community-based alternative sentencing sanctions. For example, a "sentencing to service" project in Minnesota takes inmates from prison out on supervised crews where they learn new occupational skills while helping to build energy-efficient homes for low-income families. Another project in Oregon features individuals cutting firewood for elderly residents. Alternative sentencing policies should be developed by examining the profile of women offenders and the etiology of their crimes to generate options that could hold women accountable for their offenses and address some of the social structural issues that many report led to their illegal choices.

For women exiting incarceration, practices that emphasize community reconnection can promote the restoration of offenders. Social workers can facilitate offender connections to community members through mentoring programs, spiritual or religious ministries, and involvement in community projects with nonoffender participants. A recent needs assessments of the unique needs of incarcerated women informed by both institutional and program administrators and women offenders (Koons et al., 1997) provides a starting point for creating a continuum of services to support women's postincarceration success.

Finally, social workers could work with correctional staff to promote the inculcation of a "free world" attitude within prison facilities. This shift in attitude would challenge correctional institutions to examine their policies and practices that shape the day-to-day experience of incarcerated inmates and look for ways to widen the array of reparative services to address the multiple needs of incarcerated women during a potential time for transformative change. As Sadie eloquently stated, "We [exinmates] are your neighbors, your coworkers, your friends, and your family members." Programs must be developed with an appreciation for women's relational capacity to learn from others about how they can manage the challenges of returning to the free world. If we can build a response to crime based on relationships rather than fear, we can enter this new century with stronger communities that promote movement toward health and well-being.

CONCLUSION

The increasing numbers of women entering and exiting prison today provide unique opportunities for practice at all levels of social systems. An empowerment, strengths-based orientation to practice emphasizes the capabilities and potential of individuals to make growth-enhancing choices for their lives and for social workers to work in partnership with clients to do so. Empowerment practice also involves assessing the nature and consequences of the social conditions in which people live, and policies such as the war on drugs and the overreliance on incarceration as social control.

Former Supreme Court Chief Justice Warren Burger stated in the 1970s that one way to tell the character of a society was in how it treated those who had transgressed against it. It is time to begin a constructive dialogue in our schools of social work, in our neighborhoods, and in our media that reflects our belief in solutions that challenge women's criminality or their disposability. These narratives of the lives of women as they strive to "make it" after release from incarceration offer a starting point for this dialogue and suggest new directions for responsive and restorative public policy changes.

REFERENCES

Adler, F. (1975). *Sisters in crime: The rise of the new female criminal.* New York: McGraw-Hill.

American Correctional Association (1990). *The female offender: What does the future hold?* Washington, DC: St. Mary's Press.

Arnold, R. A. (1990). Process of victimization and criminalization of black women. *Social Justice, 17*(3): 153-66.

Bandura, A. (1992). Exercise of personal agency through the self-efficacy mechanism. In R. Schwarzer (Ed.), *Self-efficacy: Thought control of action* (pp. 3-38). Washington, DC: Hemisphere Publishing Corporation.

Beck, A. J. and Karberg, J. C. (2001). Bulletin. Prison and Inmates at Midyear 2000. Bureau of Justice Statistics. Washington, DC: U.S. Department of Justice.

Beck, A. J. and Mumola, C. (1999). *Prisoners in 1998.* Washington, DC: U.S. Government Printing Office.

Beck, A. J. and Shipley, B. E. (1989). *Recidivism of prisoners released in 1983.* Washington, DC: U.S. Government Printing Office.

Belknap, J. (1996). *The invisible woman: Gender, crime, and justice.* Belmont, CA: Wadsworth.

Bloom, B. (1987). Families of prisoners: A valuable resource. Paper presented at the annual meeting of the Academy of Criminal Justice Sciences. St. Louis, MO.

Bonta, J., Pang, B., and Wallace-Capretta, S. (1995). Predictors of recidivism among incarcerated female offenders. *The Prison Journal 75*(3): 277-294.

Brownell, P. (1997). Female offenders in the criminal justice system: Policy and program development. In A. R. Roberts (Ed.), *Social work in juvenile and criminal justice settings,* Second edition (pp. 325-349). Springfield, IL: Charles C Thomas.

Burke, C. (1992). *Vision narratives of women in prison.* Knoxville, TN: University of Tennessee.

Carlen, P. and Worrall, A. (Eds.) (1987). *Gender, crime and justice.* Philadelphia: Open University Press.

Chapman, J. R. (1980). *Economic realities and the female offender.* Lexington, MA: Lexington Books.

Chesney-Lind, M. (1991). Patriarchy, prisons, and jails: A critical look at trends in women's incarceration. *The Prison Journal, 71*(1): 51-67.

Chesney-Lind, M. and Rodriguez, N. (1983). Women under lock and key: A view from the inside. *The Prison Journal, 63*(2): 47-65.

Daly, K. (1994). Criminal law and justice system practices as racist, white, and racialized. *Washington and Lee Law Review, 51:* 431-464.

Daly, K. and Immargeon, R. (1998). The past, present, and future of restorative justice: Some critical reflections. *Contemporary Justice Review, 1*(1): 21-46.

Danner, T. A., Blount, W. R., Silverman, I. J., and Vega, M. (1995). The female chronic offender: Exploring life contingency and offense history dimensions for incarcerated female offenders. *Women and Criminal Justice, 6*(2): 45-66.

Devine, K. (1997). *Family unity: The benefits and costs of community-based sentencing programs for women and their children in Illinois.* Unpublished report. Chicago: Chicago Legal Aide to Incarcerated Mothers.

Ditton, P. M. (1999). *Mental health and treatment of inmates and probationers.* Washington, DC: U.S. Government Printing Office.

Dressel, P. L. (1994). And we keep on building prisons: Racism, poverty, and challenges to the welfare state. *Journal of Sociology and Social Welfare, 21*(3): 7-30.

Erez, E. (1992). Dangerous men, evil women: Gender and parole decision making. *Justice Quarterly, 9*(1): 105-126.

Fesseler, S. R. (1991). *Mothers in the correctional system: Separation from children and reunification after incarceration.* Unpublished doctoral dissertation, State University of New York at Albany.

Field, G. (1998). From the institution to the community. *Corrections Today, 60*(6): 94-97, 113.

Flanagan, L. W. (1995). Meeting the special needs of females in custody: Maryland's unique approach. *Federal Probation, 59*(2): 49-53.

Fletcher, B. R., Shaver, L. D., and Moon, D. G. (1993). *Women prisoners: A forgotten population.* Westport, CT: Praeger.

Gilfus, M. (1992). From victims to survivors to offenders: Women's routes of entry and immersion into street crime. *Women and Criminal Justice,* 4(1): 63-89.

Glaser, B. and Strauss, A. (1967). *The discovery of grounded theory.* Chicago: Aldine.

Greenfeld, L. A. and Snell, T. L. (1999). *Women offenders.* Washington, DC: U.S. Government Printing Office.

Hairston, C. E. (1991). Mothers in jail: Parent-child separation and jail visitation. *Affilia, 6*(2): 9-27.

Harlow, C. W. (1999). *Prior abuse reported by inmates and probationers.* Washington, DC: U.S. Government Printing Office.

Jurik, N. C. (1983). The economics of female recidivism. *Criminology, 21*: 603-622.

Koons, B. A., Burrow, J. D., Morash, M., and Bynum, T. (1997). Expert and offender perceptions of program elements linked to successful outcomes for incarcerated women. *Crime and Delinquency, 43*(4): 512-526.

Laird, J. (1989).Women and stories: Restorying women's self-constructions. In M. McGoldrick, C. M. Anderson, and F. Walsh (Eds.), *Women in families: A framework for family therapy* (pp. 427-449). New York: W. W. Norton.

Lambert, L. R. and Madden. P. G. (1976). The adult female offender: The road from institution to community life. *Canadian Journal of Criminology and Corrections, 18*: 319-331.

Lincoln, Y. S. and Guba, E. G. (1985). *Naturalistic inquiry.* Beverly Hills, CA: Sage.

Maruschak, L. M. (1999). *HIV in prisons 1997.* Washington, DC: U.S. Government Printing Office.

McCarthy, B. R. (1980). Inmate mothers: The problems of separation and reintegration. *Journal of Offender Counseling, Services and Rehabilitation, 4*(3): 199-212.

O'Brien, P. (2001). *Making it in the "free world": Women in transition from prison.* Albany, NY: State University of New York Press.

Phillips, L. and Votey, H. L. (1984). Black women, economic disadvantage and incentives to crime. *American Economic Association Papers and Proceedings, 74:* 293-297.

Pinderhughes, E. (1994). Empowerment as an intervention goal. In L. Gutiérrez and P. Nurius (Eds.), *Education and research for empowerment practice* (pp. 17-30). Seattle, WA: Center for Policy and Practice Research.

Pollock-Byrne, J. M. (1990). *Women, prison, and crime.* Belmont, CA: Brooks-Cole.

Qualitative Solutions and Research Ltd. (1995). *QSR NUD IST.* Thousand Oaks, CA: Scolari.

Reinharz, S. (1992). *Feminist methods in social research.* New York: Oxford University Press.

Richie, B. E. (1996). *Compelled to crime: The gender entrapment of battered black women.* New York: Routledge.

Robinson, E. B. (1971). *Women on parole: Reintegration of the female offender.* Unpublished doctoral dissertation, Ohio State University.

Rose, S. M. and Black, B. L. (1985). *Advocacy and empowerment: Mental health care in the community.* Boston: Routledge and Kegan Paul.

Schulke, B. B. (1993). *Women and criminal recidivism: A study of social constraints.* Unpublished doctoral dissertation, The George Washington University.

Severson, M. (1994). Adapting social work values to the corrections environment. *Social Work, 39*(4): 451-456.

Snell, T. L. (1994). *Women in prison: Survey of state prison inmates, 1991.* Washington, DC: U.S. Government Printing Office.

Sobel, S. B. (1982). Difficulties experienced by women in prison. *Psychology of Women Quarterly, 7*(2): 107-117.

Visher, C. (1983). Gender, police arrest decisions, and notions of chivalry. *Criminology, 21*(1): 22-23.

Watterson, K. (1996). *Women in prison.* Boston: Northeastern University Press.

Wilson, M. K. and Anderson, S. C. (1997). Empowering female offenders: Removing barriers to community-based practice. *Affilia, 12*(3): 342-358.

Young, D. S. (1996). Contributing factors to poor health among incarcerated women: A conceptual model. *Affilia, 11*(4): 40-46.

Zamble, E. and Quinsey, U. L. (1997). *The criminal recidivism process.* New York: Cambridge University Press.

Chapter 8

Supporting the Strengths of Older Women

Rosemary Chapin

Attainment of the status of "older woman" is a testament to the capacity to survive, to individual resiliency, to personal strengths. The woman who lives to be sixty-five or older has done so despite inattention to her health care needs as different from those of men, despite discrimination in employment and educational opportunities, and despite the intolerable rates of violence against women still present in our society. For women of color who face the interlocking forces of ageism, sexism, and racism, the feat is even more remarkable. How, then, do we chart an agenda for the new millennium that helps to build on the strengths and resources of older women so that the years after sixty-five, eighty-five, even 100 are good years to be alive? Poverty, loneliness, and inadequate health care should not be the reward for survival. Social workers engaged in interpersonal and policy practice can help to develop and implement this strengths-based agenda.

The resources of older women and the supports they need are most clearly understood in the context of their life cycle. The woman who has been poor all of her life, who was denied educational and employment opportunities, and who received inadequate health care will bring that legacy of poverty and discrimination to her later years. Similarly, strong ties to family, friends, church, and community created and nurtured over a lifetime may continue to provide needed support. Heterogeneity in life experiences will influence mightily the life of the older woman; age is not the great equalizer. Any agenda charted must take into account these individual differences.

Social work practice from the strengths perspective initially focuses on listening carefully to people's recounting of their strengths
as well as needs. Research and practice-focused articles can give
voice to women's stories. These stories can reflect the diversity of
older women's lives, including women of color, women who are lesbians or bisexual, women who are sixty-five as well as women who
are 113, and women with both adequate and inadequate incomes. The
paradigm of midlife decline must be replaced with one that creates
expectation of continued growth and development through all stages
of life. Focus on physiological measures where decline can be documented, and then extrapolation of that decline to all areas of life,
needs to be reframed. The stories of women who have lived life fully
until their deaths, despite physiological decline, need to be heard
again and again.

As we move from a paradigm of midlife decline and begin to explore the lives of women who found opportunities for continued
growth and experienced a positive quality of life in old age, increased
attention to the environmental and social supports that undergird
these lives can help us chart policy and practice strategies so that
more older women can have these opportunities. Economic security,
health care, and social interaction—including the chance to make
choices, to set individual goals, and to work to attain them—are fundamental to a positive quality of life in old age. Selected historical
and current issues for women in these arenas are explored in this
chapter. The examination of each arena is used to frame a strengths-
focused practice and policy agenda to enhance the quality of life for
older women.

ECONOMIC SECURITY

Women can expect to live a greater number of years than can men.
Greater longevity makes economic security in old age a key issue for
women. By age sixty-five, the gender ratio favoring women is clearly
reflected (Bern-Klug and Chapin, 1999). Currently, there are approximately 20 million American women and 14 million men sixty-five
and over (U.S. Bureau of the Census, 1999). The gender ratio increases until at age ninety-five, when American women outnumber
American men by a ratio of nearly four to one (Alliance for Aging
Research, 1998). By 2030, U.S. Census Bureau projections indicate

there will be approximately 39 million American women and 31 million American men sixty-five and over (U.S Bureau of the Census, 2000).

Over 3 million people sixty-five and over are below the poverty level. The majority of poor elders are women. For women over eighty-five, the risk of poverty increases to the point that 51 percent are in or near poverty (Devlin and Arye, 1997). The risk of poverty is even greater for older women of color. Conditions for older African-American women are particularly troubling. African-American women over seventy-five experience a poverty rate of 43 percent, higher not only than white women but also women from Spanish-speaking backgrounds (Devlin and Arye, 1997). Since our primary income support program for older adults, Old Age, Survivors, and Disability Insurance (OASDI), first established as part of the Social Security Act of 1935, is employment based, and has its roots in the male breadwinner family model, women have historically been disadvantaged by this system. Most women's retirement income is, in large part, determined by the wages earned during their own or their spouse's present or past employment. Since older women have experienced gender inequality in educational and employment opportunities over a lifetime, they often enter old age with a shorter, inconsistent, and lower paid employment history. Although the policy of providing coverage for a spouse in the amount of half of the worker's earnings does partially recognize the role of the spouse in supporting the worker, this amount varies not by the contribution of the spouse but by the earning of the worker. In addition, a couple in which both spouses work outside of the home may pay more taxes and receive lower yearly Social Security benefits at retirement than will a one-earner couple with the same income (Quadagno, 1999).

Since Social Security credits are not earned for the unpaid labor necessary to care for children and frail older adults, women, who have traditionally been expected to assume these duties, are disadvantaged initially by lack of payment for their work and later by lack of recognition of their contributions at the time of retirement. In fact, the time women spend as unpaid caregivers currently penalizes them under all three of the major ways that are open to supporting them in old age. They do not get credit in the public pension scheme, Social Security, because they are hindered from taking paid employment. Since they are not paid, the potential for private savings and investment for retirement is diminished. Private savings schemes, including Individual Development Accounts and Individual Retirement Accounts, are of little value to an unpaid caregiver unless a way is found to value caregiving through monetary contributions not directly made by the caregiver. Private pension funds have a role to play, but the danger is that if they are given a central role, they can lead to social exclusion, particularly of poor women caregivers. Women who do not do paid work outside of the home, women who move in and out of the workforce to accommodate caregiving responsibilities, and divorced women—in short, a great many women—are not adequately covered by a private pension system.

Even among working women, most working women still lack private pension coverage; working women under the age of thirty are the least likely to have pension coverage (Older Women's League, 1998). It is obvious that, given the role of caregiver and the insecurities of a postmodern working life, many women will be unable to secure adequate retirement income based on privately funded schemes. Women who have also experienced racial discrimination during their work life are even more likely to have inadequate retirement income.

An additional major public program, Supplemental Security Income (SSI), provides income to older people in poverty. This public assistance program is also administered by the Social Security Administration and benefits are not dependent on work history or marital status. Women comprise 74 percent of the beneficiaries for old age assistance under SSI (Taeuber and Allen, 1993). However, benefits are so low that beneficiaries are still in poverty, and poor women have low usage rates for SSI.

The demand side of the retirement income issue also merits further consideration. Women are now having fewer children, are experiencing more divorces, and many never marry. These different life patterns create differential learning experiences from those of women now in their seventies and eighties. Employment experience, particularly technological competence, can make it possible for women to work at older ages if given the chance. Policies that support retraining opportunities and investment in education for women and policies to help reduce age discrimination are also key to creating economic security for young and older women alike.

However, before effective policy to support women as workers and in retirement can be developed, much more research focused specifically on women's work and retirement patterns is needed. Aging research has been criticized for focusing primarily on women in explorations of family life and loss of spouse and primarily on men in retirement research. When women are included as subjects in research, the conceptual model used is one based on men's experiences (Quadagno, 1999). Lack of research means we do not yet have the information necessary to understand the needs of future women retirees, particularly women of the baby boom era who will soon become part of the elder boom.

Beyond the dimensions of economic security discussed thus far, ways of reframing our understanding of the aging of the baby boomers has important implications for considering the economic security of older women. For example, one partial explanation for the economic expansion underway as we enter the twenty-first century surely must be the fact that men and women of the baby boom generation (the 76 million Americans born between 1946 and 1964) are now in their most economically productive years. Women of that era are better educated and much more likely to be employed than any previous generation of American women. The part played by American women in fueling growth in economic productivity needs far greater attention. By concentrating on the aging of the baby boomers and framing the process as a catastrophic problem especially for older women, again opportunities to recognize and support strengths are overlooked. Work in the information age is such that many employment opportunities for older adults could be created given policies and programs that support such development. Budget surpluses accumulating during this time of unparalleled economic productivity should logically be considered resources available to finance reforms to Social Security and Medicare so that they more equitably support the unique needs of older women.

Women are the primary recipients of both Social Security and Supplemental Security Income. When reform or expansion of these programs is considered, it must be remembered that the brunt of any reform will fall on older women. Needed policy reforms are discussed in detail in the Contemporary Policy Issues segment of this chapter.

HEALTH CARE

Historically, women's health has been synonymous with reproductive health. Research on women's health, as distinct from men's health in other arenas, has been given inadequate attention. Although women have a longer life expectancy than men, men can expect more years with no disabling conditions (Quadagno, 1999). Poorer health and higher levels of disability for women than men are consistently reported in studies of comparative health status (George, 1996). Although a variety of factors, including more contact with health providers and thus more likelihood of women reporting ailments, may contribute to this disparity, adequate home and community-based long-term care services are crucial for older women with disabilities. Since women who do marry typically outlive their spouses, older women are more likely to live alone, with the accompanying complexity of meeting health care needs.

Lifestyle differences between women now seventy-five and over and younger women may increase disability rates in future cohorts of older women. Increased rates of smoking, alcoholism, and obesity among younger women will exacerbate this problem. Health promotion initiatives have been designed to help women make lifestyle changes. However, unless women can actually assume control of their health care, demand more research focused on women, and press for increased access to health care for women at all stages of life, disability rates for older women are likely to remain high.

Poorer socioeconomic status is also a risk factor for poorer health at all ages, for reasons that are incompletely understood but are at least partly due to environmental factors, behavior, and access to health care services. Older women (13 percent) are more likely to live in poverty than older men (7 percent). Minority elders of both genders are more likely to live in poverty than older whites. Nationally, more than one in four black and Hispanic women live in poverty compared to one in ten white women and one in twenty white men.

Fair to poor health is also associated with minority racial status, widowhood, lower levels of education, retirement, and lower household income. Seniors at highest risk of poor health are also likely to be those who are poorer, less educated, unmarried, and living in a rural area, placing them at higher risk of nursing facility admission and needing to reduce their assets to be financially eligible for Medicaid. Among current boomers, higher divorce rates, larger numbers of never-married people, and smaller families can also be expected to weaken informal support systems and provide fewer informal caregivers.

Health care costs impact women of color and poor elders disproportionately. In 1994 through 1996, 20 percent of whites and 39 percent of African Americans over eighty-five had no private or supplemental insurance beyond Medicare (U.S. Department of Health and Human Services, 2000). In 1993, 36 percent of all elderly persons admitted to nursing facilities incurred catastrophic financial expenses, defined as expenditures equal to or greater than 40 percent of income and non-housing assets (National Academy on Aging, 1997).

Researchers are currently trying to determine whether aging boomers can be expected to be healthier than their parents and grandparents. The direction of disability trends is a matter of debate (Manton, Corder, and Stallard, 1997). Medical breakthroughs may revolutionize health care for older adults. But even if fewer people are disabled, the greater number of elders by itself will put a severe strain on the health and long-term care systems. Indeed, if more seniors are healthy and live to experience the functional declines of very old age, they will still need significant amounts of personal care. Even experts who predict declining disability rates predict that demand for long-term care will increase rapidly, even though the types and amounts may be different than today (Manton and Stallard, 1996).

Long-term care will also be affected by changes elsewhere in the health care system. Current trends include shorter hospital stays, the shift from institutional to community settings (for both acute and long-term care), and steep increases in health costs. The Medicare program will be in economic jeopardy, and Medicaid reform of some type also seems likely.

The total cost of nursing facility and home health care in 1995 was estimated at $106.5 billion. Of this amount, $34.6 billion, or about one-third, was paid out of pocket (National Academy on Aging, 1997). Long-term care costs impose a heavy burden on older women, who often rapidly exhaust their savings. The United States does not have a program that provides universal coverage for long-term care expenses. Contrary to popular opinion, Medicare covers only a small part of long-term care, and then only for "skilled" services (i.e., ones involving a licensed medical professional, such as a nurse, physical therapist, etc.). In 1996, less than 15 percent of total Medicare expenditures went for either nursing facilities or home health care. Only 12 percent of all nursing facility costs are paid by Medicare (Health Care Financing Administration, 1999). Private insurance also plays a minor role—only about 6 percent of expenditures for nursing facility and home- and community-based services are paid by private insurance.

The risk of nursing facility admission rises with age, from about 1 percent between ages sixty-five and seventy-four, to about 5 percent between ages seventy-five and eighty-four, to nearly 20 percent at eighty-five and over (Kramaroe, Lentzner, Rooks, Weeks, and Saydah, 1999). Nationally, over half of all older residents of nursing facilities are eighty-five and over, three-quarters of whom are female. Unmarried persons have a higher risk of nursing facility admission than married persons. Nearly two-thirds of all current nursing facility residents are widowed. Living alone increases the risk of nursing facility admission. Cultural factors impact living arrangements. White, non-Hispanic women seventy-five and over are 1.2 times as likely as black women and 1.7 times as likely as Hispanic women to live alone, while black and Hispanic women are more likely to live with other relatives (U.S. Department of Health and Human Services, 2000).

Medicare, a national health insurance program for all people sixty-five or older who are eligible for Social Security and certain categories of younger disabled people, was enacted in 1965. Medicare focuses primarily on acute care and provides little coverage for long-term care. Medicare Part A is hospital insurance paid through payroll taxes. Medicare Part B is an optional program that requires beneficiaries to pay a premium. Part B covers a portion of the costs of physician's office visits. Because so many health care expenses are not covered by Medicare, many older people pay privately for yet another policy, a Medigap policy. It is not surprising to find that poor women and particularly poor women of color are less likely to have this coverage and therefore face additional barriers to access to medical care. Medicare has provided much-needed access to health care for many older adults. However, the costs of copays, deductibles, and items not covered by Medicare, such as prescription drugs and most long-term care, mean that most older women pay a high proportion of their income for health care, and those costs are rising. It has been estimated that Medicare pays for only 40 percent of the total health care costs of people sixty-five and over.

The Medicare Trust fund is currently projected to run out of money in 2023. Options for containing the costs of Medicare generally fall into one of three categories: limiting services, raising the age of eligibility, and shifting costs onto the elderly by increasing out-of-pocket costs (Quadagno, 1999). All of these options will disproportionately affect older women because of their relatively lower income in old age. Unlike Social Security, where costs per beneficiary are determined by law and can be known, Medicare costs in large part are determined by the type and amount of health care received by beneficiaries and the costs of providing it (Binstock, 1999). Consequently, between 2010, when the first of the baby boomers, the cohort of 76 million persons born between 1946 and 1964, begins turning sixty-five, and 2030, when all baby boomers will be sixty-five or over, Medicare costs as a percentage of gross domestic product (GDP) are projected to rise by 73 percent (Binstock, 1999). Before that time, methods of controlling health care costs as well as the remedies outlined above will need serious national attention. In addition, the lack of coverage for prescription drugs and long-term care under Medicare are glaring omissions that put older women at great risk of impoverishment, inadequate care, and institutionalization. Given current policies, impoverished older women with long-term care needs may have to enter nursing facilities where Medicaid will cover costs for care including prescription drugs.

In the area of health and mental health, major programs are biased in not meeting the different needs of women. For example, Medicare policy contains a gender bias. Medicare provides coverage for acute illness and rehabilitation. However, chronic illness necessitating long-term care is not covered. Women disproportionately experience chronic illness and find themselves without protection from the high costs of long-term care. This bias must be corrected if women are to have the opportunity to live out their lives without becoming destitute and thereby qualifying for Medicaid benefits.

Medicaid, a program of health insurance for the poor, was enacted in 1965. It is financed jointly by federal and state dollars. Medicaid pays more than half of nursing home costs, nationally. However, a person must be impoverished in order to receive this benefit. Although Medicaid waivers have made home- and community-based services available for some older adults, the home- and community-based services are not an entitlement and a number of states have long waiting lists. As discussed in the following section, emphasis on home- and community-based services is both a blessing and a dilemma for women.

A 1997 study done by the National Alliance for Caregiving found that most of the care recipients are women, most of the caregivers are women, and that the average age of the care recipient is seventy-seven years (1997). Policies that encourage home- and community-based care are often structured around informal family care. Family typically means women, and the assumption is that women will shoulder the burden of providing care for frail elders without financial or community support. Until adequate means are found to redress this inequity, women will continue to face economic and health jeopardy in old age as a consequence of being caregivers.

The 1975 amendments to the Community Mental Health Act, in combination with the Medicare provisions of the Social Security Amendments of 1965, changed the availability of mental health services to older adults (Tice and Perkins, 1996). Medicare provided the financial vehicle for at least limited access to mental health services for this population. Funding through the Older Americans Act of 1965 and services provided through some community mental health centers and senior centers also helped to increase availability. However, a combination of reluctance on the part of many community mental health centers to do outreach; cultural barriers; overriding needs for basic resources such as clothes, food, and shelter; and elders' negative stereotypes about receiving mental health services has resulted in inadequate access to mental health services for many older women.

Finally, any discussion of health care and older women must address end-of-life planning so that older women can live out their lives, free of unnecessary pain. The majority of older women in the United States die outside of the home, in nursing homes or hospitals (Alliance for Aging Research, 1998). If elders are to make informed decisions about when to shift from life prolonging care to palliative care, more research needs to be done on the impact of chronic disease and disability on older women at the very end of life. Preliminary studies have found that older women are at heightened risk for the undertreatment of pain (Ahronheim, 1997). Older women need to be supported in reclaiming power over life's end so that humane and compassionate end-of-life care is provided.

SOCIAL INTERACTION

Positive social interaction is a key element of successful aging. Social isolation is a risk factor for deteriorating health status and increases the chance of institutionalization for older women. Social interaction, including the chance to make choices, to set individual goals, and to work to attain them, are integral to a positive quality of life. Historically, the strengths and capacities of women to control their own lives have not been valued. However, in old age, many women are faced with the necessity of now assuming control. Alternatively, they can again cede control to health professionals or family who may or may not be guided by the older person's best interests, and certainly cannot know the older woman's hopes and desires as well as she herself does. Support for assumption of this new role must be strong if older adults are to gain confidence in their capacities for self-determination. At the same time, life conditions may necessitate more emphasis on interdependence. Capacity for self-determination is not antithetical to interdependence. In all relationships there is room for self-determination.

Social exchange theorists argue that decrease in social interaction for older adults is the result of lessening economic, political, and social power, thus making interaction less rewarding (Bernheim, Shleifer, and Summers, 1985; Bould, Sanborn, and Reif, 1989; Dowd, 1980). These theorists suggest that aging can be viewed as an exchange. Social interaction is maintained because it is found to be rewarding. Economic, psychological, and employment issues in aging are linked to loss of social interaction because as social resources are lost, so is the capacity to engage in mutually rewarding social interactions. Viewed from this perspective, the loneliness and social isolation of older adults cannot be adequately addressed unless ways are found to overcome barriers to access social resources such as economic security, adequate transportation, and meaningful roles that allow for continuing contribution to the community.

In addition to loss of social resources as an inhibitor of social interaction, many women of all ages have absorbed the widespread cultural belief that women are less valuable than men and that older people are less valuable than the young. These cultural biases create yet more impediments to positive social interaction for older women.

The Older Americans Act (OAA), passed in 1965, contains a number of provisions designed to promote social interaction and enhance independent living. The OAA provides funding for senior centers, meal programs, personal care and nursing services, day care, and chore services. There has never been sufficient funding to fully implement the OAA, and so many older women who need these services have not been able to obtain them. Since state and local money are often additional sources of public funding for these services, availability of services varies widely from state to state and community to community.

Communities are now beginning to direct attention to creating "age sensitive community infrastructures" in preparation for the coming elder boom. For example, the need for universal housing codes that enhance accessibility in residential construction is receiving greater support in many communities. State transportation departments are beginning to test visibility of road sign paint with sixty-five-year-old drivers rather than twenty-five-year-old males. It is clear that support for older people's strengths will be an important component of planning for the increasing number of older men and women in the future, so that they can remain an active and contributing part of the community.

Strategies that enhance social interaction and reduce social isolation must be promoted. The most damaging and incorrect strategy for charting our future agenda is to build on intergenerational conflict. It is a false dichotomy. If we are lucky, all of us, including the young, will become old someday. Children are not poor because older adults receive Social Security. Poor children disproportionately live in single-parent homes headed by women. These women receive lower wages than do men. These lower wages result in poverty for their young family and will contribute to inadequate income in old age because they inhibit savings and pension fund contributions.

Social programs that helped to support low-income families, such as AFDC, have been dismantled. These programs were not dismantled so that Social Security could be funded. Rather, the push to eliminate the safety net for young families was fueled by many of the same forces that press to dismantle the Social Security Retirement Fund. What is needed is even greater support for programs, such as Foster Grandparents and intergenerational school programs, that build on the natural interdependence of generations. Young and old people need to understand that any practice or policy that implies people are less valuable because they are old is antithetical to social justice. Just as we have come to know that discrimination based on skin color, gender, or sexual orientation is wrong, we must now scrutinize any implication that devaluing of old people is acceptable, unmask incorrect assumptions, and point out the injustice. Lack of opportunities to develop empathy with the very old and our own fear of aging must not result in inattention to the needs and strengths of older women. Specific practice and policy strategies, as outlined in the following section, merit careful consideration as we attempt to strengthen supports for older women.

CONTEMPORARY PRACTICE ISSUES

Social workers who practice with older adults will typically be working with older women. Approximately 75 percent of people age seventy-five and older are women. They often have outlived their support system. These women today represent a diverse background. They may be facing life as a widow who is for the first time being called on to handle life tasks such as financial management and transportation. Conversely, they may be women, married or single, who have experienced a long work life and who now have survived their siblings and friends. They also may be women who have contended with inaccurate stereotypes based on their sexual orientation. Stereotypes of older lesbian women as alone and lonely have been researched and found to be inaccurate (Berger and Kelly, 1986). Older lesbian women often have a lifetime of strong supports from friends. Practitioners must recognize and support the diversity older women bring to the helping process.

The historic hesitancy of practitioners to embrace therapeutic work with older people was bolstered by the belief that older people were unwilling to change, that they were not intellectually or emotionally able to take part in a therapeutic process, and that time was better spent with younger people who could enjoy the benefits of the change for a longer period. This attitude is also fostered by the words used to describe treatment of older adults. For example, the term "senescence" is still being used in some social work texts to encompass mental health issues of older adults, and the word "senescence," we are told, is interchangeable with the term "late life" (Farkas, 1999, p. 174). Senescence has obvious negative connotations and so before practitioners even begin to absorb specific content, all of late life has been cast in a negative light. As Tice and Perkins point out, "Older adults are not victims of senescence but survivors of life" (1996, p. 5). It is hoped that negative attitudes will lessen as more and more people are living to old age, are healthier, have more money, and as therapists experience firsthand the dramatic changes older people can and do make.

In order to build on strengths of older women, social workers must begin by examining their own attitudes about aging. A simple exercise can help practitioners begin this process. I ask practitioners to imagine they are seventy-five and write a life reminiscence that includes a description of their own lives at seventy-five. If the description of themselves at seventy-five consists of a list of problems, life in an institution, and lots of rocking, resting, and ruminating over their past lives, I know they have absorbed the stereotypes rampant in our society today. Most troubling, some practitioners portray themselves at seventy-five as so useless to society that they should commit suicide because they have already used up more than their share of the earth's resources. They obviously have absorbed the dominant paradigm, that old people are only problems or takers rather than contributors.

However, this exercise also provides a wonderful starting place to help practitioners begin to reframe the possibilities and potential for hopeful and joyful living at every stage of life. Having older adults who continue to live life joyfully and fully at seventy-five, eighty-five and even ninety-five take an active part in educating practitioners is key to opening minds to a new vision of aging. The older adults' stories of how they have faced chronic illness and disabilities without letting those conditions define them, and most important, discussion of their current hopes, dreams, and passions, support this new vision for practitioners. Educational materials designed to help social service professionals identify and build on strengths of older adults can also help build skills necessary to effective practice with older women (Cox and Parson, 1994; Fast and Chapin, 1996; Fast and Chapin, 1997; Fast and Chapin, 2000; Tice and Perkins, 1996).

In addition to ambivalence on the part of practitioners, there are many older adults and families who may be reluctant to seek help because they think depression, dementia, and loss of functioning are normal adjuncts to aging and not amenable to change. When they do seek help, most often older adults want help with specific needs such as loss of income due to death of spouse, help with activities of daily living, or issues of grief and depression. Chronic health problems disproportionately impact older women. When health issues become overwhelming, it is the physician who is often sought out as the initial contact. It is important to work to educate physicians and other members of the health care team to recognize and build on strengths rather than focusing solely on issues of problems and compliance.

Practice with older women does raise some very distinct challenges. First of all, health problems do not always but often increase with age. Therefore, the biopsychosocial perspective must be carefully employed. A comprehensive medical exam with careful attention to physiological conditions and drug interaction or reactions that may be contributing to emotional and psychological issues is basic to effective practice. Lifestyle issues leading to lack of exercise and hydration problems must be considered. This information should form the cornerstone of the assessment process with older women. The assessment of older women needs to include careful attention to needs and strengths of the older woman in the areas of physical health and lifestyle. The role of spirituality in her life should be explored. Her methods of coping with life's challenges in the past should be highlighted and acknowledged. The sheer volume of experience that a person who is sixty-five, seventy-five, or eighty-five brings can surely provide ample stories of successful coping.

Implementation of the strengths model of social work practice begins by learning how people have learned to survive and perhaps even thrive despite difficult circumstances (Fast and Chapin, 2000). Listening carefully to the stories women tell about themselves, and being particularly attuned to how stories shape women's lives rather than merely reflect it, allows the practitioner to help women explore alternative meanings of their stories and to emphasize capacities and strengths. This approach is particularly suited to work with older women, survivors all. This emphasis on exploring strengths in the context of unique life experiences is a focus that is appropriate across ethnic, cultural, and income groups. Social workers can listen to narratives and help older women to reframe their stories so that structural as well as personal issues are examined, focusing not only on decline but also on past successes that can build a platform for future goal setting. The task is to form a partnership with the older woman so that, in collaboration, individual and communal resources are found to meet their needs. The client is supported in assuming an active role in determining the course of the helping encounter, recognizing goals as attainable, and learning to find and secure needed resources.

The importance of assessing people in relation to their environment is particularly valuable when working with older women. Practitioners see older women in dual roles, that of the customer or patient and that of the caregiver for an older person. In all relationships, there is room for self-determination, but oppressive social conditions may have obscured the possibility of self-determination for the older woman. When assessing older women, it is important to be alert to dementia, depression, and thoughts of suicide and to explore whether depression due to oppressive environmental conditions has been mislabeled as dementia. When working with caregivers, burnout and violence may be issues. Older women with whom social workers practice may have experienced a series of losses of loved ones, often in a short time period. The changes that have occurred in their lives as a result of those deaths must to be explored. Besides changes in caregiving and companionship, older women may have suffered a drastic loss in income with the death of their spouse. Inadequate income is an antecedent of social stress that can lead to depression and anxiety. Loss, change, and the meaning of the changes from the point of view of the older woman are central to the use of a strengths perspective with older women.

Discussion of change should include a focus on opportunities to build new supports and explore new ways of living. Emphasis on the opportunities inherent in change should be stressed. Older women have faced a multitude of changes by the time they reach age sixty-five. How they coped in the past can provide clues to the strengths they have traditionally used. Hispanic, African-American, and Asian women have experienced differential treatment all through their work histories and thus arrive at retirement with very different skill sets. Strategies to deal with racism that these women developed early in life may help them cope more effectively with age-based discrimination.

The practitioner's affirmation of possibilities for living joyfully and fully is critical. The belief that old age is a time of decay and loss with little possibility of joy and fulfillment is one that has traditionally underpinned the treatment of older adults (Chapin, 1999). Focusing on strengths, possibilities, hopes, and dreams, rather than on loss, will provide support for the older person's own capacities to cope. It is the strengths and resources of individuals and their environment that are the building blocks for meeting life's challenges at each stage of life. These women may need help to focus on their strengths and capacity for self-determination as they look for ways to meet their needs in areas including health and housing. They may also need help in navigating the difficult emotional and legal issues surrounding end-of-life decision making.

Although older adults are increasingly seeking out therapeutic services through mental health centers, case management through public agencies and managed care organizations is a more common form of social work service to the older adult. Providing information, referral, and brokering services are central tasks of case managers. Case managers have the opportunity to be most effective when they support the strengths of older adults. Case managers often have access to information that older adults lack. For example, finding ways to help older women access the information necessary to accurately assess Medicare managed-care options is essential. The expansion of choice and the concomitant reduction of service makes informed choice that much more crucial.

In working with older women, their contributions as caregivers in terms of time, money, and emotional energy should be recognized. It is particularly important, if people are to have the choice of remaining in the community and not entering nursing facilities, that older adults as caregivers be supported. Older women may need support as they struggle to find the balance between taking care of others and paying adequate attention to their own aspirations.

Helping older women develop and maintain supportive relationships is key to successful aging. Upcoming generations of older women who were born during the baby boom era are more likely to be childless or single when they retire. Also, the delay in childbirth for many women means their children are less likely to be in positions where they can be depended on during crises or old age. Longer life and fewer children point to the need to develop more intergenerational relationships that extend beyond the nuclear family. More careful study of the ways in which older lesbian women have built strong informal support systems, not based on the traditional nuclear family model, may yield important insights into how such relationships may be fostered (Berger and Kelly, 1986).

Strengths and independence should not be considered synonymous. Many of women's strengths lie in the area of relationship building and resource acquisition that undergird systems of interdependence. Indeed, older women's historic support of their children and grandchildren in coping with the challenges of child rearing and childhood illnesses is recognized. Reciprocity is obvious. These systems of interdependence can be the source of support during episodic periods of need for increased care common to many chronic illnesses.

Discussion of this interdependence, particularly the contributions that older adults can and often do make, helps to reframe relationships so that their reciprocal nature is emphasized. For example, older women are the repositories of rich historical memories of their families and their communities. Local area agencies on aging can help elders find intergenerational programs where young and old work together to build historical records of their communities.

Many older women are in excellent positions to make major contributions to their families because ability to type was considered a basic survival skill for women who were young adults during World War II. Work as a secretary was one of the limited number of employment possibilities open to women without access to a college education. Renaming this talent "keyboarding skills" and reframing the ability as opening the door to the Internet, e-mail, online shopping, and the latest medical information can create many new opportunities for intergenerational reciprocity and communication. Spending time looking up needed information on the Web is a valuable contribution even frail, homebound older women may provide to their children and grandchildren. Many local senior centers now offer courses designed to help older adults build computer skills. These centers can often put social workers in touch with businesses or programs that can help low-income seniors acquire needed computer equipment. Computer abilities can either be another way that the old are differentiated and segregated or they can be an avenue for building intergenerational communication and reciprocity. Many older women have a head start because they already have "keyboarding skills." Practitioners should make sure that these abilities are not devalued or overlooked, and that the potential for lifelong learning is supported.

Although recognition of the strengths and contributions of older adults is building in the professional literature, once people begin to experience disability as well as old age, stigma and loss of expectation of capacity for self-determination again becomes widespread. Disabilities such as loss of hearing and blindness lead to institutionalization at far greater rates for older adults than for younger people. Older women who also have serious disabilities are at particular risk, and a strengths approach that supports capacity to make choices is crucial. Social workers should carefully assess the extent to which individuals can still be involved in decision making about their own lives and support those capacities. They should also advocate for the older adult with other members of the professional team caring for the older adult, if the older adult's capacities are being ignored. The social worker's support in accessing adequate spiritual and legal guidance, as well as hospice care when necessary, can help the older woman retain dignity and choice until the end of life.

Community practice is key to developing preventive programs that help older adults identify the strengths and resources necessary for a fulfilling late life. Whether older women are black, Hispanic, Native American, white, or Asian, communities will need social workers who are sensitive to the ethnicity of their older clients. Programs such as those funded under the Older Americans Act that develop at the local level using local providers will be important in tailoring service to community. New community structures, both formal and informal, need to be developed. Access for people with disabilities is an area where alliances between the young disabled community and older adults have been forged and need to be nurtured. Disabilities are still allowed to define people age sixty-five and over in ways that younger people with disabilities no longer tolerate. The proposition that loss of sight or hearing or need for a wheelchair justifies institutionalization is rejected by the younger disabled community. The older disabled community, disproportionately women, has not sufficiently mobilized. Surely support of attempts to do this important grassroots work should be high on the social work agenda.

CONTEMPORARY POLICY ISSUES

The growing numbers of older women in our society underscore the importance of reexamination of policies that influence their capacity to age successfully. As discussed previously, women with low incomes and women of color are at particular risk. It is projected that minority elders will represent 25 percent of the elderly population in 2030, up from 15 percent in 1998 (AARP, 1999). Public policy must refocus programs to include minority elders. Three policy areas are especially germane to the lives of older women. They are: economic security; health, including mental health and long-term care; and support for productive aging.

Given the heterogeneity of the life experiences of younger women, the policy issues related to economic security in old age must begin with a focus on diverse needs and strengths. Savings, continuing to work either full- or part-time, and pensions, both public and private, are the major sources of income for older women. Policies and programs that encourage all women to become educated about investing and saving are crucial. Programs such as Individual Development Accounts, which provide matching dollars for low-income women who are able to save, represent an innovative approach to building economic security for women (Boshara, Scanlon, and Page-Adams, 1998).

Public and private pensions also provide economic security for older women. Women who have been married to men receiving pensions will be best served by policies that assure them the right to share in the decision of whether they will be able to continue to receive the pension when they become widows. Richardson (1999) also indicates the need to change pension policies that pay women lower benefits or require them to pay more into the system because they often live longer.

Portability of pensions is a key policy issue for working women. Job changes due to changes in caregiving duties, corporate downsizing, and increasing mobility of the workforce result in women being disproportionately disadvantaged by nonportable private pension systems. In fact, social insurance programs undergirded by the principles of risk pooling and portability, particularly if they are modernized to minimize exclusions and to maximize the sense of individual ownership, seem even better suited to today's labor market than when such programs were first introduced in Europe (Walker, 1999). Our Old-Age, Survivors, and Disability Insurance, better known as Social Security, is such a program.

It is important also to consider the demand side of the pension equation. More support for part-time work, less age discrimination in the labor market, and encouraging employers to recruit and retrain older women all will help women who wish to remain employed to do so. Policies that support lifelong educational programs as well as remedial programs for older workers who need to catch up with new technology are important. Programs to support the health of workers and to help prevent disability will make it possible for older women to remain in the workforce.

Conversely, to raise the age of eligibility for pensions without dealing with age discrimination in the workplace is to exclude older workers, and consign them to low incomes and eventually reduced pensions. Research needs to focus on employment policies that support older women if they wish to remain in the workforce. For example, elder care policies that establish on-site care for older disabled family members and provide information and referral for needs related to caregiving for elders, have begun to be developed in some corporations. Evaluations of their efficacy need to be completed and disseminated.

As Richardson (1999) points out, for retired women to ever achieve parity with retired men, policies need to be crafted that will help eradicate discriminatory and unjust gender and ethnic differences in wages and promote comparable wages for women who work in female-dominated professions. It is also necessary to devise policies that will at least allow women caregivers to receive Social Security retirement credits for performing caregiving duties. Social Security rules that penalize married working women are also in need of reform.

Improving the economic status of very low-income older women may best be achieved by reform of the Supplemental Security Income program, a public assistance program administered by the Social Security Administration (Browne, 1998). This programs targets older people in poverty, and benefits are not dependent on work history or marital status. Raising SSI benefits to 110 percent of poverty and lowering the age of benefit eligibility from 65 to 62 would help a great many older women escape poverty. However, poor women have low usage rates for SSI. It is incumbent on social workers to make sure older women know about this resource and can get help in filling out the complicated application form. Beyond expanding actual benefits, the barriers to accessing benefits under the current policy, such as complicated forms and inadequate staffing, need to be addressed.

Low-income older women who did not work forty quarters and thus do not qualify for Social Security and Medicare also are at risk in meeting their health care needs. When health care needs develop, they often become dependent upon Medicaid, a program jointly funded by federal and state taxes available only if the older woman is impoverished. Both Medicare and Medicaid have been a boon to older women and have created health care access for many people who would have had no other means to pay for needed care. However, throughout the life span, as discussed in the Health Care section of this chapter, women experience needless dependency and loss of power to self-determine because current policies and programs, particularly Medicare, do not provide services and funding for a range of medical and nonmedical services necessary for people with chronic health problems. Financing must be available for more than medical and acute care. Different sources of payment for long-term care must be coordinated, and families who provide long-term care need emotional and financial support. The bias in funding that results in a disproportionately large share of public funds being spent to support nursing-facility rather than community-based care needs to be corrected. Coverage of prescription drugs and controlling of health care costs via a national health program that also includes long-term care benefits are needed in order to adequately address women's health care needs. Medicare reform efforts should include these elements.

How do we develop mental health and social services policies to support older adults? Nationally, many community mental health centers have not offered specialized services for older adults and have not invested resources in services to older adults proportional to their numbers in the community (Tice and Perkins, 1996). This imbalance must be corrected. The Older Americans Act created a national network made up of federal, state, and local agencies to plan, organize, and provide services to older adults. These functions are more important than ever as we prepare for the coming elder boom. Increased funding and policies that clearly focus on outcomes, particularly inclusion of minority elders, are needed to implement more fully the intent of this legislation. This network, with its emphasis on home- and community-based services and flexibility to address local needs could potentially provide leadership in ameliorating housing, health, and social interaction concerns of older women.

Pensions, retirement, and health and social service policies must be considered jointly to promote productive aging. As Quinn states, social policies are typically written in gender-neutral language, but their effects are very different for women than men (1996). Her analysis of the impact of the Community Mental Health Center Act of 1963, designed to support deinstitutionalization and foster community treatment, points out the tremendous cost to women as unpaid caregivers when institutions were closed and people were returned to communities unprepared to care for them. Although the stated goal of initiatives to keep people in the community is not also to keep women in precarious financial positions, too often that is the outcome. Informal care is essential for mental health and long-term care for older adults in the community. If this care is to continue, policies must begin to take into account the gendered effects of caregiving, particularly as it relates to capacity for women to have adequate income in old age. Policies must be analyzed from the standpoint of how outcome differs for women and men. Policies should no longer be built on the assumption that women are available, able, and willing to provide unpaid care. Caregiving is not only a private issue; as Hooyman and Gonyea (1999) assert, it should be a public policy issue as well. Adequate public funding for long-term care is long overdue, and caregiving must be valued and compensated. Men must share responsibility for caregiving, and women should have the right to choose whether they will do the caregiving. Any caregiver benefits that are developed should be available regardless of gender. The value of a caregiver's allowance and the time spent caregiving for dependents should be counted in an individual's work history in determining eligibility and amount of Social Security benefits. Alternatively, the child tax credit could be expanded as a refundable Care Credit for all caregivers, regardless of the age of the person with disabilities receiving sustained care. In pushing caregiving into the community and emphasizing family, the clear message is that it is women who will be doing more unpaid caregiving whether as volunteers or family. Policies should be evaluated in terms of their impact on women, as well as on other family members.

We are entering a unique time of history when four and five generations of many families will be alive at the same time. Policies need to ensure that the generations continue to live in harmony. Exaggerating the economic impact of population aging risks threatening the intergenerational social contract. The fundamental importance of intergenerational solidarity needs to be underscored in policy decisions. The moral obligation of one generation to another can be combined with enlightened self-interest in crafting viable policies. Investing in intergenerational approaches, such as Foster Grandparents, where the contributions of elders are clear, can help avoid conflict and build on the older woman's considerable strength in fostering alliances between generations. Churches, Boy Scouts and Girl Scouts, and other voluntary organizations have developed policies and programs to build intergenerational cooperation, and such efforts should be encouraged and expanded.

If our society is to forge new policies that support successful aging for older women, it is important to ask, "What would policies look like that are more responsive to the needs of older women?" Beginning answers to that question have been provided in this article. However, in order to craft fuller answers, efforts first to engage women across economic and racial groups in defining common interests must be initiated and supported. For example, information on Social Security reform that focuses on potential common interests needs to be widely disseminated and discussed. Ways of mobilizing older women to support needed policy change must be developed. Groups such as the Older Women's League are working to forge these coalitions. The new century will provide ample opportunity for social workers educated to be effective policy practitioners to join with older women to create effective policy.

Analysis of needed policy initiatives to support the strengths of older women is at best an imprecise undertaking. No one has a crystal ball. However, a vision of the future is fundamental to policy development. The challenge is to develop policies that are sufficiently flexible so that "surprise events," such as medical breakthroughs and wide economic fluctuations, can be accommodated. Policies and programs, particularly entitlement programs, must be crafted that are not so expensive or rigid that little room is left for new opportunities or innovation. Contrary to the widely publicized misperception that the coming elder boom will surely have disastrous consequences, if moderate economic growth can be sustained, financial support for the coming elder boom is clearly within our capacity as a society (Friedland and Summer, 1999).

CONCLUSION

A model for growing old that focuses on strengths as well as needs can be the basis for effective practice and planning with young and older women alike and can help them gain a sense of their ability to influence their lives and a sense of empowerment. A worldview that questions existing social policies and considers issues from a trans-generational perspective can aid in conceiving policies and developing best practice strategies that support the strengths of women. All women need a view of possibilities in old age that energizes our life's journey until its end.

REFERENCES

AARP (1999). *A profile of older Americans.* Washington, DC: Author.

Ahronheim, J. (1997). End-of-life issues for very elderly women: Incurable and terminal illness, *Journal of the American Medical Women's Association, 52*(3): 147-151.

Alliance for Aging Research (1998). *One final gift: Humanizing the end of life for women in America.* Washington, DC: Author.

Berger, R. and Kelly, J. (1986). Working with homosexuals of the older population. *Social Casework, 67*(4): 203-210.

Bernheim, B. D., Shleifer, A., and Summers, L. H. (1985). The strategic bequest motive. *Journal of Political Economy, 93:* 1045-1076.

Bern-Klug, M. and Chapin, R. (1999). The changing demography of death: Implications for human service workers. In B. deVries (Ed.), *End-of-life issues: Interdisciplinary and multidimensional perspectives* (pp. 265-280). New York: Springer.

Binstock, R. (1999). Challenges to United States policies on aging in the new millennium. *Hallym International Journal on Aging, 1*(1): 3-13.

Boshara, R., Scanlon, E., and Page-Adams, D. (1998). *Building assets for stronger families, better neighborhoods and realizing the American dream.* Washington, DC: Corporation for Enterprise Development.

Bould, S., Sanborn, B., and Reif, L. (1989). *Eighty-five plus: The oldest old.* Belmont, CA: Wadsworth.

Browne, C. (1998). *Women, feminism, and aging.* New York: Springer.

Chapin, R. (1999). It is expected by the year 2000: Using lessons from the past to plan for the elder boom. *Journal of Gerontological Social Work, 32*(2): 21-40.

Cox, E. and Parson, R. (1994). *Empowerment-oriented social work practice with the elderly.* Monterey, CA: Brooks/Cole.

Devlin, S. and Arye, L. (1997). The Social Security debate: A financial crisis or a new retirement paradigm? *Generations, 21*(2): 27-33.

Dowd, J. (1980). Aging as exchange: A preface to theory. In J. Quadagno (Ed.), *Aging, the individual and society* (pp. 103-121). New York: St. Martin's Press.

Farkas, K. (1999). Senescence. In F. Turner (Ed.), *Adult psychopathology: A social work perspective* (pp. 174-193). New York: The Free Press.

Fast, B. and Chapin, R. (1996). The strengths model in long-term care: Linking cost containment and consumer empowerment. *Journal of Case Management, 5*(2): 51-57.

Fast, B. and Chapin, R. (1997). The strengths model with older adults: Critical practice components. In D. Saleebey (Ed.), *The strengths perspective in social work practice* (pp. 115-130). New York: Longman.

Fast, B. and Chapin, R. (2000). *Strengths-based case management for older adults.* Baltimore: Health Professions Press.

Friedland, R. and Summer, L. (1999). *Demography is not destiny.* Washington, DC: National Academy on an Aging Society.

George, L. (1996). Social factors and illness. In. R. Binstock and L. George (Eds.), *Handbook of aging and the social sciences* (pp. 229-268). San Diego: Academic Press.

Health Care Financing Administration (1999). *Nursing home care expenditures aggregate and per capita amounts and percent distribution, by source of funds: Selected calendar years 1960-98.* Retrieved April 27, 2000, from the World Wide Web: <http://www.hcfa.gov/stats/nhe-oact/tables/t7.htm>.

Hooyman, N. and Gonyea, J. (1999). A feminist model of family care: Practice and policy directions. *Journal of Women and Aging, 11*(2-3): 149-169.

Kramaroe, E., Lentzner, H., Rooks, R., Weeks, J., and Saydah, S. (1999). *Health and Aging Chartbook: Health, United States, 1999.* Hyattsville, MD: National Center for Health Statistics.

Manton, K., Corder, L., and Stallard, E. (1997). Chronic disability trends in elderly United States populations: 1982-1994. *Proceedings of the National Academy of Sciences of the United States of America, 94*(6): 2593-2598.

Manton, K. and Stallard, E. (1996). Changes in health, mortality, and disability and their impact on long-term care needs. *Journal of Aging and Social Policy, 7*(3-4): 25-52.

National Academy on Aging (1997). *Facts on long-term care.* Retrieved April 27, 2000, from the World Wide Web: <http://gsa/iog.wayne.edu/NAA/ltc.html>.

National Alliance for Caregiving and the American Association of Retired Persons. (1997). *Family caregiving in the U.S.: Findings from a national survey.* Washington, DC: National Alliance for Caregiving and the American Association of Retired Persons.

Older Women's League (1998). *Women, work, and pensions: Improving the odds for a secure retirement.* Washington, DC: Author.

Quadagno, J. (1999). *Aging and the life course: An introduction to social gerontology.* Boston: McGraw-Hill College.

Quinn, P. (1996). Identifying gendered outcomes of gender–neutral policies. *Affilia, 11*(2): 195-206.

Richardson, V. (1999). Women and retirement. *Journal of Women and Aging, 11*(2-3): 49-66.

Taeuber, C. and Allen, J. (1993). Women in our aging society: The demographic outlook. In J. Allen and A. Pifer (Eds.), *Women on the front lines: Meeting the challenge of an aging America* (pp.11-45). Washington, DC: Urban Institute Press.

Tice, C. and Perkins, K. (1996). *Mental health issues and aging: Building on the strengths of older persons.* Pacific Grove, CA: Brooks, Cole.

U.S. Bureau of the Census (1999). *Population Estimates.* Washington, DC: U.S. Government Printing Office.

U.S. Bureau of the Census (2000). *Population Projections.* Washington, DC: U.S. Government Printing Office.

U.S. Department of Health and Human Services (2000). *Health, United States, 1999. Health and Aging Chartbook.* Hyattsville, MD: Centers for Disease Control and National Center for Health Statistics.

Walker, A. (1999). The future of pensions and retirement in Europe: Toward productive aging. *Hallym International Journal on Aging, 1*(2): 3-15.

Chapter 9

Beyond Women of Color, Welfare, and Identity Politics

Faye Y. Abram
Jeanette Mott Oxford
Angela H. Roffle

The three authors of this chapter have strong ties to the Reform Organization of Welfare (ROWEL), a statewide community-based organization of poor women and their allies who use education, advocacy, and social action to fight poverty and prejudice. Two of us are African American. One of us is lesbian. One of us received AFDC. Our lives consist of very different realities. In reply to questions about policy concerns of women of color, however, we respond with clearly different voices to say similar things: The concerns of women of color and others who are marginalized are our concerns. Moving beyond such a generalization, we find we have very different ideas about "women's issues" and "race matters." Nevertheless, we have nearly identical views of welfare policy as the "Bermuda Triangle" that lies at the intersections of racism, sexism, and class oppression. It is the big sinkhole in U.S. public policy in which nonwhites, women, children, and the poor enter and may disappear or die without a trace. Thus, for us, welfare is the mother of all policy issues. Welfare is the hugely complex and significant issue that cuts across race, gender, and class lines. And we agree that it is the policy issue that must be understood and targeted for real reform, serious action, and consistent change if we are to realize greater social and economic justice.

In this chapter, we look at welfare history and recent welfare policy developments primarily from the eyes of African-American women and poor women—not to be exclusionary, but to add a perspective that is often missing (Johnson, 1991; Jimenez, 1999) and that may make the whole picture more inclusive. To demonstrate why millions of women and children as well as a disproportionate number of African Americans have experiences with the welfare system that leave them stranded or lost, we include a case vignette. We intend to amplify voices muffled by a media snow of "welfare-to-work" success stories. Against the backdrop of racist and sexist thinking that continues to shape social welfare policy in the United States, we assert that our voices, the voices of other marginalized groups, and the voices of those who have disappeared off welfare must be heard to move us all beyond the confines of gender, race, welfare, and "identity politics" toward liberation and systemic change.

Appeals to vote for only women or only pro-life candidates or a black slate epitomize the shortsighted logic of identity politics (i.e., the exploitation of people's identification with a racial, gender, religious, or other membership group to elicit an emotional reactionary response for political gain or advantage). John Anner (1996) notes how identity politics has worked in the past. However, he and Marable (1993) assert that we now need to move beyond simplistic identity politics to win progressive victories, as a number of social justice movements in communities of color have done. Both authors argue that identity politics—whether in the guise of nationalism, feminism, or some other form of political expression—is too narrow and isolating to be effective in addressing the needs of groups that have been marginalized by the rest of society. The major criticism is that for the most part identity movements lack a political program beyond making things better for their particular constituents. Anner shows that when Americans of African, Asian, Latino, and Indian ancestry and others break out of socially constructed identities, they find some new, more inclusive identity. New and collectively shaped identities help members of these groups recognize binding issues and concerns and enable them to forge successful multiracial, multiclass, multigender, and even multinational coalitions against conservative, right-wing, reactionary corporate and political powers.

Although we agree with Anner and Marable, we focus here on African-American women and poor women as "outsider" sisters (Lorde, 1984) because the voices of those affected must be heard in policy debates that determine their fate. The leadership of past struggles has come from these groups whose voices also offer promise for the future. More often than not, women of color and notably "black women who are conscious of their double disadvantage are especially likely to seek political remedy . . . and to believe in the efficacy of political action (Wilcox, 1997, p. 89). Admittedly, a focus on women of color and poor people narrows our view, but we ask practitioners to explore the extent to which practice principles emphasized here are relevant to other groups, particularly gays and lesbians, white women, and men of color. We recognize the term "women of color" not only embraces women of many population groups, but also tends to minimize differences within and among African-American, Asian-American, Latina, and Native American women and to obscure bridgework needed within and between genders, classes, and other groups.

To realize racial justice and economic progress for all, we must forge new connections. Chief among those connections should be joining movements led by (or at least informed by) poor people and women of color. This is needed because most Americans are insulated from the poor and they do not look into the faces of women and children on welfare (Berrick, 1995). Similarly, the voices, views, and realities of American women of African, Asian, Indian, Hispanic, and Latin descent are not well represented in accounts of past decades. Recent social work practice and feminist literature, however, include important contributions by and about women of color (e.g., hooks, 1984; Collins, 1990; Bricker-Jenkins, Hooyman, and Gottlieb, 1991; Morris, 1993; Comas-Diaz and Greene, 1994; Suarez, Lewis, and Clark, 1995; Van Den Bergh, 1995; Wilcox, 1997; Carlton-LaNey, 1999; Gutierrez and Lewis, 1999; and Julia, 2000). A few works note the involvement of women of color in social policy. Ruth Brandwein (1995), for example, identifies Mary McLeod Bethune, Sara Fernandis, and Beatriz Lassalle as women of color who were key political actors into the 1940s. Most recently, Icard, Jones, and Wahab (1999) relate the story of Sherry Harris, who in 1991 was elected to the city council of Seattle and became the first publicly elected, openly lesbian African American in the United States. Her story shows not only efforts to combat oppression based on race, gender, and sexual orientation but also her transformation from individual empowerment to political advocacy. Continuing in this line, we aim to give voice to our collective lived experiences as women representative of a diverse group and to share understandings derived from our work as welfare advocates, social work practitioners, and educators.

We assert that feminists cannot successfully combat sexism or other forms of oppression without joining women of color and the poor to reconstruct welfare because racism impairs efforts to bring women and members of diverse groups together. Both racism and sexism undermine our thinking, actions, and policies regarding welfare in the United States (Dressel, 1994; Quadagno, 1994; Abramovitz, 1995, 1997; Rose, 1995; Rowan, 1996; Williams, 1997). Similarly, welfare policies are often off base because

> rarely have the voices of poor women been heard in the debate over their fate. . . . Until poor women are heard, they and their children will remain hostages to contemporary feminism and the most tragic commentary on feminists' failure to achieve real social justice. (Jimenez, 1999, p. 291)

WELFARE HERSTORY: HISTORY RETOLD

Using the corrective lenses of outsider women to look at history, we see ample evidence that welfare was established and is being dismantled despite the needs of marginalized people, not in response to their needs. Basically, the U.S. welfare system was created in 1935 at a time when the Great Depression threatened the lives of millions of white citizens. Similar poverty conditions had long threatened slaves and descendants of slaves, recent immigrants, Native Americans, and others marginalized groups. However, it was agitation by whites in poverty that led to the creation of our welfare system.

The first three decades of welfare were marked with blatant and legal discrimination based on race and marital status. Women who had children outside marriage were not entitled to aid.

> When Aid to Dependent Children (ADC) was created by Congress in 1935, women were conspicuously left out of its financial provisions; stipends were provided for children, not their caretakers. Those who designed and supported the policy, including social workers, were convinced that including mothers (many of whom were divorced and some of whom were single) would risk provoking a substantial amount of hostility from pol-

iticians and the public, thereby dooming it. (Jimenez, 1999, p. 290)

The fear of encouraging single-parent families and weakening men's role in families were the most important reasons ADC provided no stipends for mothers. Similarly, many county welfare agency directors felt justified in rejecting women of color for welfare payments, saying that black and Latina women could readily find employment in farm fields or as domestics (Williams, 1997). Then, as now, there was no acknowledgment that women could not provide adequately for their children with wages from the jobs available to them.

Politicians such as Huey Long opposed welfare for black women, claiming that they would become lazy and dependent if aid were offered. Ironically, when civil rights legislation made it illegal to bar aid from any woman meeting the income and eligibility guidelines, these politicians changed their tune to claim that whole generations of black women were welfare loafers. "The cycle of welfare" or "generational welfare" is still a commonly cited demon even though the findings are mixed as to the number of welfare daughters who return to AFDC later on, and it is unclear whether the cause is welfare, poverty, or something else (McLanahan and Garfinkel, 1989; U.S. House of Representatives, 1993). Such manipulation of the facts and use of welfare myths and stereotypes have fueled welfare reform debates throughout the decades. Ronald Reagan's use of the "welfare queen" as a symbol for the decline of the United States is perhaps the pinnacle of media chicanery on this issue. Ironically, after gaining access to the welfare system, women of color have often been prevented from leaving the welfare system because the only jobs available to them pay too little to allow them to care for their children, access transportation and health care, and cover the additional work-related expenses. The layers of inequalities are based on past and present disadvantages and discrimination.

In 1988, Congress passed the Family Support Act (FSA) that called for investment in case management, child care, and transportation in order to move women to work. Because any welfare system that calls for interaction with clients is vastly more expensive than simply mailing a check to a family, the FSA never sought to serve all families on welfare. Instead, states were to work up until a goal of 25 percent was reached with the Job Opportunities and Basic Skills program (JOBS, called FUTURES in Missouri). States were slow to implement even pilot projects of the new programs.

For example, it took Missouri until 1990 to begin implementing FUTURES with a two-county pilot, and the new system was not available statewide until 1992. FUTURES was known to provide opportunities to attend college and to get extensive job training. Flying in the face of the myth of the unwilling, lazy welfare recipient, Missouri's waiting list of recipients wanting to get into the FUTURES program rose to 7,000.

In 1994, the GOP gained the majority in Congress and opened a full-scale attack on the welfare system, again pointing to the supposed immorality of welfare recipients. The bashing of welfare recipients is ongoing and chronic in our society as evidenced by Minister Joe Wright's statement in a prayer at a recent opening session of the Kansas Legislature: "We have rewarded laziness and called it welfare" (Hobson, 1996). Reverend Wright ignored the fact that it takes hard work just to survive on a welfare grant, with cash aid averaging roughly one-third of the federal poverty level. Later, welfare became a target of the Contract with America put forward by far-right legislators. After three years of constant attacks on all programs serving the poor ("a hundred fronts war" as termed by Marian Wright Edelman of the Children's Defense Fund), the entitlement to aid for needy families was lost in 1996 with the passage of the Personal Responsibility and Work Opportunity Reconciliation Act of 1996 (PRWORA). The new law included time limits and required recipients of Temporary Assistance to Needy Families (TANF) to participate in "work activities" in order to receive full benefits. The message was clear: if you are poor in the United States, that is your personal responsibility.

Three years into the vast social experiment of PRWORA, some pronounce it a success due to steep declines in welfare caseloads. Advocates of the poor and others attribute many of the changes to ten years of "growth" in the U.S. economy and record low unemployment. A decline in the poverty rate would be a better indicator of real success, but the percentage of persons living in poverty has increased over these years. Unfortunately, if caseload reduction is the measure of success, it is possible to create welfare programs that are so chaotic, unwelcoming, and unhelpful that no one will access them. Recent studies show those leaving welfare for work often remain in poverty like many low-income workers, although some achieve incomes slightly higher than those who remain on or return to welfare (Gallagher et al., 1998; Sherman et al., 1998; Loprest, 1999). Studies also show that many families are leaving welfare but not maintaining employment (Greenberg, 1999) and that children in those families are often living at or below 50 percent of the federal poverty level, sinking into the deepest child poverty seen in decades.

In the meantime, welfare-to-work programs continue to press welfare recipients to change, to blame them for their decisions, and to create punishments for their shortcomings. In 1998, the head of one such program invited a staff member from ROWEL to come out to talk with a class of welfare recipients about voter registration. Revealing his patriarchal mind-set, he said, "I'd like these young women to learn to act normal and vote." While he was obsessed with blaming the victim and asking what is to be done to change them, we demand an answer to more fundamental questions. How should society change to support the needs of mothers and children and to provide appropriate and realistic opportunities to participate in the economy and move out of poverty? Can public policy increase the likelihood that no worker lives in poverty and prevent injustices such as racial discrimination, educational inequalities, and domestic violence that have often led to the need to access welfare? The prejudice and discrimination of a clueless privileged group exacerbates the already tall challenges facing those who struggle on the edge of survival.

CASE ILLUSTRATION: VANESSA

Vanessa, a mandatory welfare-to-work participant, is African American, twenty-five years of age, and a mother of four (ages two to ten). She and the other women targeted for special training and services in a neighborhood center program have received TANF benefits for thirty months or more. Like them, Vanessa will hit a time limit and exhaust her lifetime benefits in 2002. She lives with her mate, her mother, and her children in a four-room apartment in a poor, crime-ridden area of the city.

Since Vanessa started the welfare-to-work program, she has lost three jobs. In one instance it was because her "man came on the job and started acting crazy and threatening folks." With another employer, she was informed that the maintenance contractor could no longer use her because it was clear that she could not read or understand the instructions for using certain cleaning products. She lost her third job following a bout with depression.

Vanessa now works at a chicken-processing factory from 11:00 p.m. to 7:00 a.m. in a rural area that is more than an hour's drive from the city. She does not know how long she can continue to do this job because she now has a problem with "aching joints due to the type of work" she does in the factory. She also has difficulty catching rides and paying someone to drive her out there. Vanessa fears that this job will be another that does not work out for her. She is starting to feel that she is a failure and that she is never going to make it in the work world. To make matters worse, she says that financially she is "no better off working" and now she is not there for her kids.

Vanessa wishes she could have remained at home with her children because, according to her, she is "really good at taking care of [her] kids." She reports with pride that her kids were always neat, clean, and well behaved, that she made it to all of their school activities and parent-teacher meetings, and that they did okay with the added money from her "doing hair" in her kitchen and cooking for other people. Vanessa hates that she now has to leave her kids with her mother because "Mom has seizures and sometimes passes out," but she cannot afford any other child care. It is also harder for her to deal with her man, who now gets jealous and beats her about who she might be seeing when she is at work. He gets angry when he sees her dressed for work and looking presentable. He wants to know where she is going looking like that and whom she might be meeting at the bus stop. Vanessa has suggested that she might have to leave the program, check into a safe house, and draw an order of protection against him.

When officials remind Vanessa that she only has two years left before her lifetime TANF benefits run out, she looks back with a blank stare. Clearly, the magnitude of this deadline escapes her. Given her past, the future is unimaginable and unpredictable. For ten years, she has been getting "stingy but dependable" welfare. Now, she says, "You can't count on anything, not a job, not welfare, not your man or family, not anything. It's crazy. It's making me crazy." Vanessa decides to "go home and smoke a little weed so as not to worry about all this stuff, so [she] won't get too depressed." She says, "weed is like a cigarette; it's calming." But employers treat marijuana like cocaine or heroin; because it is in her system, she would test positive for drugs, which effectively eliminates her from other employment opportunities. Vanessa has just received a letter stating she is ineligible for certain benefits, but she "can't make heads or tails of it" and she does not know what to do. So, for now she decides to do nothing.

Vanessa's "caseworker," herself an African-American woman, recalls when people would push her about why she was not working because she was obviously intelligent and had some skills. She recalls how tired she got explaining over and over that she could get jobs, but that did not mean that she could take care of her three kids, one with serious health problems. The caseworker is also annoyed by the questions of many of the professional "helpers," including several who also are African Americans. They want to know, "Why can't they keep jobs? Why are so many unemployed when there are so many more opportunities than there were in the past? With all the advances in birth control, why do they keep having babies? If I have children and I work, why aren't they working? Why don't they have husbands? Why don't they change?" But what bothers this caseworker most is that she is expected to "help" Vanessa and other women like her without attacking the host of structural barriers to their employment.

The above vignette illustrates a case situation of a woman who is but a small part of the diverse population of women of color to which the principles and strategies of feminist social work practice are applicable. We use this vignette both to pay homage to the rich narrative traditions from which each of us has emerged and to show how storytelling and the narrative voice is used in feminist and culturally sensitive practice (Gutierrez and Lewis, 1999; Lamphere, 1992; Holland and Kilpatrick, 1993; Comas-Diaz and Greene, 1994; and Lum, 1999). This vignette is a composite of women drawn from our own practice experiences. The strengths assessment and planned interventions that follow are the sum of our pooled understandings, skills, and values.

Vanessa's Strengths

Stories as well as policy statements about poor women on welfare often explore and provide more information about problems or difficulties than about the strengths and competence of women and their families. The Personal Responsibility Act of 1996 and its supporters,

for example, repeatedly use the labels of "welfare loafers" "drug felons," "unnaturalized immigrants," "illegitimate children," and "illegal
aliens" to refer to welfare recipients who need to take personal responsibility for the decisions they make. However, problems are associated
with focused attention on what is wrong, deficient, or pathological in
their families and environment. Dennis Saleebey (1997) notes that the
accentuation of problems tends to undermine clients' self-esteem; to
create a web of negative expectations about clients, their environment,
and problem-solving capacities; and to foster the victim mind-set and
contribute to conflict between clients and workers.

In contrast to a problem-focused approach, a strength perspective
provides an alternative point of view. It capitalizes on personal assets
and resources that support wellness amid distress and foster understanding of unrecognized potential as well as the power and capacity
of women to continue to learn, grow, and change (Saleebey, 1992,
1997). Similarly, it shifts attention from environmental deficiencies,
hazards, and obstacles to existing community resources that can be
mobilized to combat social, political, and economic factors that make
life difficult. For these reasons, a strengths perspective is the preferred approach for work with persons who are distinguished by their
gender, race, poverty, or welfare status.

Although both problems as well as strengths exist within Vanessa,
her family system, and the environment, it is important to identify
and list her particular strengths and resources, some obvious and
some less obvious. Vanessa is:

1. A mother who is "really good at taking care of her kids"
2. Resourceful, able to "do hair" and "cook for others" to make
   ends meet
3. Proud of her neat, clean, and well-behaved children
4. Age twenty-five, generally considered middle-aged, not too
   old or too young
5. Resilient, seems willing to keep trying after losing jobs and
   experiencing other setbacks
6. Living in an intergenerational household, not isolated, alone,
   or homeless
7. Generally healthy, complains only of "aching joints" since
   working at chicken-processing factory

8. Concerned about ways to protect herself from violence, considering a safe house and an order of protection
9. Familiar with the welfare system, has good relationship with her caseworker, and has won back benefits when she appealed adverse action regarding her eligibility
10. Aware of racism, has some understanding of systemic factors that affect her life as well as some attitudes and skills needed to confront individual as well as institutional racism (e.g., assertiveness/militancy, superior effort, perseverance)

As for her family and community, she may have resources that are commonly found in African-American families or those of single mothers (Hill, 1972; Marlow, 1994; Logan, 1996). These may include:

1. Strong kinship bonds
2. Strong work orientation
3. Flexible family roles
4. Emphasis on educational and occupational achievement
5. Engaged spirituality or faith
6. Greater responsiveness and utilization of extra familial support systems
7. Early independence training for youth

But what does Vanessa need and what do women like her need to succeed? Core concepts of feminist practice suggest and we assert that the following interventions are needed: (a) development of a critical consciousness; (b) reinforcement that the personal is political; (c) empowerment; (d) involvement in diverse groups for collaboration and collective action; and (e) validation/affirmation of positive "truths" about self.

Practitioners can help Vanessa and poor women like her develop *critical consciousness* by engaging her in a power analysis of the historical, social, and political influences shaping her past and present experiences. Such awareness enables her to understand that historically and economically women of color are farther behind because of the legacy of slavery as well as past and ongoing discrimination. A consciousness-raising intervention aims not only to get Vanessa working but also to heighten her understanding of gender and racial inequality as well as the need for work that pays a living wage.

By taking the stance of an advocate and ally, a practitioner working with Vanessa can make the *connection between the personal and the political.* Together they can discover that individual troubles are at least partly due to political decisions and the actions of policymakers. Active members of ROWEL, for example, recognize that their individual efforts to problem-solve the chaos of the welfare system cannot take the place of the policy-level changes that are needed. They now know that policy proposals to expand and refund Earned Income Tax Credits, to increase housing subsidies, and to raise the minimum wage and adjust it for inflation are "bread and butter" policy matters that can made a tangible differencce in their daily lives.

With greater political awareness, *empowerment* interventions enable women of color and poor people—once victimized by structured inequality—to increase their personal, interpersonal, and political power. In this lifelong process, they develop new skills and greater confidence in their capacity to affect change. ROWEL, for example, provides advocacy training and support to women who are fighting for their rights to benefits and services. They later use that knowledge to advocate for others, moving from personal empowerment to peer advocacy and leadership.

Women such as Vanessa, her worker, and others frequently gain a heightened *respect for diversity through involvement* in organizations that intentionally unite people from different races, ethnic groups, and socioeconomic and political backgrounds. Successful organizations provide antiracism training that they see as critical to the organization's success. Such training serves to eliminate false dichotomies and prejudice, to foster appreciation of the special talents and unique contributions of members, and to motivate people to fight common enemies and not one another. Just as labor unions have often found ways to provide for families of striking workers, those of us with resources must find creative ways to support women in poverty so that they and their children have stability while involved in organizing efforts.

Validation and affirmation of positive truths about self occur when we provide accurate information that refutes welfare myths and stereotypes which welfare recipients often learn and internalize. Part of this process involves the deconstruction of stigma and the reconstruction of new terms, meanings, and associations in place of old labels (Mills, 1996).

BEYOND RACE OR GENDER ISSUES

Groups and advocates routinely avoid the Bermuda Triangle of welfare policies, often pursuing other, minor issues that appear more winnable or less hopeless. Many feminist practitioners identify a particular cluster of concerns as "women's issues" and seek to develop a woman's agenda for social work (e.g., Norman and Mancusio, 1980; Freeman, 1990; Davis, 1994; Segal and Brzuzy, 1995). Similarly, the phrase "race matters" (West, 1993) refers to a set of selective concerns about race and issues that affect African Americans. However, the pressing concerns of poor women—often closely resulting from the converging inequalities of class, race, and gender—seem more urgent and far-reaching than many circumscribed gender or race issues. This is not to say that we are unconcerned about issues that many women's groups or race caucuses identify as "their" issues but to acknowledge that we have a decidedly different perspective on many of these topics.

Take, for example, the issue of pay equity. Although the wage gap between men and women has narrowed in the past ten years (due in part to a decrease in men's earnings, an increase in the minimum wage, and an increase in women's earnings), some see the fight to ensure equal pay for equal work as an obvious approach to decrease the wage gap. Others advocate for equal pay for different types of work that require similar skills, effort, and responsibility as an obvious way to address wage gaps due to gender segregation of occupations. Unequal pay is certainly a problem. Women continue to earn less than men, even in the same occupations, and women of color earn the least. White women earn an average of seventy-one cents for every dollar earned by white men. Black women earn an average of fifty-four cents for every dollar earned by black men, and Hispanic women earn an average of fifty-four cents for every dollar earned by Hispanic men (National Committee on Pay Equity, 1995). But what will pay equity policies deliver to women and children in poverty's Bermuda Triangle? For women of color, it is obvious that the men who earn less are our men; we who work longer hours and several part-time jobs are still poor; a gender-segregated and race-stratified labor market ensures inequality. In addition, the work we do is often unhealthy, unnecessarily dehumanizing, stressful, depressing, and without medical benefits.

Mired in such circumstances, "pay equity" will do nothing to improve conditions in the workplace for women nor help unemployed women of any class find jobs. For these reasons, worker-protection and job-creation policies, especially for those expected to leave welfare for the workforce, demand our attention and are more important than wage equity proposals. Pay equity will not benefit the millions of women who remain in poverty, combining part-time and low-wage work with welfare benefits or the millions who remain poor while working full time in minimum wage jobs. In contrast, if we address issues of importance to women of color and poor people, the changes initiated may significantly improve the lives of all in the United States. One mother who still uses some welfare programs sees hope in the possibility of attacking broader issues that transcend economic or racial privilege: "I have hope because I have seen issues of health care and child care become issues for not just poor white women and poor black women, but also for middle-income, and even higher-income women. There are some things that are just basic and that we can get together on."

Another policy issue that politically active women and persons of color advocate for is increasing representation in positions of power. Chafetz (1990) argues that the only way to change the system of gender inequality is to increase the number of women occupying elite power positions. But Segal and Brzuzy (1995) point out that "equality of results is not simply more women in positions of political power. . . . Having more women in Congress may not improve gender equity unless policy changes supportive of women's equality is realized" (p. 149). Moreover, it seems that as women strategize to reduce gender inequality they, knowingly or not, sanction other systems of inequality based on class or race.

Cornell West (1993) analyzed the 1991 Clarence Thomas confirmation hearings and his subsequent placement on the Supreme Court following the challenge on grounds of sexual harassment by Anita Hill. West's analysis of this political controversy reveals the limitations of racial reasoning. He accused black leadership of resorting to a "vulgar form of racial reasoning" by rendering an opportunity to critically discuss race and gender in the black community to a "crude discourse" void of substance and tangential to important policy issues (pp. 23-24). According to West, racial reasoning presumes a racial consensus and makes an appeal to (1) black authenticity, (2) black closing-ranks mentality, and (3) "black male subordination of black women in the interest of the black community in . . . a racist country" (p. 24).

The three previous elements in combination seem to operate when Democratic Washington, DC, Mayor Marion Barry calls for mandatory Norplant injections for welfare recipients and that call goes unchallenged. Because of the allegiance required by principles of identity politics, poor people and people of color often hold back criticism of "their" elected officials. This can be found all over the country. The black community in St. Louis, for example, has not done a good job of holding black male elected officials accountable. If poor women target a black official to demand more work on their issues, they get accused of "trying to tear that brother down," when that would have been unnecessary if he had been more responsive to his "sistahs' needs." One activist and mother breaks the silence, asking, "Why didn't black elected officials across America fight harder against the welfare bill? Surely they knew how it would play out in their districts." Despite the pressure to be lenient towards black elected officials or women in office, we refuse to remain silent. What West particularized as "racial reasoning" is another form of identity politics—a generalized appeal to simple-minded political decision making based on gender, a candidate's position on a single policy issue, such as abortion or some other emotional identity trigger. The silence that protects elected officials who are not dedicated to real change for poor women and women of color contributes to the isolation and hopelessness that descends on anyone who lands in poverty and in the sinkhole of welfare policies.

To attain true equality and real reform, we ask people to strain to hear the voices of women and children in poverty. We direct attention to the margins where all women of color face racism and poor women of color face barriers that are structured around economics. A poor woman may know the strengths she has to offer, but when she looks out her front window, she may see only deficits: low-paying jobs, a neighborhood with no programs or activities for her children, lack of health care for her extended family, unsafe child-care options, schools that fail to educate her sons and daughters, the disappearance of affordable housing created by urban renewal. Programs that are designed to "move" people from welfare to work have that "lift yourself up by your bootstraps" mentality. The programs do not really address—are not designed or funded to address—the problems women face in trying to find and keep a good job in this economy. The loss of the entitlement to a social safety net can place whole families in jeopardy. The focus may be on getting one woman to change, but the opportunities and traps around her are not changing, and those women and children are at increasing risk.

The protective stance of identity politics demands silence about many critical issues. Two other problems poor women often face are substance abuse and illiteracy. The educational systems in inner-city schools have failed to educate many people, and some are not at a math or reading level where they can carry out written directions. This can be a problem even in low-wage housekeeping jobs; the label may say do not mix this chemical with that one. Technology has advanced until almost all jobs require the ability to read messages and carry them out. In addition, jobs that actually can help the family out of poverty require training for technical skills, and literacy is absolutely necessary. These problems reveal structural reasons many women (as well as men) continue to be disadvantaged in the work world and within competitive institutions. Similarly, a woman whose family deals with substance abuse may be unable to get treatment because of health care policies and the "cost controls" of Medicaid since managed care. If her first step is to deal with her addiction—or an addiction within her immediate family—she is utterly stalled. Policies that do not acknowledge systemic problems such as unavailability of treatment for substance abuse will surely leave these people out.

The binds poor women of color find themselves in emerge not only from policies, but also from the assumptions of some social work practitioners and other professionals. Too many of the welfare-to-work providers, even trained professional staff, counselors, and therapists, say to women, "You just need to get a job." Speaking from middle-class values, they want poor women to behave in middle-class ways, yet poor women live in very different neighborhoods, in circumstances that are very different. Such programs do not realistically look at the context of the poor women's lives. Welfare-to-work programs do not even begin to address deep-seated problems such as

domestic violence, a reason many women are unable to finish training or utilize job placement programs. When we tinker with one part
of a family system, we tinker with all of it. Welfare reform policy, just
as advocacy for pay equity, is based on privileged perspectives of the
lives of families in poverty. Policy based on that vantage point often
harms the families they are supposed to help.

In addition to ignoring the context of poor women's lives, programs that serve poor families are often spoiled with the same inequalities that converge to place women of color and their children in
poverty. Susan Tinsley Gooden's examination of workfare programs
nationwide disclosed that there are stark differences in the treatment
of black and white women in these programs (Grass Roots Innovative
Policy Program, 1999). Under the new TANF guidelines, local departments of social services, specifically their caseworkers and staff
who determine eligibility, exercise more authority and discretion in
making decisions about welfare applicants and program participants.
This marks a return to discretion. Before welfare became a federal
program, states and localities decided who was deserving or not deserving of benefits. A number of states and local communities used
such discretion to systematically exclude whole groups of people
(predominately persons of color) they judged to be ineligible for welfare. In fact, one of the main reasons welfare and social security were
federalized and standardized was to eliminate known practices of discrimination and unequal distribution of benefits at the state level.
Have we forgotten this? Sadly, in addition to hard evidence of
present-day housing and labor market discrimination, it now seems
discrimination is a reoccurring problem in county welfare offices.
Gooden's evaluation of a Virginia workfare program revealed systemic discrimination. No black woman interviewed in the study received discretionary transportation support, nor knew of its existence, while white women routinely got the aid. When discrimination
based on race, sex, and class is allowed to operate, poor women of
color and their families are not only pushed off welfare and over the
"welfare cliff" (Hagen, 1999) but also out of decent jobs and out of
sight and mind.

Some of the proposed solutions to poverty create new problems.
As the right wing has moved to replace inadequate government assistance and services with the "compassionate conservatism" of private
charity and "charitable choice" that provides direct funding to faith-

based organizations (FBO) to run welfare-to-work programs, poor women and women of color are put at risk. The sinkhole expands to another area. Nowhere is it outlined that program participants may not be discriminated against on the basis of religion. No protection exists to prevent or discourage countless comments from well-meaning "social service" providers that cast poverty as a personal sin and moral flaw and suggest who is good, who is bad, who is deserving, and who church folk may choose not to help. One worker in a faith-based community service organization describes the experiences of a lesbian mother in the program. This mother has had to face criticism about her right to be a parent from "helpers" in the system and from other women in the class. Yet she must depend on these services if she hopes to get training and beat time limits. What happens when prejudice leads to unmerited hotline calls? What about the woman who is a nonbeliever, or wishes to have an abortion, or is already clinically depressed and riddled with shame and self-hate? Women keep butting up against this wall about what is not right with them, and some lives are destroyed by the sanctions imposed. Linda Kessler with the Center for Faith Action and Response (a federally funded FBO) tells the story of a woman in the program who had failed part of her GED. She came out of the testing site crying hysterically, convinced she was doomed to fail. She soon disappeared from the program, not to be found. Many others like her exist. Where is she? Where are they? It is not okay not to ask or care—even though an array of labels have been used to place these people outside the circle of human compassion.

But because we see our future as inextricably connected to their futures and because we share a critical understanding of the welfare system, we call on women of all colors to build bridges across racial, class, and cultural boundaries and to work, not for the reduction of welfare, but to end poverty. Such work will require us to avoid playing identity politics as usual and to rename and reclaim people, rights, services, and opportunities that are due to all citizens of a democratic society. We, therefore, invite you to join with us and others in the movement to end poverty, organized and led by poor people (those who best know about poverty) which grows today. We recite in unison the personal pledge of Mary Bricker-Jenkins (2000) to stand with those who are living in poverty and with social workers and others who stand with them on ethical principles and values that say

we must not implement policies and programs that harm people.
. . . Together we can refuse and resist and we can create ways to
live our commitments to economic justice as we erase the line
between social worker and activists (p. 5)

and, we add, the lines between ourselves and all who are oppressed.

REFERENCES

Abramovitz, M. (1995). Welfare and women's lives: Toward a feminist understanding of the reform debate. *Democratic Left, 23*(3) (May/June): 5-8.
Abramovitz, M. (1997). Temporary Assistance to Needy Families. In R. L. Ed-
wards (Editor-in-Chief), *Encyclopedia of social work: 1997 Supplement*, Nine-
teenth edition (pp. 311-330). Washington, DC: NASW Press.
Anner, J. (1996). *Beyond identity politics: Emerging social justice movements in
communities of color.* Cambridge, MA: South-End-Press.
Berrick, J. D. (1995). *Faces of poverty: Portraits of women and children on welfare.*
New York: Oxford University Press.
Brandwein, R. A. (1995). Women in social policy. In R. L. Edwards (Editor-in-
Chief), *Encyclopedia of social work,* Nineteenth edition. Volume 3 (pp. 2552-
2560). Washington, DC: NASW Press.
Bricker-Jenkins, M. (2000). March of the Americas [October 1, 1999, Opening
rally/comments]. *BCR Reports, 11*(2): 5.
Bricker-Jenkins, M., Hooyman, N. R., and Gottlieb, N. (Eds.) (1991). *Feminist so-
cial work practice in clinical settings.* Newbury Park, CA: Sage.
Carlton-LaNey, I. (1999). African-American social work pioneers' response to
need. *Social Work, 44*(4): 311-321.
Chafetz, J. (1990). *Gender equity: An integrated theory of stability and change.*
Newbury Park, CA: Sage Publications.
Collins, P. H. (1990). *Black feminist thought: Knowledge, consciousness, and the
politics of empowerment.* Boston, MA: Unwin Hyman.
Comas-Diaz, L. and Greene, B. (Eds.) (1994). *Women of color: Integrating ethnic
and gender identities in psychotherapy.* New York: Guilford Press.
Davis, L. V. (1994). Why we still need a woman's agenda for social work. In L. V.
Davis (Ed.), *Building on women's strengths: A social work agenda for the
twenty-first century* (pp. 1-26). Binghamton, NY: The Haworth Press.
Dressel, P. L. (1994). And we keep building prisons: Racism, poverty and chal-
lenges to the welfare state. *Journal of Sociology and Social Welfare, 21:* 7-30.
Freeman, M. L. (1990). Beyond women's issues: Feminism and social work. *Affilia,
5*(1): 72-89.

Gallagher, L. J., Gallager, M., Perese, K., Schreiber, S., and Watson, K. (1998). One year after federal welfare reform: A description of state Temporary Assistance for Needy Families (TANF) decisions as of October 1997. *Assessing the new federalism* [Occasional Paper Number 6]. Washington, DC: The Urban Institute.

Grass Roots Innovative Policy Program of the Applied Research Center (1999). The secret truth about race and welfare. *GRIPP News and Notes, 1* (Spring: 1-2, 5. [Interview with Susan Tinsley Gooden, Assistant Professor in the Center for Public Administration and Policy at Virginia Tech University.]

Greenberg, M. (1999). *The disconnected.* Presentation at the Center for Law and Social Policy, St. Louis, Missouri, August 20.

Greene, B. (1994). Diversity and difference: Race and feminist psychotherapy. In M. P. Mirkin (Ed.), *Women in context: Toward a feminist reconstruction of psychotherapy* (pp. 25-47). New York: Guilford Press.

Gutierrez, L. (1990). Working with women of color: An empowerment perspective. *Social Work, 35:* 149-154.

Gutierrez, L. M. and Lewis, E. A. (Eds.) (1999). *Empowering women of color.* New York: Columbia University Press.

Hagen, J. L. (1999). Time limits under Temporary Assistance to Needy Families: A closer look at the welfare cliff. *Affilia, 14*(3): 294-314.

Hill, R. (1972). *Strengths of black families.* New York: Emerson Hull.

Hobson, G. (1996). Prayer provokes passions: Wichitan's message upsets Kansas house. *The Wichita Eagle,* January 24, p. A1.

Holland, T. P. and Kilpatrick, A. C. (1993). Using narrative techniques to enhance multicultural social work practice. *Journal of Social Work Education, 29*(3): 302-308.

hooks, B. (1984). *Feminist theory: From margin to center.* Boston, MA: South End Press.

Icard, L., Jones, T., and Wahab, S. (1999). Empowering lesbian and bisexual women of color: Overcoming three forms of oppression. In L. M. Gutierrez and E. A. Lewis (Eds.), *Empowering women of color* (pp. 208-225). New York: Columbia University Press.

Jimenez, M. A. (1999). A feminist analysis of welfare reform: The Personal Responsibility Act of 1996. *Affilia, 14*(3): 278-293.

Johnson, A. E. (1991). The sin of omission: African-American women in social work. *Journal of Multicultural Social Work, 1*(2): 1-15.

Julia, M. (2000). *Constructing gender: Multicultural perspectives in working with women.* Belmont, CA: Wadsworth.

Lamphere, L. (1992). *Structuring diversity: Ethnographic perspectives on the new immigration.* Chicago, IL: University of Chicago Press.

Logan, S. L. (Ed.) (1996). *The black family: Strengths, self-help, and positive change.* Boulder, CO: Westview Press.

Loprest, P. (1999). How families that left welfare are doing: A national picture. [Series B. No. B-1.] *Assessing the new federalism: National survey of America's families*. Washington, DC: The Urban Institute.

Lorde, A. (1984). *Sister outsider*. New York: Crossing Press.

Lum, D. (1999). *Culturally competent practice: A framework for growth and action*. Pacific Grove, CA: Brooks/Cole.

Marable, M. (1993). Beyond racial identity politics: Toward a liberation theory for multicultural democracy. *Race and Class, 35(1)*: 113-130.

Marlow, C. (1994). Ex-partner, family, friends and other relationships: Their role within the social network of long-term single mothers. *Journal of Applied Social Psychology, 24:* 60-81.

McLanahan, S. and Garfinkel, I. (1989). Single mothers, the underclass and social policy. *Annals of the American Academy of Political and Social Science, 501* (January): 92-104.

Mills, F. B. (1996). The ideology of welfare reform: Deconstructing stigma. *Social Work, 41(4)*: 391-406.

Morris, J. K. (1993). Interacting oppressions: Teaching social work content on women of color. *Journal of Social Work Education, 29(1)*: 99-110.

National Committee on Pay Equity (1995). *Questions and answers on pay equity*. Washington, DC: Author.

Norman, E. and Mancuso, A. (Ed.) (1980). *Women's issues and social work practice*. Itasca, IL: F. E. Peacock.

Quadagno, J. S. (1994). *The color of welfare: How racism undermined the war on poverty*. New York: Oxford University Press.

Rose, N. E. (1995). *Workfare or fair work: Women, welfare, and government work programs* (pp. 150-185). New Brunswick, NJ: Rutgers University Press.

Rowan, C. T. (1996). *The coming race war in America: A wake-up call* (pp. 159-182). Boston, MA: Little, Brown and Company.

Saleebey, D. (Ed.) (1997). *The strengths perspective in social work practice*, Second edition. New York: Longman.

Segal, E. and Brzuzy, S. (1995). Women actors for women's issues: A new political agenda. In N. Van Den Bergh (Ed.), *Feminist practice in the 21st century* (pp. 143-157). Washington, DC: NASW Press.

Sherman, A., Amey, C., Duffield, B., Ebb, N., and Weinstein, D. (1998). *Welfare to what: Early findings on family hardship and well-being*. Washington, DC: Children's Defense Fund and National Coalition for the Homeless.

Suarez, Z. E., Lewis, E. A., and Clark, J. (1995). Women of color and culturally competent feminist social work practice. In N. Van Den Bergh (Ed.), *Feminist practice in the 21st century* (pp. 195-210). Washington, DC: NASW Press.

U.S. House of Representatives, Committee on Ways and Means (1993). *1993 green book: Overview of entitlement programs*. Background material and data on programs within the jurisdiction of the Committee on Ways and Means, July 7, Washington, DC: U.S. Government Printing Office.

Van Den Bergh, N. (Ed.) (1995). *Feminist practice in the 21st century.* Washington, DC: NASW Press.

West, C. (1993). *Race matters* (pp. 21-32). Boston, MA: Beacon Press.

Wilcox, C. (1997). Racial and gender consciousness among African-American women: Sources and consequences. *Women and Politics, 17*(1): 73-94.

Williams, L. (1997). *Decades of distortion: The right's 30-year assault on welfare.* Somerville, MA: Political Research Associates.

Chapter 10

Lesbians and Bisexual Women: Relevant Policy and Practice Issues

Sandra C. Anderson

Historically, most lesbians and bisexual women in this society have led lives of secrecy and have been overlooked or pathologized in research endeavors. In her review of forty years of research on lesbians, Tully (1995) notes that most of the research between the 1960s and 1980s compared samples of lesbians with heterosexual women, seeking to determine whether lesbianism constituted pathology and/or focusing on the problematic and "dysfunctional" aspects of lesbianism. Interestingly, many of these studies have revealed, instead of psychopathology, evidence of lesbians' extraordinary strengths.

Comparative studies conducted since the 1980s show either no consistent differences between lesbians and heterosexual women in degree of mental health or illness (Bell, Weinberg, and Hammersmith, 1981) or exceptional psychological and social functioning by lesbians. Lesbians have a greater sense of autonomy and independence (Hopkins, 1969; Nichols and Lieblum, 1986), a higher capacity for self-confidence, self-sufficiency, and assertiveness (Thompson, McCandless, and Strickland, 1971; Wilson and Greene, 1971), and a greater sensitivity to op-

Portions of this chapter are adapted or excerpted from Anderson, S. (1995), Addressing heterosexist bias in the treatment of lesbian couples with chemical dependency. *Journal of Feminist Family Therapy, 7*(3/4), pp. 87-113; and Anderson, S. and Sussex, B. (1999), Resilience in lesbians: An exploratory study. In J. Laird (Ed.), *Lesbians and lesbian families: Reflections on theory and practice* (pp. 305-329). New York, Columbia University Press.

pression and the need for social change (Pharr, 1988). Rothblum (1988) notes that lesbians have always been in the "vanguard of social change" (p. 10), initiating alternative health care, feminist therapy collectives, violence against women programs, and grassroots organizations.

Given the distinct cultural disadvantages of lesbian couples, it is interesting that they report significantly higher levels of cohesion, adaptability, and satisfaction than do heterosexual couples (Zacks, Green, and Morrow, 1988). Lesbian couples want more time with their partners and place more value on equitable distribution of household duties (Blumstein and Schwartz, 1983; Patterson, 1996; Peplau, 1991). Overall, studies indicate that the majority of lesbian couples view their relationship as extremely close, personally satisfying, and egalitarian (Peplau et al., 1978). In an attempt to explain the "superior functioning" of lesbian couples, Zacks, Green, and Morrow (1988) note that lesbians have fewer sanctions against ending unhappy relationships. The egalitarian nature of lesbian relationships enhances the competencies of both partners, and "the superior relational skills of two women enable them to form better-functioning relationships" (p. 480).

A study on lesbian families by Levy (1992) showed that lesbian parents have high self-esteem, and family functioning is characterized by balanced levels of family cohesion and family organization. Levy notes that the lesbian parents in her study developed coping mechanisms that "challenged societal norms, asserted their human rights, and provided support for their lesbian identities" (p. 29). The children of lesbian parents do not differ on most variables from children raised by heterosexual parents and may, in fact, be less rigid, more tolerant of diversity, more flexible in their own gender identities, and have a greater sense of well-being (Patterson, 1992).

Lesbian mothers are more concerned than are single heterosexual mothers that their children have male role models and usually have more adult male family and friends participating in the lives of their children (Hare and Richards, 1993; Kirkpatrick, 1987). When compared to divorced heterosexual mothers, lesbian mothers tend to have more congenial relations with their previous husbands, and their children are more likely to have contact with their father (Golombok, Spencer, and Rutter, 1983). It is interesting that lesbian couples with children feel more accepted as a family by their own families of origin and friends than by the lesbian community (Hare, 1994).

As noted by Laird (1996a, 1996b), lesbians and their families are quite diverse. In spite of stereotypes in the popular and professional literature, most lesbians are not cut off from their families of origin and do have role models (who may be straight, lesbian, or bisexual). They receive fairly high degrees of support from their biological family members and assume extensive family caregiving responsibilities (Fredriksen, 1999).

The literature on bisexual women has not kept pace with that on lesbians. Although some studies of lesbians contain bisexual participants, there are few studies focusing on bisexual women. For that reason, most of the material in this chapter relates to lesbians and may or may not be generalizable to bisexual women. It is also important to recognize probable sources of bias in all existing research on lesbian and bisexual women. It is almost impossible to obtain random or representative samples when studying a stigmatized population. Possible sources of bias are related to chronology, race and ethnicity, social class, and degree of disclosure. Research conducted many years ago probably reflects less overall societal acceptance, hence those willing to self-identify and participate in these earlier studies are very likely a different population than those who are studied currently. In addition, research on lesbians has focused primarily on white, middle-class respondents. It is likely that many less-well-educated, unemployed, or ethnic minority lesbians have not been available for study, perhaps in part because they are "passing" as heterosexual. All of these potential sources of bias must be kept in mind when attempting to make meaning of existing research.

SOCIOCULTURAL CONTEXT

Lesbians have historically been labeled as sinful, criminal, and mentally ill. They have been institutionalized, burned as witches, hanged, beheaded, and starved to death. Prior to 1973, the American Psychiatric Association (APA) regarded homosexuality as a psychopathology, and it is still a diagnosis in the international classification of diseases (World Health Organization, 1997).

Although there continues to be great interest in discovering the causes of homosexuality, heterosexuality is assumed and apparently requires no explanation. Current psychoanalytic theories of lesbianism focus primarily on deficits in development; feminist revisions of object relations theory stress difficulties in intimate relationships (for a comprehensive critique of dynamic theories of lesbianism, see Glassgold, 1992). In general, these theories assume that normal psychosocial development always results in heterosexual adults and that individuals are influenced only by biology and family dynamics. They are monocultural in nature, reflecting white Northern European paradigms.

Biological theories of homosexuality have been tested most frequently on samples of gay men. The few studies using lesbian samples have not found significant evidence that female sexual orientation has a genetic component, but this research is in its infancy. The only empirical research to date suggesting a biological component to lesbianism found greatly increased numbers of lesbian or bisexual sisters of a group of lesbians compared to a matched sample of heterosexual women (Bailey and Benishay, 1993).

Both dynamic and biological models fail to explain the fluidity of sexual identity experienced by many women. As suggested by Chodorow (1992), there may be many differing homosexualities. It is clear that women's sexuality is flexible and can change throughout life (Golden, 1987; Loewenstein, 1984/1985). It is not uncommon for a woman to recognize or change her sexual orientation late in life or to change her preference several times over her lifetime (Kinsey et al., 1953). D'Augelli (1994) points out that patterns of sexual identity may be quite complex, fluid during certain phases of the life span and more constricted at others. He also notes that "there is no methodologically sound longitudinal research on lesbian/gay development in the social science literature" (p. 129).

According to Marmor (1998), from a scientific perspective, the etiology of homosexuality is neither more nor less significant than that of heterosexuality. From a sociopolitical perspective, however, it becomes quite important since prejudice and discrimination are based in large part on lack of knowledge. Individuals who believe that homosexuals "were born that way" are significantly less homophobic than those who do not have this belief (Ernulf, Innala, and Whitam, 1989). In addition, Laird (1993) notes the important legal and political implications:

> If homosexuality is seen as biologically or genetically caused, homosexuals may be considered a protected class under the United States Constitution. However, if homosexuality is seen

by the courts as voluntary, it is a practice less clearly protected under the law. (p. 287)

The existence of fluidity in the sexual orientations of women is also central to the issue of bisexuality. Burch (1993) found that "primary lesbians" never clearly self-identified as heterosexuals and wondered about being lesbian in their adolescence or early twenties. "Bisexual lesbians" often self-identified as heterosexual early in life and as lesbian or bisexual later in life. Rust (1992) notes that many lesbians question whether bisexuals actually exist or view bisexuality as a personal and political threat; bisexuals are portrayed as "sexual opportunists, fickle lovers, traitors, political cowards, or fencesitters" (p. 368). In her sample of 365 lesbian and bisexual-identified women, the vast majority of lesbian respondents preferred to relate socially and politically to other lesbians rather than bisexuals; three-quarters refused to date bisexual women at all. Although exclusively homosexual feelings were unique to lesbian respondents and predominantly heterosexual feelings were unique to bisexual respondents, most respondents of both groups shared a nonexclusive preference for women. A heterosexual history was common to both groups, with 90 percent of lesbian and 100 percent of bisexual respondents having been involved in heterosexual relationships. Rust concludes that it is this similarity of experiences in the two groups that aggravates their sociopolitical differences. In essence, she argues that "preservation of an essentialist and dichotomous construction of sexuality is critical to modern lesbian politics" (p. 382). Bisexuality threatens lesbian politics by raising doubts about the essential nature of lesbianism and by blurring the boundary between homosexuality and heterosexuality, between the oppressed and oppressor. In essence, many lesbian feminists do not view bisexual, gay male, or transsexual "concerns" as supportive of a feminist challenge to male dominance. Their antagonism toward bisexuals has only increased in response to popular discourses on AIDS. According to Ault (1996):

Increasingly stigmatized and politicized by these discourses, women locating themselves as bisexuals have begun to organize for two competing purposes: to achieve "bi rights" through increased social recognition on the one hand; to subvert the binary identity paradigm, on the other. (p. 453)

Clearly, bisexuality challenges the rigid lesbian/heterosexual dichotomy which assumes mutually exclusive categories of sexual orientation (Shuster, 1987). In spite of the Kinsey researchers' delineation of seven points along a continuum of sexual orientation, the predominance of a dichotomous view has constrained the development of theoretical and research literature on bisexuality. Now some research supports the notion that bisexuality is a distinct, unique sexual orientation (Blackford, Doty, and Pollack, 1996; Fox, 1995), not just a transition to or denial of another orientation. Klein (1993) describes four kinds of bisexuality: transitional, a stage in coming out as lesbian; historical, the experience of both same and opposite gender attractions in the past; sequential, relationships with only one man or woman during a particular period of time; and concurrent, relationships with both men and women during the same time period. Research on nonclinical samples of bisexual women has found no evidence of psychopathology or maladjustment (La Torre and Wendenberg, 1983). Within the sexual minority community, lesbians hold higher status because of bisexual women's closer relationships with two dominant out-groups, men and heterosexuals. In addition, the resources of the bisexual community are inferior to those of the lesbian community. Only recently have bisexual women asserted that they have unique needs that are not being met by either heterosexual or lesbian communities (Rust, 1993b).

HOMOPHOBIA AND HETEROSEXISM

Homophobia is the irrational fear, hatred, and intolerance of homosexuals (Margolies, Becker, and Jackson-Brewer, 1987) which leads to the denial of civil rights to lesbians, bisexuals, and gay men. Internalized homophobia occurs when lesbians accept society's negative attitudes about themselves and other homosexuals (Fassinger, 1991). As defined by Falco (1991), heterosexism is "the assumption that heterosexuality is in any way better than homosexuality" (p. 7). Rich (1980) argues that heterosexuality is a powerful political institution of patriarchy and that lesbians are the most serious challenge to patriarchy. As summarized by Laird (1995):

> That some women might choose or prefer to love and to spend their emotional and sexual lives with other women is unthink-

able in patriarchal discourse. The lesbians' very existence gives testimony to the notion that women do not need men to become complete, to survive, to succeed, to live in families, to raise children. (p. 197)

Studies continue to show that both social work professionals and students display homophobic and heterosexist attitudes. Wisniewski and Toomey (1987) found that almost one-third of MSW social workers were homophobic, and De Crescenzo (1984) found that social workers were more homophobic than psychologists and other mental health professionals. A more recent study of MSW social workers (Berkman and Zinberg, 1997) found that 10 percent of respondents were homophobic and a majority were heterosexist. Homophobia was greater in relation to gay men than lesbians, and there was a negative association between homophobia/heterosexism and knowing a gay man or lesbian. Women were significantly less heterosexist than men, but there was no association between attitudes and amount of education on topics related to homosexuality. Religiosity was associated with higher levels of homophobia and heterosexism, and having been in psychotherapy was associated with more positive attitudes toward gay men and lesbians.

A recent study of undergraduate and graduate social work students (Black, Oles, and Moore, 1998) found a significant relationship between homophobia and sexism, with male students more homophobic and sexist than female students. These findings support earlier ones noting the association between homophobia and an individual's endorsement of traditional gender roles (Herek, 1994).

These findings are alarming in that social workers with homophobic attitudes can be ineffective or harmful in their work with gay, bisexual, and lesbian clients. Rudolph (1988) reported that dissatisfaction with treatment is often attributed to the heterosexist bias of the counselor.

COMING OUT AND "PASSING"

Many writers continue to equate disclosure of lesbianism ("coming out") with good mental and physical health and authentic interpersonal relationships (Coleman, 1982; Falco, 1991; Garnets and Kimmel, 1991; Gonsiorek and Rudolph, 1991; Lewis, 1984; Scasta,

1998). Jourard (1958) concluded that a nondisclosing person could never love or receive love from another person, and others (Cass, 1979; Gartrell, 1984; Moses, 1978; Murphy, 1989; Ponse, 1978) have concluded that coming out is crucial for self-acceptance and self-esteem. Coming out has been characterized by Krestan (1988) as "a highly specialized instance of differentiation" (p. 119) and by Kleinberg (1986) as "a rite of passage into adulthood for lesbian women" (p. 1).

It is certainly true that being closeted involves constant vigilance, denying and concealing true feelings, and being viewed as single and available to males. On the other hand, coming out can also be risky. As summarized by Greene, Causby, and Miller (1999), coming out "may result in ostracism by one's friends; alienation from one's family; the loss of one's job, housing, or child custody; and subjection to gay bashing or other forms of harassment and abuse" (p. 80).

Most work on the coming-out process neglects bisexual identity. One exception is a recent study of over 400 lesbian and bisexual women (Rust, 1993a) which found that bisexuals came out later than lesbians and exhibited less "stable" identity histories. The average lesbian and bisexual woman experienced coming-out events in the same order, but bisexuals experienced each event at an older age. Lesbians were first sexually attracted to women at age fifteen and bisexuals at eighteen on average. About two years after this experience, both groups began questioning their heterosexual identities. When lesbians were twenty-two and bisexuals twenty-five, they adopted their current identities. However, both groups continued to wonder about their identities for a number of years, undergoing periods of alternative identification or uncertainty about their identities. The major difference between the two groups was that most lesbians maintained their original lesbian identity while bisexual women tended to change their sexual identities more rapidly and frequently than lesbians. Rust (1993a) concluded that, "Outdated developmental models can be replaced by an understanding of sexual identity formation as an ongoing dynamic process of describing one's social location within a changing social context" (p. 74).

Before discussing what is known about the consequences of self-disclosure, it is informative to examine the *language* of coming out. Healy (1999) examines the verbal and behavioral language of self-disclosure and concludes that behavior often speaks louder than words. Language affirming or negating lesbian identity can be expressed and received in both verbal and behavioral forms. For example, talking about one's partner as significant, buying a home together, and bringing your partner to family, work, and social events represents self-affirming behavioral language. Denial or rejection of lesbian identity through silence or not bringing one's partner to special occasions represent self-negating behavioral language, consistently associated with uncomfortable feelings. Healy found that choices about verbal and behavioral disclosure are highly context sensitive. Some degree of self-censoring was pervasive even when a lesbian was generally "out" in her life. Interestingly, lesbians did not claim being "out" in their families without direct verbal disclosure. As noted by Laird (1996b):

> Certainly, there can be serious costs to silencing and censoring oneself and being silenced by others. But all of us make choices about what we will share or not share about ourselves every day. In every sentence, we select what we wish to bring into the conversation—in our body language, through dress, in the ways we organize our homes, and in other uses of the said and the unsaid. . . . There are always rules and strategies for conversation in any family. . . . (p. 111)

Families of origin go through a parallel process of coping with the coming out of a lesbian family member (Healy, 1999). The family's response to self-disclosure is often unpredictable. They may be accepting immediately, deny the revelation, or reject the lesbian temporarily or permanently (Browning, Reynolds, and Dworkin, 1991; Rosen, 1992). LaSala (1998), summarizing several surveys, notes that 23 to 50 percent of those disclosing to their parents report adverse reactions. Murphy (1989), on the other hand, noted that her small sample of lesbians did not report one instance of total parental rejection and that any negative consequence of parental disapproval was overshadowed by the benefits to the couple of coming out. Green, Bettinger, and Zacks (1996) found that satisfaction of lesbian couples was entirely unrelated to whether partners were out to their mothers, fathers, siblings, or a combination of the three.

Erving Goffman's concept of "passing" is very helpful in understanding lesbian identity management. In passing, an individual is endowed with some kind of personally discrediting information about self, and this information is undisclosed to others who observe or interact with her (Goffman, 1963). Passing is facilitated by the assumption that women are heterosexual unless demonstrated to be otherwise. Newman and Muzzonigro (1993) found that 85 percent of lesbian and gay adolescents pretend to be heterosexual some of the time. Others have found that three-quarters of the lesbians studied had not disclosed their identity to the world at large (Eldridge and Gilbert, 1990; Moses, 1978). More than one-third of lesbians have been married and one-fifth have had children by men (Rothberg and Ubell, 1985), but it is not known how many of these women have passed as heterosexual or how many currently married women are passing as heterosexual. There has been little research on how lesbians think about their potentially conflicting identities of wife and lesbian or how they decide to disclose or not disclose to their husbands (Strommen, 1989).

In the first in-depth study of the concept of passing in lesbians, Kanuha (1998) characterizes passing as learned resistance to heterosexist domination. Her subjects reported four types of passing strategies: (1) dissociating, behaving as if one is not part of the stigmatized group; (2) omission, responding directly to an inquiry but omitting some key clarification that would disclose the stigma; (3) mutual pretense, whereby accomplices collude with the passer to conceal the stigma; and (4) playing with the audience, in which respondents are passing as a caricature of their stigma. She concluded that "passing is essentially a strategy of resistance to oppression" (p. 18), and that lesbians must continually engage in a decision-making process to determine the cost-benefit analysis of social encounters. This process involves lesbians' assessment of the situation and those interacting in it, with a subsequent determination of how participants would deal with their being lesbian in this context.

Kanuha's (1998) major finding was that lesbians construct and enact multiple self-representations ("selves") that are grounded in particular social contexts. They were comfortable and self-accepting in calling themselves different things in different settings. Passing is always an intentional performance, accepted as a fact of life of being lesbian. And contrary to what one might expect from the dire predictions about nondisclosure in the clinical literature, most lesbians did not report any substantive negative effects of passing in a variety of encounters. They were able to experience a sense of continuity and wholeness in spite of multiple, inconsistent, and sometimes conflicting partialized selves. These findings support earlier ones by Crocker and Major (1989) that prejudice against members of stigmatized groups (minority racial, ethnic, or sexual) generally does not result in lowered self-esteem, and by Eldridge and Gilbert (1990) that non-disclosure is as adaptive for some lesbians as disclosure is for others.

SOCIAL POLICY ISSUES

It is still legal in thirty-nine states to discriminate on the basis of sexual orientation, and there has been no success in including sexual orientation in federal civil rights legislation. As pointed out by Hartman (1996), a central issue is the definition of the family embedded in social policy. For example, the Bureau of the Census defines the family as two or more people living together and related by blood, marriage, or adoption (Poverny and Finch, 1988). The exclusion of gay and lesbian couples from this definition means that they are not eligible for certain benefits such as tax breaks, family leave, social security benefits, or family rates on health, auto, or home insurance.

Laws governing invasion of privacy (sodomy laws) are still in effect in almost half of the states, leading to harassment and arrest for engaging in sexual acts that heterosexuals can do without fear (Swan, 1997). Since February 1994, "Don't ask, don't tell" has been the U.S. government's policy on the hiring and retention of lesbians in the military.

Although housing and employment discrimination is still allowed in most states, the move to offering domestic partner benefits appears to be growing. Unfortunately, these benefits will not be fully utilized as long as sexual orientation is excluded from job protection policies. Contrary to data used to claim that homosexuals are seeking "special rights," lesbians do not earn more than heterosexuals. Married couple households and male same-sex couples have roughly equal household incomes, while female same-sex couples bring home 18 to 20 percent less (Badgett, 1998b). This is true in spite of the fact that the most comprehensive study on U.S. lesbians to date found that most lesbians work, 69 percent have college degrees, and almost one-third have advanced degrees (Bradford, Ryan, and Rothblum, 1994). Burgess (1997) found that lesbians who work in organizations with lesbian sensitive programs are more "out" to their co-workers, socialize more with them, and use fewer prescription drugs. It seems clear that lesbian sensitive policies in the workplace may result in lower health expenditures and increased bonding, teamwork, and productivity.

Concurrent with the move toward domestic partner benefits is the drive to legalize same-sex marriage. In anticipation of legalization in Hawaii, the Defense of Marriage Act (DOMA) was signed into law by President Clinton, effectively denying federal benefits to same-sex couples and permitting states to ignore such marriages performed legally in other states. Congress and the far right have continued to be extremely reactive to the idea of same-sex marriage. Interestingly, gays and lesbians are themselves divided on the issue. Supporters include those who view marriage as the best avenue to attain the privileges and protections afforded to heterosexual couples and gay conservatives who argue that marriage supports mainstream values. The case has even been made that allowing same-sex marriages would be of considerable fiscal benefit to states (Badgett, 1998a). On the other hand, many recognize marriage as a sexist institution that could destroy the continued development of lesbian culture. For an interesting discussion of the pros and cons of "hitching the lesbian and gay agenda to the same-sex marriage star," see Hartman (1999, pp. 112-117).

Closely related to the issue of same-sex marriage is that of child custody. Although almost all states now allow adoption and fostering by same-sex couples, the process is often unnecessarily difficult. Lesbians continue to lose custody of their children on the basis of their sexual orientation, and the rights of coparents are not legally protected in most states. Many coparents who have not adopted their child are denied custody and visitation rights in the event of separation (Rothblum, 1988). Finally, many unresolved policy issues exist regarding pregnancy by alternative insemination (Barrett, 1997). Whether the donor is known or unknown, profound psychosocial issues are involved and, according to Hartman (1996), ". . . the mother, the co-parent, and the donor are embarking on a journey through a legal minefield" (p. 82).

Any discussion of social policy issues relevant to lesbian and bisexual women would be incomplete without addressing hate crime. Although data collection is quite unsophisticated, reports of physical attacks on gay men and lesbians in 1998 increased significantly over the 1,081 reported the previous year (Bull, 1999). Forty-two states have some kind of hate-crimes legislation, and twenty-one states, plus the District of Columbia, specify sexual orientation as a category for protection (Bull, 1999; Otis and Skinner, 1996). Proponents of hate-crime laws view them as deterrents while opponents note that they are difficult to prove in court, pose bothersome civil liberties issues, and can cause as much harm as good to the oppressed group.

Tremendous progress has been made in the social policy arena in the past twenty-five years, but much is yet to be accomplished. Most state legislative victories are difficult and time consuming, often complicated by well-funded antigay groups. In spite of these barriers, advocates have continued to organize for civil rights laws, recognition of homosexual family relationships, repeal of sodomy laws, increased penalties for hate crimes, and benefits for domestic partners. These efforts have resulted in an increase in the number of gay-favorable bills introduced between 1996 and 1998. In 1996, there were 61 favorable bills introduced versus 132 in 1998 (National Gay and Lesbian Task Force, 1998). It is hoped that, with time, the lesbian and bisexual women communities will be able to unite in a common struggle against heterosexist society.

PRACTICE ISSUES

Lesbians

Mental Health

Some lesbian feminists have raised concerns about all psychological therapies with lesbians. Perkins (1991) argues that, while paying lip service to the need for sociopolitical change, psychotherapy with any lesbian aims to change her and her interactions with others. Perkins views this focus on "the oppressor within" as pathologizing and victim-blaming. By reducing problems to the personal level, the powerful roles of patriarchal society and male supremacy are ignored, and energy is diverted from political activism. Contrary to this notion, Eliason and Morgan (1996) found that lesbians who had been in therapy were actually more politically oriented than lesbians who had not been in therapy. Many viewed therapy as having made them more aware of oppression as lesbians and women.

Issues presented by lesbians need to be viewed in the context of sex-role socialization, internalized homophobia, and societal oppression (Buhrke and Douce, 1991). When a lesbian in a couple relationship presents herself for treatment, couple therapy may not even be considered, although it is usually the therapy of choice; this is because lesbian clients are typically considered single and their relationships considered transient and insignificant.

Once a lesbian is in treatment, heterosexism can impede change in a number of ways (Long, 1996). Therapists may assume that all presenting problems were created by the client's sexual orientation, with little recognition of the role of societal homophobia, sexism, or other issues. They may encourage lesbians to move toward heterosexuality or may perceive lesbianism as a symptom of an underlying psychiatric problem. Some may be preoccupied with the causes of lesbianism (Riddle and Sang, 1978). Clients' self-denigrating comments about lesbians may go unchallenged. The therapist may collude with the client to "make the best of it," accept certain limitations without question, and treat same-sex relationships as though they could never be as valid or healthy as heterosexual ones (Cabaj, 1988). Therapists who are uncomfortable with a couple's closeness may label it as immature and pathological (McCandlish, 1982). Therapists concerned about establishing themselves as liberal may divert attention from clients' treatment needs by assuring them repeatedly of their positive views about lesbianism. Others may point out all the supposed lost opportunities being lesbian causes, emphasize the positive aspects of clients' heterosexual relationships and the negative aspects of their lesbian relationships, and discourage coming out to family and friends (De Crescenzo, 1984). It is not known how prevalent these behaviors are among contemporary therapists. As discussed previously, however, a recent study did indicate that a majority of social workers are heterosexist.

The attitude that sexual orientation makes no difference ignores the significance of a rejecting society (Tievsky, 1988), and being too accepting may lead to missing important issues and romanticizing the couple's out relationship. McCandlish (1982) points out that lesbian therapists are particularly prone to "idealizing the relationship, over-identifying with the couple, and becoming invested in the therapy outcome" (p. 74). The lesbian therapist may attribute all problems to societal and internalized homophobia, losing sight of important family of origin and relational issues. It is critical to recognize that age, social class, ethnicity, and race make every relationship unique.

As long as therapy is consistent with feminist ideas, collaborative, and nonhierarchical, it is likely that whatever models have proved successful in work with heterosexuals will prove helpful in work with lesbians. Certainly all therapists need to be aware of the sexist, heterosexist, and homophobic biases in the theories and models they use (Laird, 1999). It is critical to discuss with lesbian clients the relationship between oppression and psychosocial functioning. Some therapists maintain that lesbian couples should be treated by "out" lesbian therapists (Gartrell, 1984; McDermott, Tyndall, and Lichtenberg, 1989; Riddle and Sang, 1978). Bradford, Ryan, and Rothblum (1994) found that 89 percent of lesbians preferred to see a woman counselor and 66 percent preferred to see a counselor who was lesbian or gay. A recent analogue study of the effects of sexual orientation similarity and counselor experience level on perceptions by lesbians found that experienced therapists, both lesbian and heterosexual, were rated as more expert (Moran, 1992). It was suggested that the sexual orientation of the counselor may be of less concern when the therapeutic issue is not primarily related to sexual orientation. Because of the analogue nature of the study, however, the usual precautions about generalizations to actual therapy sessions must be exercised. Stein (1988) concludes that what the therapist communicates about sexual orientation is more important than actual sexual orientation and that "a therapist's unwillingness to acknowledge a personal sexual orientation may be viewed as a statement that the patient should also continue to keep his or her sexual orientation hidden from others" (p. 86).

Many issues presented by lesbian clients are identical to those presented by heterosexuals. One issue, however, the ongoing coming-out process, is unique. It is important to recognize that equating lesbian mental health with disclosure can be quite damaging to some lesbians. Severe negative consequences of coming out still exist for many lesbians, and their reluctance to do so does not necessarily reflect internalized homophobia (Hartman, 1996; Healy, 1999). It is a mistake to push clients to come out before they are ready to do so (Hartman and Laird, 1998), before they have explored all possible consequences and considered appropriate timing (Zitter, 1987). Despite the assumption that coming out to family is the most difficult, nothing indicates that lesbians come out to their families last or to siblings before parents (Radonsky and Borders, 1995). It is important that clients recognize that family members' initial responses are not necessarily their final positions (Roth and Murphy, 1986).

The decision not to disclose can also be adaptive (Kleinberg, 1986); many ways exist to achieve differentiation from one's family of origin. Some well-differentiated clients will choose not to come out to their families; their decision in this matter must be respected. Even in these cases, however, the therapist should avoid comments that could serve to solidify distance from family and preclude future connections. The life stories of lesbians are often very negative and indicative of oppression. As Laird (1994) notes, clients who are lesbian need to recognize the sources and contexts of their stories, construct new stories, and develop new interpretations of old self and social stories.

When clients are out to their parents and less reactive to them, I prefer to invite parents in for at least one session during the final stage of treatment. The purpose of such sessions is to challenge the family mythology by asking the parents to tell stories about their lives. As Freeman (1992) notes, these stories inform adult children about how events shaped their parents' responses to them and can be used as positive legacies.

It is clear that many lesbian couples get significantly more of their support from friends than from family members. This close network of friends, "families of choice," are regarded as extended family and often assume family roles with children of the lesbian couple (Erera and Fredriksen, 1999). The support of families of choice may explain, in part, the finding that the amount of family of origin support is not related to the psychological adjustment of the lesbian family member (Kurdek and Schmitt, 1987).

Historically, it has been widely accepted by researchers and clinicians that lesbians have higher rates of suicide attempts and substance abuse than heterosexual women. Saunders and Valente (1987) reported that Caucasian lesbians were two and a half times more likely to attempt suicide than were heterosexual women. And the National Lesbian Health Care Survey (NIMH, 1987) found suicide rates among black and Latina lesbians to be 27 and 28 percent respectively, higher than the 16 percent rate of white lesbians. Although studies in the 1970s and 1980s found that lesbians reported rates of alcohol consumption and problems that were significantly higher than those of heterosexual women, all of these studies were limited by serious design and methodological problems (Anderson and Henderson, 1985, 1995, 1996a, 1996b; Hughes and Wilsnack, 1997).

These findings become even more questionable in light of those showing that lesbians do not differ significantly from heterosexual women on measures of general psychological adjustment. Lesbians and heterosexual women appear to have similar rates of mental illness and childhood histories of physical and sexual abuse (Cabaj, 1988; Ross, Paulsen, and Stalstrom, 1988; Thompson, McCandless, and Strickland, 1971). It also appears that alcohol and other drug problems are decreasing in the lesbian and bisexual populations. Two recent studies found no significant differences between heterosexual and lesbian/bisexual women in drug or alcohol consumption and problems (Bloomfield, 1993; Saulnier and Miller, 1997).

Health Care

Unfortunately, many lesbians avoid routine health care because of neglect or abuse from health care providers. Out of fear, one-third do not disclose their sexual orientation to providers (Hepburn, 1988; Rothblum, 1994; Saulnier, 1999). This avoidance of care is significant because lesbian and bisexual women, like all other women, are at risk for cervical cancer and should receive routine cytological screenings. The quality of their interactions with physicians strongly influences whether they will seek this care (Mathieson, 1998; Rankow and Tessaro, 1998).

Although female-to-female sexual transmission of HIV is extremely rare, some lesbian and bisexual women engage in high-risk sexual behaviors (Perry, 1995). One study in California found that 1.2 percent of lesbians and bisexual women were infected with HIV, 10 percent reported injecting drugs on a long-term basis, and 40 percent had unprotected vaginal or anal sex with males (including males who were gay, bisexual, or injection drug users) (Lemp et al., 1995). Another study of lesbian and bisexual women found that participants were aware of the risk of contracting HIV but responded with increased testing rather than safer sex practices (Einhorn and Polgar, 1994). Lesbian and bisexual women should be aware that although Immunoglobulin A in saliva neutralizes HIV, other STDs such as herpes, hepatitis, chlamydia, syphilis, and gonorrhea can be transmitted by oral sex (Munson, 1996).

In addition to engaging in high-risk sexual behaviors, some lesbians avoid seeking essential, often lifesaving social services due to homophobia. For example, fewer than half of the abused lesbians in one study sought help from shelters for abused women; these shelters were viewed as unresponsive to the needs of lesbians (Browning, Reynolds, and Dworkin, 1991; Schilit et al., 1991). This is not an insignificant problem in the lesbian community; a recent study (Scherzer, 1998) found that 17 percent of lesbian respondents reported experiencing physical abuse during their current or most recent relationships, and 31 percent reported experiencing emotional abuse. No differences were evident between racial groups in seeking help for the abuse.

Lesbian Couples

Much of the clinical literature on lesbian couples focuses on the concepts of fusion, merging, or enmeshment (Burch, 1982, 1986, 1987; Decker, 1984; Krestan and Bepko, 1980). Mencher (1990) notes how patterns of intimacy in lesbian couples have been pathologized as fusion and reviews theories about the sources of these dynamics. (For more information, see Anderson, 1994; Berg-Cross, 1988; Bograd, 1988; Elise, 1986; Goodrich et al., 1988; Green, 1990; Laird, 1993; Lindenbaum, 1985; McKenzie, 1992; Pearlman, 1989; Roth, 1989; Slater and Mencher, 1991; and Zacks, Green, and Morrow, 1988.)

Mencher concludes that the relationship characteristics most valued by lesbian couples are those that would be labeled as "fused" and that enduring lesbian relationships are characterized by fusion. She quotes Benjamin (1988) on how psychoanalytic thought may have distorted our understanding of intimacy: "The classic psychoanalytic viewpoint did not see differentiation as a balance, but a process of disentanglement. Thus it cast experiences of union, merger, and self-other harmony as regressive opposites to differentiation and self-other distinction. Merging was a dangerous form of undifferentiation" (pp. 46-47).

Bowen (1978) has been unfairly criticized for devaluing the "feminine" relationship orientation and overvaluing separateness and autonomy. In fact, he repeatedly emphasized the importance of balance, viewing a fused and reactive emotional position, not a relationship orientation, as problematic. As Walsh and Scheinkman (1989) point out, poorly differentiated people are dominated by their emotions and are overdependent on others, either too closely fused, reactively distanced, or cut off from their families. Differentiation always involves the maintenance of self in *relation to* one's family, being *both* separate and connected. Autonomy and intimacy are equally valued and not mutually exclusive (Nelson, 1989).

Pearlman (1989) believes that intense emotional bonding occurs in most relationships to varying degrees. In some, it is present mainly during sexual or emotional closeness. In others, "it is a normative preference for intense connection which can include some loss of individuality" (Pearlman, 1989, p. 78). In still others, it is more permanent and includes excessive dependency and loss of self. Intense bonding may occur more easily in lesbian relationships because of similar socialization, joining forces against a hostile world, or many other reasons. When it is excessive, couples complain of feeling trapped, bored, or overwhelmed by conflict or involvement in outside affairs. But extreme closeness is not in itself pathological (Falco, 1991), and it is even possible that what is normative for lesbian couples may be healthy for all couples (Brown, 1989). In my experience, the intense emotional connection experienced by lesbian couples is indeed the most valued aspect of their relationship.

Recent studies cast doubt on the widespread belief that lesbians are more prone to fusion in relationships than are heterosexual women. Pardie and Herb (1997) found that nonclinical samples of lesbians and heterosexual women did not differ significantly on dependency, autonomy, or similar sharing behaviors believed to be linked to merger. And Greene, Causby, and Miller (1999) found that no differences existed between lesbian and heterosexual women's levels of fusion and that fusion was strongly related to both dependence and satisfaction.

Another myth specific to lesbianism is the reputed drop-off in sexual activity between couples knows as "lesbian bed death." Iasenza (1999) notes, "I find it interesting how, just as we got over the merging problem, we suddenly got the 'bed death' problem. Do we have a problem not having a problem?" (p. 9). She notes that there are inevitable shifts in sexual passion in many long-term relationships, that this is not a lesbian phenomenon. In summarizing the research in this area, Iasenza finds little evidence that lesbian sexuality is less active or fulfilling than gay or heterosexual sex. Lesbian couples value nongenital contact, such as touching and hugging, as not only part of other sexual activity but as ends in themselves. Lesbian couples take more time having sex and are more orgasmic than heterosexual women. Overall, lesbians are more sexually assertive, more sexually arousable, more communicative about their sexual needs and desires, and more satisfied with the quality of their sexual lives than are heterosexual women (Iasenza, 1999).

Bisexual Women

The literature pertaining to practice with bisexual women is extremely limited. Some women who are just beginning to face their bisexuality may enter counseling because of their confusion and only need permission and support to accept their authentic self and create a lifestyle that fits their unique needs (Matteson, 1996). The coming-out process may be particularly difficult, and they may eventually be excluded from lesbian communities. They are a very diverse group—some come out as lesbians and then as bisexuals, some change from a heterosexual to bisexual identity, and some have always identified as bisexual. Some have sexual relationships exclusively with women or men, but identify as bisexual on the basis of their desires. Still others may be celibate or have ongoing relationships with both women and men concurrently. Bisexual women of color face the added burden of fighting racism as well as discrimination on the basis of their bisexuality (Weasel, 1996).

Lesbian Women of Color

As mentioned previously, research on lesbians has focused primarily on white middle-class respondents. According to Hartman and Laird (1998):

> . . . there are enormous differences within and between sexual minorities. Differences exist on the basis of gender, race, ethnicity, locality, age, life experience, and the extent of involvement in a sexual minority community or subculture; there are, in fact, multiple lesbian and gay cultures and communities with very different characters. (p. 272)

These differences must be kept in mind when attempting to work with lesbians of color in culturally sensitive ways. There are relatively few empirical studies which include ethnic minority lesbians;

they include primarily those who are African American, Native American, Asian American, and Latina.

In summarizing studies to date that include African-American lesbians, Greene and Boyd-Franklin (1996) state that, when compared to their white counterparts, African-American lesbians are more likely to have children, maintain closeness to their families, and have more contact with men and heterosexual peers. They are also more reluctant to seek professional help. Many view their African-American community as extremely homophobic. This may be due to the perceived threat of nonreproductive sexual practices (Kanuha, 1990), the selective interpretations of biblical scripture, the need to hold on to heterosexuality as their only privileged status, or other factors. Conflicting loyalties between African-American and mainstream lesbian communities are complicated by the racial discrimination experienced in the latter.

Native American lesbians also experience racism in the mainstream lesbian community. Because of colonization, genocide, and loss of traditional values and customs, their own community is also less accepting of them than were their ancestors. When younger lesbians leave the reservation to find other lesbians, the loss of support from their family and community can be devastating. They report higher rates of heterosexual experiences, demonstrating a more fluid notion of sexual expression, than their white and other ethnic counterparts (Tafoya, 1992).

Asian-American lesbians come from many different ethnic groups, but most research has been done on those of Japanese and Chinese ancestry. Women from these cultures derive status from their roles as dutiful daughters, wives, and mothers—and are blamed if their daughters do not conform. Sexual orientation is viewed as volitional, with a lesbian or bisexual identity seen as a conscious choice to shame the family or, at best, a temporary disorder that will be outgrown. Asian-American lesbians have loyalty conflicts similar to those observed in other ethnic groups; interestingly, many see their primary identification as lesbian rather than Asian American (Chan, 1992).

Latina lesbians are part of a culture in which women are expected to be sexually naive and extremely submissive to men (Espin, 1987; Morales, 1992). Morales (1992) suggests that the heterosexist oppression in Latin culture is extreme and that lesbianism is experienced as a betrayal of the culture and family. Trujillo (1991) states that most Chicano heterosexuals see Chicana lesbians as a threat to male dominance. They fear that lesbians could raise the consciousness of other Chicana women such that they could begin to question female subordination. Although families may deny or tolerate a lesbian orientation, they rarely accept it. In spite of this, Latina lesbians remain deeply attached to their families and communities (Espin, 1987).

Lesbians of color, according to Greene (1994b), ". . . frequently experience a sense of never being part of any group completely, leaving them at greater risk for isolation, feelings of estrangement, and increased psychological vulnerability" (p. 414). The prejudice they experience from health care providers regarding sexual orientation, race, gender, and sometimes class, serves to intensify their vulnerability (Stevens, 1998). But as Greene (1994b) points out, they bring considerable resilience to this challenge. Unlike white lesbians, they have learned valuable coping mechanisms against racism which can be called on as needed to deal with homophobia and heterosexism.

CONCLUSIONS

Bisexuals and lesbians who are of color, poor, or disabled are extremely under researched (Greene, 1994a). Mallon (1998) makes the point that:

> It takes a substantial budget to conduct research, and many of us use our own money to fund it. It's no wonder that white, middle-class, gay men, who are more likely to have money than lesbians or queers of color, are doing most of the research, and that the research we have often reflects our biases. (p. 25)

It is critical that future research continues to inform social policy, practice, and social work education. A great need exists for more training and education about gay and lesbian issues for social workers (Berkman and Zinberg, 1997; Greene, Bettinger, and Zacks, 1996), and, in fact, the Council on Social Work Education's (CSWE) Curriculum Policy Statement requires all accredited schools of social work to include such content (CSWE, 1994). The reader is referred to Stein and Burg (1996) for a discussion of relevant knowledge, skills, and attitudes that students must master in this area. The effectiveness of professional education in reducing homophobic attitudes is not clear. Some studies show no association between education and attitudes (Berkman and Zinberg, 1997), whereas others suggest that classes do reduce homophobia (Cramer, Oles, and Black, 1997). Cramer (1997) found that social work students' attitudes influenced their anticipated professional behavior (APB) toward gay and lesbian clients but found no significant differences in APB between students who received an educational intervention on attitudes and those who did not. Oles, Black, and Cramer (1999) found that having gay or lesbian friends exerted a significantly positive effect on APB. They conclude that:

> . . . social work education should not be satisfied with attitude change as an educational outcome in and of itself. Attitude is, at best, a necessary precondition for professional behavior with gay men and lesbian clients, but it is not sufficient to ensure such behavior. Social work education should focus on changing behavior as well as changing attitudes . . . the profession needs to develop standards for practice with gay men and lesbian clients. (p. 97)

The high use of counseling by lesbians has been noted in a number of studies (Bradford, Ryan, and Rothblum, 1994; Morgan, 1992). Thus, an even greater imperative exists for social workers to learn about the diversity, special issues, and resiliencies of the lesbian population. A focus on resiliency, empowering people to discover their strengths and resources, is consistent with a feminist worldview and provides a useful paradigm to guide work with lesbians and other oppressed groups (Levy, 1995). As a result of oppression, many lesbians have developed strong resiliencies over time (Anderson and Sussex, 1999). As Stewart (1994) notes, no one is ever only oppressed. Finally, social work educators would do well to incorporate the findings of Kanuha's (1998) study into their human behavior and practice courses. Her research raises serious questions about linear stage models of identity development and challenges us to integrate multiple self-representations into various human development models. For many lesbian clients, "passing" can be reframed as a stigma management strategy, an act of resistance rather than a reflection of assimilation, passivity, or internalized homophobia. Kanuha's study demonstrates that lesbians are inherently resourceful and resilient in the face of oppression. She concludes by stating:

> If in ten years another study is conducted on stigma, identity, and passing that suggests gay men, lesbians, women, the poor, immigrants, people with disabilities and so many others at the margins need not conceal, omit, dissociate, distance or play with the audience to protect themselves from social sanctions, we will have accomplished the promise of what social workers and the profession can and always should be: agents for social change. (p. 263)

REFERENCES

Anderson, S. C. (1994). A critical analysis of the concept of co-dependency. *Social Work, 39:* 677-685.

Anderson, S. C. (1995). Alcohol abuse. *Encyclopedia of social work.* (pp. 203-215). Washington, DC: NASW Press.

Anderson, S. C. (1996a). Addressing heterosexist bias in the treatment of lesbian couples with chemical dependency. *Journal of Feminist Family Therapy,* 7(3/4): pp. 87-113.

Anderson, S. C. (1996b). Substance abuse and dependency in gay men and lesbians. *Journal of Gay and Lesbian Social Services,* 5(1): 59-76.

Anderson, S. C. and Sussex, B. (1999). Resilience in lesbians: An exploratory study. In J. Laird (Ed.), *Lesbians and lesbian families* (pp. 305-329). New York: Columbia University Press.

Ault, A. (1996). Ambiguous identity in an unambiguous sex/gender structure: The case of bisexual women. *Sociological Quarterly, 37:* 449-463.

Badgett, M. V. L. (1998a). The fiscal impact on the state of Vermont of allowing same-sex couples to marry. *Institute for Gay and Lesbian Strategic Studies,* Technical Report 98-1 (pp. 1-8). Amherst, MA: IGLSS.

Badgett, M. V. L. (1998b). Income inflation. *Institute for Gay and Lesbian Strategic Studies* (pp. 1-23). Amherst, MA: IGLSS.

Bailey, J. M. and Benishay, D. S. (1993). Familial aggregation of female sexual orientation. *American Journal of Psychiatry, 150:* 272-277.

Barrett, S. E. (1997). Children of lesbian parents: The what, when and how of talking about donor identity. *Women and Therapy,* 20(2): 43-55.

Bell, A., Weinberg, M., and Hammersmith, S. (1981). *Sexual preference: Its development in men and women.* Bloomington, IN: Indiana University Press.

Benjamin, J. (1988). *The bonds of love: Psychoanalysis, feminism and the problem of domination.* New York: Pantheon.

Berg-Cross, L. (1988). Lesbians, family process and individuation. *Journal of College Student Psychotherapy, 3*(1): 97-112.

Berkman, C. S. and Zinberg, G. (1997). Homophobia and heterosexism in social workers. *Social Work, 42:* 319-332.

Black, B., Oles, T. P., and Moore, L. (1998). The relationship between attitudes: Homophobia and sexism among social work students. *Affiliate, 13*(2): 166-189.

Blackford, L., Doty, S., and Pollack, R. (1996). Differences in subjective sexual arousal in heterosexual, bisexual, and lesbian women. *The Canadian Journal of Human Sexuality, 5*(3): 157-167.

Bloomfield, K. (1993). A comparison of alcohol consumption between lesbians and heterosexual women in an urban population. *Drug and Alcohol Dependence, 33:* 257-269.

Blumstein, P. and Schwartz, P. (1983). *American couples: Money, work, sex.* New York: William Morrow.

Bograd, M. (1988). Enmeshment, fusion or relatedness? A conceptual analysis. In L. Braverman (Ed.), *Women, feminism, and family therapy* (pp. 65-80). Binghamton, NY: The Haworth Press.

Bowen, M. (1978). *Family therapy in clinical practice.* Northvale, NJ: Aronson.

Bradford, J., Ryan, C., and Rothblum, E. D. (1994). National lesbian health care survey: Implications for mental health care. *Journal of Consulting and Clinical Psychology, 62:* 228-242.

Brown, L. S. (1989). New voices, new visions: Toward a lesbian/gay paradigm for psychology. *Psychology of Women Quarterly, 13:* 445-456.

Browning, C., Reynolds, A. L., and Dworkin, S. H. (1991). Affirmative psychotherapy for lesbian women. *The Counseling Psychologist, 191:* 177-196.

Buhrke, R. A. and Douce, L. A. (1991). Training issues for counseling psychologists in working with lesbian women and gay men. *Counseling Psychologist, 19:* 216-234.

Bull, C. (1999). The state of hate. *The Advocate* (April): 23-31.

Burch, B. (1982). Psychological merger in lesbian couples: A joint ego psychological and systems approach. *Family Therapy, 9:* 201-208.

Burch, B. (1986). Psychotherapy and the dynamics of merger in lesbian couples. In T. S. Stein and C. J. Cohen (Eds.), *Contemporary perspectives on psychotherapy with lesbians and gay men* (pp. 57-71). New York: Plenum.

Burch, B. (1987). Barriers to intimacy: Conflicts over power, dependence, and nurturing. In Boston Lesbian Psychologies Collective (Ed.), *Lesbian psychologies: Explorations and challenges* (pp. 126-141). Urbana, IL: University of Illinois Press.

Burch, B. (1993). *On intimate terms: The psychology of difference in lesbian relationships.* Chicago, IL: University of Chicago Press.

Burgess, C. A. (1997). The impact of lesbian/gay sensitive policies on the behavior and health of lesbians in the workplace. In W. Swan (Ed.), *Gay/lesbian/bisex-*

ual/transgender public policy issues (pp. 35-47). Binghamton, NY: Harrington Park Press.

Cabaj, R. P. (1988). Homosexuality and neurosis: Considerations for psychotherapy. *Journal of Homosexuality, 15:* 13-23.

Cass, V. C. (1979). Homosexual identity formation: A theoretical model. *Journal of Homosexuality, 4:* 219-235.

Chan, C. (1992). Cultural considerations in counseling Asian-American lesbians and gay men. In S. Dworkin and F. Gutierrez (Eds.), *Counseling gay men and lesbians* (pp. 115-124). Alexandria, VA: American Association for Counseling and Development.

Chodorow, N. (1992). Heterosexuality as a compromise formation: Reflections on the psychoanalytic theory of sexual development. *Psychoanalysis and Contemporary Thought, 15:* 267-302.

Coleman, E. (1982). Developmental stages of the coming-out process. *Journal of Homosexuality, 7:* 31-43.

Council on Social Work Education (CSWE) (1994). *Handbook of accreditation standards and procedures.* Alexandria, VA: Author.

Cramer, E. P. (1997). Effects of an educational unit about lesbian identity development and disclosure in a social work methods course. *Journal of Social Work Education, 33:* 461-472.

Cramer, E., Oles, T. P., and Black, B. M. (1997). Reducing social work students' homophobia: An evaluation of teaching strategies. *Arete, 21:* 36-49.

Crocker, J. and Major, B. (1989). Social stigma and self-esteem: The self-protective properties of stigma. *Psychological Review, 96:* 608-630.

D'Augelli, A. R. (1994). Lesbian and gay male development. In B. Greene and G. Herek (Eds.), *Lesbian and gay psychology* (pp. 118-132). Thousand Oaks, CA: Sage.

Decker, B. (1984). Counseling gay and lesbian couples. *Journal of Social Work and Human Sexuality, 2:* 39-52.

De Crescenzo, T. (1984). Homophobia: A study of the attitudes of mental health professionals toward homosexuality. *Journal of Social Work and Human Sexuality, 2:* 115-136,

Einhorn, L. and Polgar, M. (1994). HIV-risk behavior among lesbians and bisexual women. *AIDS Education and Prevention, 6:* 514-523.

Eldridge, N. S. and Gilbert, L. A. (1990). Correlates of relationship satisfaction in lesbian couples. *Psychology of Women Quarterly, 14:* 43-62.

Eliason, M. J. and Morgan, K. S. (1996). The relationship between therapy usage and political activity in lesbians. *Women and Therapy, 19:* 31-45.

Elise, D. (1986). Lesbian couples: The implications of sex differences in separation-individuation. *Psychotherapy, 23:* 305-310.

Erera, P. I. and Fredriksen, K. (1999). Lesbian stepfamilies: A unique family structure. *Families in Society, 80:* 263-270.

Ernulf, K. E., Innala, S. M., and Whitam, F. L. (1989). Biological explanation, psychological explanation, and tolerance of homosexuals: A cross-national analysis of beliefs and attitudes. *Psychological Reports, 65:* 1003-1010.

Espin, O. (1987). Issues of identity in the psychology of Latina lesbians. In Boston Lesbian Psychologies Collective (Ed.), *Lesbian psychologies: Explorations and challenges* (pp. 35-51). Urbana, IL: University of Illinois Press.

Falco, K. L. (1991). *Psychotherapy with lesbian clients: Theory into practice.* New York: Brunner/Mazel.

Fassinger, R. E. (1991). The hidden minority: Issues and challenges in working with lesbian women and gay men. *The Counseling Psychologist, 19:* 157-176.

Fox, R. C. (1995). Bisexual identities. In A. R. D'Augelli and C. J. Patterson (Eds.), *Lesbian, gay, and bisexual identities over the lifespan: Psychological perspective* (pp. 48-86). New York: Oxford University Press.

Fredriksen, K. (1999). Family caregiving responsibilities among lesbians and gay men. *Social Work, 44:* 142-155.

Freeman, D. S. (1992). *Family therapy with couples.* Northvale, NJ: Aronson.

Garnets, L. and Kimmel, D. (1991). Lesbian and gay male dimensions in the psychological study of human diversity. In J. D. Goodchilds (Ed.), *Psychological perspectives on human diversity in America* (pp. 137-192). Washington, DC: American Psychological Association.

Gartrell, N. (1984). Issues in psychotherapy with lesbian women. *Work in progress* No. 83-04 (pp. 1-12). Wellesley, MA: Wellesley College, Stone Center for Developmental Services and Studies. Monograph.

Glassgold, J. M. (1992). New directions in dynamic theories of lesbianism: From psychoanalysis to social constructionism. In J. C. Chrisler and D. Howard (Eds.), *New directions in feminist psychology* (pp. 154-164). New York: Springer Publishing Company.

Goffman, E. (1963). *Stigma: Notes on the management of spoiled identity.* New York: Simon and Schuster.

Golden, C. (1987). Diversity and variability in women's sexual identities. In Boston Lesbian Psychologies Collective (Ed.), *Lesbian psychologies: Explorations and challenges* (pp. 18-34). Urbana, IL: University of Illinois Press.

Golombok, S., Spencer, A., and Rutter, M. (1983). Children in lesbian and single-parent households: Psychosexual and psychiatric appraisal. *Journal of Child Psychology and Psychiatry, 24:* 551-572.

Gonsiorek, J. C. and Rudolph, J. R. (1991). Homosexual identity: Coming out and other developmental events. In J. C. Gonsiorek and J. D. Weinrich (Eds.), *Homosexuality: Research implications for public policy* (pp. 161-176). Newburg Park, CA: Sage.

Goodrich, T. J., Rampage, C., Ellman, B., and Halstead, K. (1988). The lesbian couple. In T. J. Goodrich, C. Rampage, B. Ellman, and K. Halstead (Eds.), *Feminist family therapy: A casebook* (pp. 143-159). New York: Norton.

Green, G. D. (1990). Is separation really so great? *Women and Therapy, 9:* 87-104.

Green, R. J., Bettinger, M., and Zacks, E. (1996). Are lesbian couples fused and gay male couples disengaged? In J. Laird and R. J. Green (Eds.), *Lesbians and gay couples and families* (pp. 185-230). San Francisco, CA: Jossey-Bass.

Greene, B. (1994a). Ethnic-minority lesbians and gay men: Mental health and treatment issues. *Journal of Consulting and Clinical Psychology, 62:* 243-251.

Greene, B. (1994b). Lesbian women of color: Triple jeopardy. In L. Comas-Diaz and B. Greene (Eds.), *Women of color: Integrating ethnic and gender identities in psychotherapy* (pp. 389-427). New York: Guilford Press.

Greene, B. and Boyd-Franklin, N. (1996). African-American lesbian couples: Ethnocultural considerations in psychotherapy. *Women and Therapy, 19:* 44-60.

Greene, K., Causby, V., and Miller, D. H. (1999). The nature and function of fusion in the dynamics of lesbian relationships. *Affilia, 14:* 78-97.

Hare, J. (1994). Concerns and issues faced by families headed by a lesbian couple. *Families in Society, 75:* 27-35.

Hare, J. and Richards, L. (1993). Children raised by lesbian couples: Does context of birth affect father and partner involvement. *Family Relations, 42:* 249-256.

Hartman, A. (1996). Social policy as a context for lesbian and gay families. In J. Laird and R. J. Green (Eds.), *Lesbians and gays in couples and families* (pp. 69-85). San Francisco, CA: Jossey-Bass.

Hartman, A. (1999). The long road to equality: Lesbians and social policy. In J. Laird (Ed.), *Lesbians and lesbian families* (pp. 91-120). New York: Columbia University Press.

Hartman, A. and Laird, J. (1998). Moral and ethical issues in working with lesbians and gay men. *Families in Society, 79:* 263-276.

Healy, T. (1999). A struggle for language: Patterns of self-disclosure in lesbian couples. In J. Laird (Ed.), *Lesbians and lesbian families* (pp. 123 -141). New York: Columbia University Press.

Hepburn, C. (1988). *Alive and well: A lesbian health guide.* Freedom, CA: Crossing.

Herek, G. M. (1994). Assessing heterosexuals' attitudes toward lesbians and gay men. In B. Greene and G. M. Herek (Eds.), *Lesbian and gay psychology: Theory, research and clinical applications* (pp. 206-228). Newbury Park, CA: Sage.

Hopkins, J. (1969). The lesbian personality. *British Journal of Psychiatry, 115:* 1433-1436.

Hughes, T. L. and Wilsnack, S. C. (1997). Use of alcohol among lesbians: Research and clinical implications. *American Journal of Orthopsychiatry, 67:* 20-36.

Iasenza, S. (1999). The big lie: Debunking lesbian bed death. *In the Family* (April): 9-25.

Jourard, S. M. (1958). Some factors in self-disclosure. *Journal of Abnormal Psychology, 56:* 91-98.

Kanuha, V. (1990). Compounding the triple jeopardy: Battering in lesbian of color relationships. *Women and Therapy, 9:* 169-183.

Kanuha, V. (1998). *Stigma, identity, and passing: How lesbians and gay men of color construct and manage stigmatized identity in social interaction.* Unpublished doctoral dissertation, University of Washington, Seattle. Used by permission of the author.

Kinsey, A. C., Pomeroy, W. B., Martin, C. E., and Gebbhard, P. H. (1953). *Sexual behavior in the human female.* Philadelphia, PA: W. B. Saunders.

Kirkpatrick, M. (1987). Clinical implications of lesbian mother studies. *Journal of Homosexuality, 14:* 201-211.

Klein, F. (1993). *The bisexual option,* Second edition. Binghamton, NY: Harrington Park Press.

Kleinberg, L. (1986). Coming home to self, going home to parents: Lesbian identity disclosure. *Work in progress* (pp. 1-16). Wellesley, MA: Stone Center for Developmental Services and Studies. Monograph.

Krestan, J. (1988). Lesbian daughters and lesbians mothers: The crisis of disclosure from a family systems perspective. In L. Braverman (Ed.), *Women, feminism, and family therapy* (pp. 113-130). Binghamton, NY: The Haworth Press.

Krestan, J. A. and Bepko, C. S. (1980). The problem of fusion in the lesbian relationship. *Family Process, 19:* 277-289.

Kurdek, L. A. and Schmitt, J. P. (1987). Perceived emotional support from family and friends in members of homosexual, married, and heterosexual cohabiting couples. *Journal of Homosexuality, 14:* 57-68.

Laird, J. (1993). Lesbian and gay families. In F. Walsh (Ed.), *Normal family processes,* Second edition (pp. 282-328). New York: Guilford Press.

Laird, J. (1994). Lesbian families: A cultural perspective. In M. P. Mirkin (Ed.), *Women in context* (pp. 118-148). New York: Guilford Press.

Laird, J. (1995). Changing women's narratives: Taking back the discourse. In L. Davis (Ed.), *Building on women's strengths: An agenda for the twenty-first century* (pp. 179-210). Binghamton, NY: The Haworth Press.

Laird, J. (1996a). Family-centered practice with lesbian and gay families. *Families in Society, 77:* 559-572.

Laird, J. (1996b). Invisible ties: Lesbians and their families of origin. In J. Laird and R. J. Green (Eds.), *Lesbians and gays in couples and families* (pp. 89-122). San Francisco, CA: Jossey-Bass.

Laird, J. (1999). Gender and sexuality in lesbian relationships. In J. Laird (Ed.), *Lesbians and lesbian families* (pp. 47-89). New York: Columbia University Press.

LaSala, M. C. (1998). Coupled gay men, parents, and in-laws: Intergenerational disapproval and the need for a thick skin. *Families in Society, 79:* 585-593.

La Torre, R. A. and Wendenberg, K. (1983). Psychological characteristics of bisexual, heterosexual, and homosexual women. *Journal of Homosexuality, 9:* 87-97.

Lemp, G. F., Jones, M., Kellogg, T. A., Nieri, G. N., Anderson, L., Withum, D., and Katz, M. (1995). HIV seroprevalence and risk behaviors among lesbians and bisexual women in San Francisco and Berkeley, California. *American Journal of Public Health, 85:* 1549-1552.

Levy, E. (1992). Strengthening the coping resources of lesbian families. *Families in Society: The Journal of Contemporary Human Services, 73:* 23-31.

Levy, E. (1995). Feminist social work practice with lesbian and gay clients. In N. Van Den Bergh (Ed.), *Feminist practice in the twenty-first century* (pp. 278-294). Washington, DC: NASW.

Lewis, L. A. (1984). The coming-out process for lesbians: Integrating a stable identity. *Social Work, 29:* 464-469.

Lindenbaum, J. P. (1985). The shattering of an illusion: The problem of competition in lesbian relationships. *Feminist Studies, 11:* 85-103.

Loewenstein, S. F. (1984/1985). On the diversity of love object orientations among women. *Journal of Social Work and Human Sexuality, 3:* 7-24.

Long, J. K. (1996). Working with lesbians, gays, and bisexuals: Addressing heterosexism in supervision. *Family Process, 35:* 377-388.

Mallon, G. P. (1998). Are some queers statistically insignificant? *In the Family (October):* 25. Reprinted by permission.

Margolies, L., Becker, M., and Jackson-Brewer, K. (1987). Internalized homophobia: Identifying and treating the oppressor within. In Boston Lesbian Psychologies Collective (Ed.), *Lesbian psychologies: Explorations and challenge* (pp. 229-241). Chicago, IL: University of Illinois Press.

Marmor, J. (1998). Homosexuality: Is etiology really important? *Journal of Gay and Lesbian Psychotherapy, 2:* 19-28.

Mathieson, C. M. (1998). Lesbian and bisexual health care. *Canadian Family Physician, 44:* 1634-1640.

Matteson, D. R. (1996). Psychotherapy with bisexual individuals. In R. P. Cabaj and T. S. Stein (Eds.), *Textbook of homosexuality and mental health* (pp. 433-450). Washington, DC: American Psychiatric Press.

McCandlish, B. M. (1982). Therapeutic issues with lesbian couples. *Journal of Homosexuality, 7:* 71-78.

McDermott, D., Tyndall, L., and Lichtenberg, J. W. (1989). Factors relating to counselor preference among gays and lesbians. *Journal of Counseling and Development, 68:* 31-35.

McKenzie, S. (1992). Merger in lesbian relationships. *Women and Therapy, 12:* 151-160.

Mencher, J. (1990). Intimacy in lesbian relationships: A critical reexamination of fusion. *Work in Progress* No. 42. Wellesley, MA: Wellesley College, Stone Center for Developmental Services and Studies. Monograph.

Morales, E. (1992). Latino gays and Latina lesbians. In S. Dworkin and F. Gutierrez (Eds.), *Counseling gay men and lesbians: Journey to the end of the rainbow* (pp. 125-139). Alexandria, VA: American Association for Counseling and Development.

Moran, M. R. (1992). Effects of sexual orientation similarity and counselor experience level on gay men and lesbians' perceptions of counselors. *Journal of Counseling Psychology, 39:* 247-251.

Morgan, K. (1992). Caucasian lesbians' use of psychotherapy: A matter of attitude? *Psychology of Women Quarterly, 16:* 127-130.

Moses, A. E. (1978). *Identity management in lesbian women.* New York: Praeger.

Munson, M. (1996). Eliminating the barriers to communication: Safer sex education for lesbians and bisexual women. *Women and Therapy, 19:* 75-84.

Murphy, B. C. (1989). Lesbian couples and their parents: The effects of perceived parental attitudes on the couple. *Journal of Counseling and Development, 68:* 46-51.

National Gay and Lesbian Task Force (1998). *Capital gains and losses: A state of the states report on gay, lesbian, bisexual, transgender, and HIV/AIDS-related legislation.* Washington, DC: Author.

National Institute of Mental Health (NIMH) (1987). *National lesbian health care survey.* Washington, DC: U.S. Department of Health and Human Services.

Nelson, T. S. (1989). Differentiation in clinical and non-clinical women. *Journal of Feminist Family Therapy, 1:* 49-62.

Newman, B. S. and Muzzonigro, P. G. (1993). The effects of traditional family values on the coming out process of gay men adolescents. *Adolescence, 28:* 213-226.

Nichols, M. and Lieblum, S. (1986). Lesbianism as a personal identity and social role: A model. *Affilia, 1:* 48-59.

Oles, T. P., Black, B. M., and Cramer, E. P. (1999). From attitude change to effective practice: Exploring the relationship. *Journal of Social Work Education, 35:* 87-100. Reprinted by permission.

Otis, M. D. and Skinner, W. F. (1996). The prevalence of victimization and its effect on mental well-being among lesbian and gay people. *Journal of Homosexuality, 30:* 93-121.

Pardie, L. and Herb, C. R. (1997). Merger and fusion in lesbian relationships: A problem of diagnosing what's wrong in terms of what's right. *Women and Therapy, 20:* 51-61.

Patterson, C. (1992). Children of lesbian and gay parents. *Child Development, 63:* 1025-1042.

Patterson, C. J. (1996). Lesbian mothers and their children. In J. Laird and R. J. Green (Eds.), *Lesbians and gays in couples and families* (pp. 420-437). San Francisco, CA: Jossey-Bass.

Pearlman, S. F. (1989). Distancing and connectedness: Impact on couple formation in lesbian relationships. *Women and Therapy, 8:* 77-88.

Peplau, L. A. (1991). Lesbian and gay relationships. In J. C. Gonsiorek and J. D. Weinrich (Eds.), *Homosexuality: Research implications for public policy* (pp. 177-196). Newberry Park, CA: Sage Publications.

Peplau, L., Cochran, S., Rook, K., and Padesky, C. (1978). Loving women: Attachment and autonomy in lesbian relationships. *Journal of Social Issues, 34:* 84-100.

Perkins, R. (1991). Therapy for lesbians? The case against. *Feminism and Psychology, 1:* 325-338.

Perry, S. M. (1995). Lesbian alcohol and marijuana use: Correlates of HIV risk behaviors and abusive relationships. *Journal of Psychoactive Drugs, 27:* 413-419.

Pharr, S. (1988). *Homophobia: A weapon of sexism.* Inverness, CA: Chardon.

Ponse, B. (1978). *Identities in the lesbian world.* Westport, CT: Greenwood.

Poverny, L. M. and Finch, W. A. (1988). Gay and lesbian partners: Expanding the definition of the family. *Social Casework, 69:* 116-121.

Radonsky, V. E. and Borders, L. D. (1995). Factors influencing lesbians' direct disclosure of their sexual orientation. *Journal of Gay and Lesbian Psychotherapy, 2:* 1737.

Rankow, E. J. and Tessaro, I. (1998). Cervical cancer risk and Papanicolaou screening in a sample of lesbian and bisexual women. *Journal of Family Practice, 47:* 139-143.

Rich, A. (1980). Compulsory heterosexuality and lesbian existence. *Signs, 5:* 631-660.

Riddle, D. I. and Sang, B. (1978). Psychotherapy with lesbians. *Journal of Social Issues, 34:* 84-100.

Rosen, W. B. (1992). On the integration of sexuality: Lesbians and their mothers. *Work in progress* (pp. 1- 12). Wellesley, MA: Stone Center for Developmental Services and Studies. Monograph.

Ross, M. W., Paulsen, J. A., and Stalstrom, O. W. (1988). Homosexuality and mental health: A cross-cultural review. *Journal of Homosexuality, 15: 131-152.*

Roth, S. (1989). Psychotherapy with lesbian couples: Individual issues, female socialization, and the social context. In M. McGoldrick, C. M. Anderson, and F. Walsh (Eds.), *Women in families: A framework for family therapy* (pp. 286-307). New York: Norton.

Roth, S. and Murphy, B. C. (1986). Therapeutic work with lesbian clients: A systemic therapy view. In M. Ault-Riche and J. C. Hansen (Eds.), *Women and family therapy* (pp. 78-89). Rockville, MD: Aspen Systems.

Rothberg, B. and Ubell, V. (1985). The co-existence of system theory and feminism in working with heterosexual and lesbian couples. *Women and Therapy, 4:* 1936.

Rothblum, E. (1988). Introduction: Lesbianism as a model of a positive lifestyle for women. *Women and Therapy, 8:* 1-12.

Rothblum, E. D. (1994). I only read about myself on bathroom walls: The need for research on the mental health of lesbians and gay men. *Journal of Consulting and Clinical Psychology, 62:* 213-220.

Rudolph, J. (1988). Counselors' attitudes toward homosexuality: A selective review of the literature. *Journal of Counseling and Development, 67:* 165-168.

Rust, P. C. (1992). The politics of sexual identity: Sexual attraction and behavior among lesbian and bisexual women. *Social Problems, 39:* 366-386.

Rust, P. C. (1993a). "Coming out" in the age of social constructionism: Sexual identity formation among lesbian and bisexual women. *Gender and Society, 7:* 50-77.

Rust, P. C. (1993b). Neutralizing the political threat of the marginal woman: Lesbians' beliefs about bisexual women. *Journal of Sex Research, 30:* 214-228.

Saulnier, C. F. (1999). Choosing a health care provider: A community survey of what is important to lesbians. *Families in Society, 80:* 254-262.

Saulnier, C. F. and Miller, B. A. (1997). Drug and alcohol problems: Heterosexual compared to lesbian and bisexual women. *The Canadian Journal of Human Sexuality, 6:* 221-231.

Saunders, J. M. and Valente, S. A. (1987). Suicide risk among gay men and lesbians: A review. *Death Studies, 11:* 1-23.

Scasta, D. (1998). Issues in helping people come out. *Journal of Gay and Lesbian Psychotherapy, 2:* 87-98.

Scherzer, T. (1998). Domestic violence in lesbian relationships: Findings of the lesbian relationships research project. *Journal of Lesbian Studies, 2:* 29-47.

Schilit, R., Lie, G. Y., Bush, J., Montagne, M., and Reyes, L. (1991). Intergenerational transmission of violence in lesbian relationships. *Affilia, 6:* 72-87.

Shuster, R. (1987). Sexuality as a continuum: The bisexual identity. In Boston Lesbian Psychologies Collective (Ed.), *Lesbian psychologies: Explorations and challenges* (pp. 56-71). Chicago, IL: University of Illinois Press.

Slater, S. and Mencher, J. (1991). The lesbian family life cycle: A contextual approach. *American Journal of Orthopsychiatry. 61:* 372-382.

Stein, T. S. (1988). Theoretical considerations in psychotherapy with gay men and lesbians. *Journal of Homosexuality, 15:* 75-95.

Stein, T. S. and Burg, B. K. (1996). Teaching in mental health training programs about homosexuality, lesbians, gay men, and bisexuals. In R. P. Cabaj and T. S. Stein (Eds.), *Textbook of homosexuality and mental health* (pp. 621-631). Washington, DC: American Psychiatric Press.

Stevens, P. E. (1998). The experiences of lesbians of color in health care encounters: Narrative insights for improving access and quality. *Journal of Lesbian Studies, 2:* 77-94.

Stewart, A. (1994). Toward a feminist strategy for studying women's lives. In C. Franz and A. Stewart (Eds.), *Women creating lives: Identities, resilience, and resistance* (pp. 11-36). Boulder, CO: Westview.

Strommen, E. F. (1989). "You're a what?": Family member reactions to the disclosure of homosexuality. In F. W. Bozett (Ed.), *Homosexuality and the family* (pp. 37-58). Binghamton, NY: The Haworth Press.

Swan, W. (1997). Workplaces, schools, partnerships, and justice: An intersection that causes confrontation. In W. Swan (Ed.), *Gay/lesbian/bisexual/transgender public policy issues* (pp. 15-21). Binghamton, NY: The Harrington Park Press.

Tafoya, T. (1992). Native gay and lesbian issues: The two spirited. In B. Berzon (Ed.), *Positively gay* (pp. 253-260). Berkeley, CA: Celestial Arts.

Thompson, N. L., McCandless, B. R., and Strickland, B. R. (1971). Personal adjustment of male and female homosexuals and heterosexuals. *Journal of Abnormal Psychology, 78:* 237-240.

Tievsky, D. L. (1988). Homosexual clients and homophobic social workers. *Journal of Independent Social Work, 2:* 51-62.

Trujillo, C. (Ed.) (1991). *Chicana lesbians: The girls our mothers warned us about.* Berkeley, CA: Third Woman Press.

Tully, C. (1995). In sickness and in health: Forty years of research on lesbians. *Journal of Gay and Lesbian Social Services, 3:* 1-18.

Walsh, F. and Scheinkman, M. (1989). (Fe) male: The hidden gender dimension in models of family therapy. In M. McGoldrick, C. M. Anderson, and F. Walsh (Eds.), *Women in families: A framework for family therapy* (pp. 16-41). New York: Norton.

Weasel, L. H. (1996). Seeing between the lines: Bisexual women and therapy. *Women and Therapy, 19:* 5-16.

Wilson, M. and Greene, R. (1971). Personality characteristics of female homosexuals. *Psychological Reports, 28:* 407-412.

Wisniewski, J. J. and Toomey, B. G. (1987). Are social workers homophobic? *Social Work, 32:* 454-455.

World Health Organization (1997). *Manual of the international statistical classification of diseases, injuries, and causes of death,* Ninth revision, Fifth edition. Geneva: Author.

Zacks, E., Green, R., and Morrow, J. (1988). Comparing lesbian and heterosexual couples on the circumplex model: An initial investigation. *Family Process, 27:* 471-484.

Zitter, S. (1987). Coming out to mom: Theoretical aspects of the mother-daughter process. In Boston Lesbian Psychologies Collective (Ed.), *Lesbian psychologies: Explorations and challenge* (pp. 177-194). Chicago, IL: University of Illinois Press.

Chapter 11

Overturning Oppression: An Analysis of Emancipatory Change

Ann Weick

INTRODUCTION

In the world of social work, the concept of oppression is hauntingly familiar. Since the origin of the profession, there has been a sometimes stark, sometimes muted awareness of social forces that crush people's life chances and rob them of the dignity and vitality our values claim for them. As with any familiar concept, the word itself can become a substitute for exploring the deeper meaning it holds. If we are to invigorate social work practice for the twenty-first century, it is important to reexamine the nature of oppression so that its dynamics and effects will not flaw our efforts. To understand fully and support women's strengths, we must remember the ways in which that strength is daily drained of its force. Only from that clear-eyed view can we create a path of wisdom into the future.

From its earliest inception, social work has recognized the importance of the social environment in shaping people's lives. Through the course of time, however, the notion of the environment has increasingly been translated into interpersonal dimensions (Weick, 1981). The context of people's lives is reduced to personal relationships and attention is paid to the history and quality of those relationships. Although attempts have been made to stretch that context beyond close, immediate relationships to include intergenerational patterns, the focus remains narrow and parochial. We are left with the unexamined assumption that an adequate understanding of people's lives rests with a detailed account of their own personal world of meaning.

A closer analysis of the concept of oppression is a useful antidote to this unfortunate myopia.

THE GENEALOGY OF OPPRESSION

Foucault's (Gordon, 1980) use of the term genealogy is an instructive place to begin the analysis. He uses genealogy to refer to the "painstaking rediscovery" of "disqualified, popular knowledge" (p. 83), which has been submerged by dominant systems of knowledge and discourse. Genealogy is an excavation of the cultural history of social practices that have maintained certain forms of knowledge and power in preference to others. The study, then, is not primarily about power itself but about the means by which a particular view retains dominance in the face of other forms of knowledge. The dynamics that create this possibility are the seedbed of oppression.

It is not difficult to describe the dynamics of the dominant model of power. In Kipnis's (1976) terms, it rests on the control of resources defined as scarce. In a capitalist society, money is the major symbol of a scarce resource, but education, physical appearance, and other personal attributes are also treated as resources. In order for power to accrue, it is important that these resources not be viewed as widely available.

Those who control scarce resources and those who want or need those resources enter into a collusive relationship. The power holder (Kipnis, 1976) sets the conditions of the relationship, and the one needing the resources adapts his or her behavior to meet those conditions. The attendant rewards and penalties, coupled with a continuing level of need, insure that there will be little change in what Baker-Miller (1976) describes as a relationship of permanent inequality.

It is important to note that those in positions of power are not a permanent cast of characters. Although historical and social patterns clearly elevate certain groups over others, individual powerholders do not have an unchanging claim to their position. Fame, wealth, and high position can all be lost. At the same time, intricately interwoven circles of power exist, so that power holders in one arena are themselves lacking some resources held by others. The circles of power and oppression thus establish multiple and overlapping constrictions.

To understand power in this way is only one obvious level of analysis. It is necessary to dig more deeply into the dynamics of power by examining some of the more subtle ways in which dominant patterns of power are connected with the control of knowledge. This relationship brings us more intimately into the world of social work practice and to the resources over which professionals exert control.

The Control of Knowledge

The power of the social work profession rests on two bases: the control of social resources and the control of knowledge. Through its policies and programs, society authorizes social workers within government programs to allocate the money, goods, and services needed by those who cannot obtain these resources with their own income. Social workers are an important conduit for the allocation of these necessities. In this capacity, they have power to give and withhold and thus can, through whim, discretion, or prejudice, affect people's fate.

This obvious form of professional power is linked with a less obvious but equally compelling aspect of professional life, namely, the control of knowledge. Examining the nature of knowledge provides some important insights about how social workers may unwittingly collaborate in knowledge systems which perpetuate oppressive practices. To understand how this happens, we need to look at the ways in which knowledge, particularly "legitimate" knowledge, is developed and preserved.

All social institutions can be viewed as mechanisms for circumscribing human experience. Over the undifferentiated chaos of stimuli experienced by infants, a certain pattern is woven. The "buzzing, blooming confusion" noted by James (1984) is made coherent through language, customs, and practices which establish a particular shape for human experience (Berger and Luckmann, 1967). Infants are literally taught to see, and in that seeing alternative views vanish. A table is no longer a structure to climb on or a place to hide under. It is given a name and a purpose, and eventually that is what a table is.

Certain social institutions have exerted powerful influence in shaping the way we see the world. Both science and religion have vied to name reality in particular ways. Both are orthodoxies in the sense that each claims to present a view which is true or right and thus deserves adherence by believers. Both attempt to interpret the "buzzin'" pattern of human experience according to certain rules. The interpretation schemes are not the same but the underlying message of both is.

Both science and religion have established formalized systems of knowledge that purport to interpret reality in a true way. Each has established a class of interpreters, either scientists or priests, who have the power to name reality in particular ways. Each has an elaborate system for insuring orthodoxy, complete with punishment for those who challenge the prevailing views. The scientific worldview, which has been in ascendance since the seventeenth century, significantly shaped the development of human service professions, including social work. The same pattern of establishing a higher authority over human experience prevailed. As professions developed, complete with rituals and elitist practices, the professional practitioner was cloaked with "powers existing beyond the reach or understanding of ordinary humans. . . . Common sense, ordinary understanding and personal negotiations no longer were the effective means of human communication in society. . . . Clients found themselves compelled to believe on simple faith that a higher rationality called scientific knowledge decided one's fate" (Bledstein, 1976, p. 94).

It is true that human beings never seem to be without systems of interpretation. The prescientific world was no less without its constructions of reality than is the scientific. However, the scientific paradigm has extended its interpretative domain to include virtually all aspects of human behavior. Where medieval religion stopped at the boundaries of moral behavior, social science disciplines and the related helping professions have intruded into the psychological, emotional, social, and physical domains of human life. Very little about human relations has not been appropriated by scientific or pseudoscientific explanation. Under the guise of professional expertise, human needs have become pathological categories, ranging from narcissistic personality to codependent.

The extent of this appropriation of everyday life by experts is staggeringly immense. Its vastness signals the broad outlines of oppression, which are at once more profound and more ordinary than one typically imagines. Creating a monopoly of knowledge, to which only a select few have access, instantaneously establishes a caste system. There will always be some whose knowledge is validated and many others whose knowledge is not credited. Foucault (Gordon, 1980) uses the term "subjugated" or "disqualified" knowledges to refer to what is thought of as "naive knowledges, located low down on the hierarchy, beneath the required level of cognition and scienticity"

(p. 82). This hierarchical system of knowledge guarantees profound alienation from people's own knowledges and experiences.

Conceptual Straitjackets

The official view of legitimate knowledge is kept in place by a set of guardian concepts. The prevalence and deep adherence to these ideas help insure that the current system of knowledge, with all of its attributes of power, will remain firmly in place. The first concept is that of "normalcy." To be normal is a descriptive category which defines accepted and expected human behavior. Under the gloss of scientific measurement, certain behaviors fit the norm because most people are observed to be doing them. Observing the maturational milestones of a young child, the social behaviors of young adults, and the physical health of elderly persons, we conclude that it is normal to walk, to be married, and to develop osteoporosis within certain age spans.

The application of a statistical approach to human behavior is particularly troublesome. At best, a normal distribution applies only to one trait or characteristic. For any specific behavior, an individual may be above, below, or within the norm. But human beings are not constituted from one characteristic. To give a global judgment of "normal" is a misapplication of a statistical method. But it does accomplish the more subtle goal of insuring that experts can subject any behavior to their tests and their judgment.

The power of the concept of normalcy is best seen in the judgment of abnormality. Since any human behavior can come under scrutiny and be judged abnormal, no one is free from intimidation. The threat of being seen as abnormal strikes a primitive fear in us, a fear of ostracism, of banishment, of rejection from the human community. This threat may account for our deep-seated fear of difference as it manifests itself in racism, sexism, homophobia, and other discriminatory ideologies. Fear of difference is fear of losing our basic grounding in the human community.

Euro-American culture has produced another concept which keeps the knowledge paradigm in place. It is the concept of individualism, which elevates the individual at the expense of the collective. As a legacy of the Enlightenment, shaped by American industrial-capitalist ideology, individualism touts people's personal initiative while requiring them to be responsible for their own welfare. At the expense of a view that values mutual cooperation and interdependence, American individualism helps ensure that people feel fundamentally estranged from the concept of common goals and shared responsibilities. Making it on one's own is viewed as the highest accomplishment, with no recognition given to the silent partners who made it possible. The result for both winners and losers is a profound alienation and the lack of any communal structure for sharing the real burdens of living in the world.

The scientific view has fostered another belief that supports the dominant paradigm, namely that a solution can be found for every problem. Both the individualistic "bootstraps" mentality and scientific methods have created the belief that problems, over time, are susceptible to solutions. Julian Rappaport (1981) draws on E. F. Schumacher's distinction between convergent and divergent reasoning to make this point. Convergent reasoning assumes that problems in the material world will ultimately yield to the right answer. No problem is unsolvable; the right solution just has not been discovered yet.

Given this type of thinking, there is little impetus to challenge the basic assumptions underlying the approach. Attention is focused solely on methods of discovery and on ways to improve methods to solve problems. Believing that a right answer exists never causes anyone to question the question.

Finally, the predominant knowledge system is supported by the two connected concepts of paternalism and patriarchy. The child-like—that is to say, powerless—status of most adults is maintained by the deeply held belief that authority figures should be benevolent parents who will take care of us and solve our problems. Because this belief is embedded in the ideology of patriarchy, the ideal parent is seen as a male, a father, who will take charge and protect us. Patriarchy maintains the illusion that white monied men are the most able and most deserving to hold such positions of power.

Each of these concepts forms the boundaries of legitimate knowledge. To accept definitions of normalcy, individualism, problem-solving approaches, and patriarchy ensures that monopolistic and hierarchical systems of knowledge and power will remain in place. The beliefs themselves subvert any challenges to the status quo, making the beliefs relatively invulnerable. When challenges occur, it is clearly the challenger whose knowledge, motives, and mental state are suspect.

HIDDEN DYNAMICS OF OPPRESSION

An examination of these guardian concepts helps explain the "what" of oppression, that is, the beliefs that hold current systems in place. It is equally important to examine the "how,"—the personal processes that act like burrs to hold people within the current net of beliefs. The starting point for this examination must be the recognition that the process of socialization is a powerful initiator into a particular worldview. The family is seen as socially useful precisely for that purpose. The dominant beliefs of the culture are imbibed with baby food, long before any possibility of independent thinking or action could occur. The process of socialization, if it is successful by social standards, puts in place two levels of belief: that there is a particular way to interpret reality and that the particular way is the only correct way. The latter level initiates the base for future oppression and subjugation.

Socialization processes work symbiotically with systems of sanctions found in society's institutional structures. Education, religion, politics, economics, and social welfare all serve to reinforce the product of socialization through subtle and coercive means of punishment and reward. Understanding the leviathan power of social institutions to maintain social beliefs is fundamental to an understanding of social oppression.

Within the context of socialization and social structures, people are kept ignorant of their own power in many subtle ways. Women's socialization provides a beginning example. As Chodorow (1978) and others (Gomick and Moran, 1971) have found, young girls must contend with a paradox whose resolution sets the stage for their identity throughout life. At the heart of their socialization is a lie. A small girl will, in the normal course of exploring her world, discover that she has certain talents and abilities. Perhaps she is good at climbing fences or running fast or fixing things. Her own experience tells her how good it is to be so capable. But at some point, social gender beliefs will intrude. She will be told that what she thinks is important or good is just the opposite: that only boys are good at or should be allowed to engage in active, physical play, as well as a host of other behaviors. Her dilemma is clear. She can either trust herself and become a very young iconoclast, or she can, given the constant chiding from adults and other peers, lie to herself and decide she does not want to do it anyway. At the heart of this denial is the important, oppressive message that she cannot trust her own experience.

Socialization sets in motion another preeminent process of disempowerment. It establishes a dynamic in which children are systematically trained to look to external authority figures to interpret their experience. Their world, including their most personal and idiosyncratic ideas and responses, is shaped by the words and actions of powerful others. Although it may be easy to rationalize this practice in the interests of their safety and well-being, it sets the stage for the lifelong habit of looking outward. It is rare for children to have the opportunity and support for validating their own experience.

Some researchers (Rotter, 1972) have argued that women are especially vexed by an external locus of control. Rather than being able to take charge of their lives based on their own needs and judgments, they tend to look to others to take care of them. Walker (1984) comes at the similar phenomenon of "learned helplessness" by saying that "externalizers" (in contrast to "internalizers") believe that most of the events that occur in their life are caused by factors outside themselves (p. 48). She used this theory to help explain why many battered women stay with abusive partners even when other options appear to be available.

Because there is a tendency to confuse description and theory, the issue of where one places control deserves some discussion. My thesis thus far is that a significant aspect of socialization is precisely to train people to rely on power outside themselves. Democratic beliefs notwithstanding, the institutional bias is toward claiming and maintaining authority. Given our sexist and racist society, it should not be surprising that women and people of color receive multiple layers of messages about their own inadequacies, making them even more reliant on external sources of authority. But socialization in the broad culture prevents everyone from recognizing his or her own power. Neither women nor men can identify and appreciate their own personal resources, talents, and strengths, although the processes of disguise are different. Males, particularly white men, associate their power with their gender status. Most women attribute power to others. In both cases, the concept of power is externalized and does not rest on one's own personal worth.

These weighty forces all combine to create a crushing burden in the struggle for personal well-being. Learning to deny one's own experience inserts a duplicity that colors all aspects of life. A basic claim for self-worth is continually denied, resulting in the "wounded dignity" (Sennett and Cobb, 1972) that so injures people's image of self. At the heart of oppression is a profound alienation from one's own power, which leads to a too-ready acceptance of the power of others. The personal costs of oppression are matched by costs to society itself. The overarching cost to society lies in wasted and untapped human resources. Maintaining oppressive beliefs and structures requires a tremendous amount of human energy, spent individually and collectively. Consider the energy required to constantly scan for and react to human differences.

When legitimate behavior is narrowly defined, society becomes hypervigilant in its attempts to search out those whose behavior does not fit. At the same time, those who are thus defined as different must expend precious energy being ever watchful for their own safety and well-being. The upshot is a tremendous loss of human initiative and human talent.

The dynamics of oppression rest on the sands of delusion and myth. To create oppressive human relations, there must be a myth about people's fundamental inadequacy and the corresponding myth that someone else (some individual, some class of people, some institution) has the power to save them. Social processes must ensure that the message of inadequacy is reinforced in multiple, daily ways so that the myth itself will not be challenged, nor, will the challengers go unpunished. In this way, the myth persists, even when its basic assumption about human beings is so flagrantly wounding. Why, one could ask, do we continue to sustain a myth whose effects rob us of our energy, our creativity, our very essence?

INTIMATIONS OF EMANCIPATION

It is a tribute to human perspicacity and wisdom that the wounding myth of human inadequacy has not been allowed to go unchallenged. Throughout all of human history, prophets and seers have recognized the tremendous potential inherent in all people, and their message, however the language varied, has tried to awaken that awareness in others. From the erudite to the ordinary, from the sacred to the secular, they focused on the talents, strengths, and resources so richly evident in people's lives and experiences. One thinks of Jesus, Mahatma

Gandhi, Martin Luther King Jr., Paulo Friere, and Mother Teresa, among many others, as stirring examples of such conviction.

We are living in a time, however, when forces of social change go far beyond the voice of individual prophets. In the past thirty years, we have witnessed a cumulative march toward human liberation, begun in the 1950s with civil rights activism, through the second women's movement, to the current push for human rights for all people of color, for lesbians, gay men, and bisexuals, senior citizens, people with physical and mental handicaps, and children. These efforts are mirrored internationally with the long struggle of blacks in South Africa, the poor in Latin America, the recent shifts in Eastern Europe, and failed attempts at democratization in China. Every continent seems to be grappling with its own profound search for freedom.

This global awakening is not confined to the political sphere. In virtually every area of human life, collective questioning of the current power paradigm is occurring. Health care and ecology stand as two prominent examples of areas where a serious critique has been raised and where the holistic health movement and the green movement offer alternative perspectives. In the academic arena, the nature of knowledge itself is being called into question, giving rise to critiques of science (Kuhn, 1962), literature (Derrida, 1976), psychology (Sampson, 1983; Gergen, 1982), anthropology (Geertz, 1973), biology (Gazzaniga, 1985; Ornstein and Sobel, 1987), and philosophy (Bernstein, 1985; Foucault, cited in Gordon, 1980). Although disparate in content and form, the critiques challenge the monopolistic model of authoritative knowledge that undergirds every discipline and profession. The control of knowledge through narrow definitions of what constitutes legitimate knowledge and its interpretation has come under full-scale attack.

Although a complete discussion of these critiques is beyond the scope of this chapter, it is important to briefly sketch the general design of an alternative way of understanding human knowledge. Sampson (1983), who draws on the work of the philosopher Habermas, is useful in this regard. Central to the work of Habermas (Sampson, 1983) and the work of other critical theorists is the notion of emancipatory knowledge, in which knowledge is seen as having a transformative quality. In Sampson's words, "People can and do reflect on the conditions of their life; the knowledge they obtain about those conditions becomes part of the base of resources which they employ to reproduce or transform those very conditions" (1983, p. 68).

This view of knowledge is directed to the larger goal of "return[ing] the subject the lost or renounced powers of self-reflection and thus [to] restor[ing] real self-direction" (Sampson, 1983, p. 69).

The process of recapturing those powers of self-reflection and self-direction is a powerful and appealing way to reconstitute the notion of human knowledge. For knowledge to have emancipatory potential, there must be the assumption that people already have knowledge of value. Their ability to recognize and "reflect on the conditions of their life" (Sampson, 1983, p. 68) is a true form of knowledge, not something to be discounted. Such an assumption runs in the face of dominant models of knowledge which assume that only objective, that is, nonpersonal, knowledge can be considered legitimate.

If personal knowledge (Polanyi, 1958) is seen to be valid, then emancipation has both personal and political dimensions. On the personal level, it requires processes in which one's own experience can be named. To name something is to give it an identity that deserves recognition. Thus, to name one's experience is to call it out of the morass of discounted knowledge. Whether one's experience involves pain or joy, insight or confusion, to claim that knowledge is to honor it as valid.

Special power is found in collective sharing of experience. The rapid rise of the self-help movement attests to the validation which comes from hearing others' experiences and sharing stories. Belenky and colleagues (1986) found many ways in which women understood their lives. Although they attempted to categorize these processes of knowing within a larger and somewhat rigid framework, their study poignantly shows the range of women's experience in naming, validating, and sharing their stories. Stories are a form of knowledge and, some would say, the only knowledge we have.

But emancipation does not get played out on the personal level alone. If people are able to achieve a radical sense of their own knowledge, they may find that the normative assumptions about knowledge in general become suspect. Borrowing again from E. F. Schumacher via Rappaport (1981), the solutions that seemed so linear and one sided give way to divergent approaches, which require an appreciation of the paradoxical nature of human situations. When a monolithic knowledge structure begins tumbling down, as current challenges would suggest, then an absolutist view of the world crumbles also. In its place is a constructionist perspective which assumes that human perception is always mediated by language, culture, and ideology. No unchanging, unequivocal reality exists "out there." Thus, the act of sharing stories can lead to transformative action. Things can be other than the way we have learned them. The emancipatory potential of human beings, particularly when they act collectively, can truly change the world.

EMANCIPATORY CHANGE IN SOCIAL WORK

Social work is heavily invested in the language of individual and social change. Implicit in its professional orientation is a belief in the possibility of human growth and change. However, this belief has tended to be interlaced with notions of instrumental change, leading to approaches that make people passive recipients of external "intervention." Social workers have traditionally seen themselves as agents who do interventions, which can bring about change. The perceived ability to cause change to happen is supported by the dominant power paradigm discussed earlier. Those in power are thought to have the power to make change happen.

This traditional notion of change runs counter to a process we are calling emancipatory change. In an emancipatory process of change, growth is seen as an inherent life force, which naturally impels people to become more fully who they are. It rests on the assumption that a power exists within individuals, as reflected in their unique strength, resilience, capacities, and energy. Emancipatory change is a process of growth which reveals personal and collective power to know and to be who we are. Because oppressive processes and structures disguise this power, emancipation requires a conscious effort to critically challenge and dispel the myth of inadequacy in all its guises.

In order to support a philosophy of emancipation, social work must reconsider some of its basic tenets. Just as individuals and communities must develop a critical stance in understanding their own oppression, professionals must be willing to make a critical assessment of the nature of professional practice, particularly its reliance on externalized knowledge and technique and its adherence to models of pathology. Within the past several decades, a growing attempt has been made to examine the crisis in the professions (Schon, 1983), and social workers have added to this dialogue. Early writers such as Goldstein (1986), Imre (1984), Saleebey (1979), and Weick (1987) have been joined by many others, including Gutierrez (1994), Witkin

(1995), Laird (1998), and Saleebey (1996). These efforts are bringing to light the manifold ways in which professional practice can unwittingly add to people's oppressive life conditions or can, when redirected, serve as a resource in people's discovery of their own abilities and strengths.

Feminist critique and practice approaches have been particularly significant in awakening practitioners to the oppression of sexist ideology and behavior. Contributions by Davis (1985) and Van Den Bergh and Cooper (1986)and more recently by such authors as Sands and Nuccio (1992) have helped heighten awareness about the insidiously pervasive aspects of sexism and the long road to emancipatory change. Feminist critique provides a salutary avenue of redress for the blindness so deeply ingrained in our culture.

Efforts to foster emancipatory change as a guiding principle of practice must be moored on more generous conceptions of human behavior than have traditionally existed. To the extent that theories of human behavior are based on rigid schemes of development or focus attention on a concept of normalcy from which all people depart to some degree, those theories will not serve an emancipatory goal. Instead, these theoretical assumptions will add oppressive layers to people's ability to grow and change. The concept of emancipatory change must be lodged in an open-ended, health-oriented view of human behavior which assumes both individual potential for transformative growth and a wide range of ways in which that potential can be expressed throughout a lifetime.

One such approach uses the concept of the lifelong growth tasks of intimacy, nurturance, productivity, creativity, and transcendence to suggest a loose model for human development (Weick, 1983). Each of these areas includes challenges which are continually reworked as one engages in life situations. Neither social roles, age, nor stages determine how those challenges will be met or in what ways lessons will be learned. The process of growth for each individual is fundamentally idiosyncratic, even though the larger social structure creates common barriers and opportunities.

Such a view of human behavior provides a resonant foundation for emancipatory practice. It unhinges human behavior from the social imperatives of roles and age-related stages and, in doing so, allows a critical assessment of their impact. Because, in the growth-task scheme, the challenges of intimacy and nurturance are not tied to

marriage or motherhood, individuals can more clearly see the limitations those role expectations impose. At the same time, they can explore the liberating goal of understanding within their own life experiences what it means to share themselves in intimate relations or care
for others who need nurturing. In this way, a growth-task model demonstrates very vividly that what one assumes at a conceptual level has
everything to do with how one practices.

There is, however, an important step between theory and practice.
Although it is crucial that theoretical assumptions provide the philo-
sophic groundwork for practice, the translation will be very rough
unless social workers experience the quality of their own oppression.
It is one thing to acknowledge intellectually that a health-oriented
model of human behavior provides a good fit for emancipatory practice. It is quite another to "stand under" (understand) the forces which
systematically hide our own powers of healing and well-being. For
women, people of color, and others who suffer discrimination because of narrow ideas of what is "normal," it is essential to recognize
and deeply experience the ways in which social messages and practices have injured us. It is from this experience that both insight and
empathy emerge.

Practice begins, then, with the awareness of our own and others'
oppression. It becomes emancipatory practice when we work with
others to explore ways in which injuring messages and experiences
can be replaced by the recognition that we are the source of our own
power. Unlike the traditional connotations of power, this type of
power is both nutritive and integrative (May, 1972), allowing us to
explore and use our own wisdom and experience to grow more freely
according to our own lights.

Practicing from an emancipatory perspective is closely linked with
principles which support people's own power. The first assumption
one makes is that individuals are experts on their own lives. They
know better than anyone what their experience means to them and
what rewards and burdens it presents. Closely allied with this belief
in their expertise is the assumption that each person exhibits multiple
strengths in living through life's challenges. Because expressions of
this personal power may not be fully recognized or acknowledged,
emancipatory practice can help in this uncovering process.

Being able to recognize one's own power usually comes as a result
of events or circumstances that challenge one to see things in a new

way. One of the most profound moments of personal change is often linked to a radical reframing, where some taken-for-granted belief is challenged and changed. For women, these moments may come when they question traditional beliefs about what it means to be a woman and find that their own experience speaks to them more powerfully and overtly than any external message or meaning.

Knowing that one has the ability to reimage one's life is a fundamental aspect of personal power. To see things differently, to name things in new ways, is a source of power that is not given by others. It is a power, however, that can be shared with others, so that the act of seeing differently moves naturally into the realm of collective action. Once it is discovered and possessed, it serves as the seedbed for all other imaginings.

CONCLUDING THOUGHTS

The twenty-first century is likely to be fraught with continuing struggles as a global awakening meets head-on resistance from traditional forces of power and privilege. The degree of challenge to the old order can be measured by the severity of repressive action, whether it is carried out against individuals or the collective. We are likely to see even more attempts to force people into the old molds provided by family, church, and government.

Thus the context of emancipatory practice is not without its snares. To help individuals and communities recognize and value their own power implicitly challenges external power systems. Because these systems rely on the practice of invalidating people's own wisdom and experience, the process of honoring and developing these attributes takes the teeth out of oppressive practices. But all who gain by oppression cannot be expected to willingly give up their teeth. It is important to recognize, then, that emancipatory practice is not glib or easy. It involves the personal struggle of closely examining our own lives, both for evidence of our own oppression and for signs of how we oppress others. It requires us to relinquish the desire to exercise power over others, even in the name of professional expertise. It calls us to imagine a more generous world, in which human strengths become the focal point for support and action. Finally, it reminds us that liberation has costs. Emancipatory change does not come easily nor are its consequences lightly felt. To see the world differently invites a struggle between the old and the new, a struggle that involves confusion and doubt, as well as joy and hope.

By anchoring our conceptions of practice in the broad themes of oppression and emancipation, social work becomes part of the global processes of change. Its purpose and its goals align with our broader vision of what it means to be fully human, bringing to our practice a more vivid appreciation of the values which lie at the heart of social work. It is from the strength of these values that we can redress the injuries of oppression and return to people's lives the dignity and honor which they should rightfully claim.

REFERENCES

Baker-Miller, J. (1976). *Toward a new psychology of women*. Boston: Beacon.

Belenky, M. R, Clinchy, B. M., Goldberger, N. R., and Tarule, J. M. (1986). *Women's ways of knowing*. New York: Basic.

Berger, P. L. and Luckmann, T. (1967). *The social construction of reality*. New York: Anchor.

Bernstein, R. J. (1985). *Beyond objectivism and relativism: Science, hermeneutics and praxis*. Philadelphia: University of Pennsylvania Press.

Bledstein, B. (1976). *The culture of professionalism*. New York: Norton.

Chodorow, N. (1978). *The reproduction of mothering: Psychoanalysis and the sociology of gender*. Berkeley: University of California Press.

Davis, L. (1985). Female and male voices in social work. *Social Work, 30:* 106-115.

Derrida, J. (1976). *Of grammatology*. Baltimore: Johns Hopkins University Press.

Gazzaniga, M. S. (1985). *The social brain*. New York: Basic.

Geertz, C. (1973). *The interpretation of culture*. New York: Basic.

Gergen, K. (1982). *Toward transformation in social knowledge*. New York: Springer-Verlag.

Goldstein, H. (1986). Toward an integration of theory and practice. *Social Work, 31:* 352-357.

Gomick, V and Moran, B. (1971). *Woman in sexist society*. New York: Basic.

Gordon, C. (Ed.) (1980). *Michael Foucault—Power/knowledge*. New York: Pantheon.

Gutierrez, L. (1994). Beyond coping: An empowerment perspective on stressful life situations. *Journal of Family Social Work, 1:* 33-46.

Imre, R. (1984). The nature of knowledge in social work. *Social Work, 29:* 41-45.

James, W. (1984). *Psychology: Briefer course*. Cambridge, MA: Harvard University Press.

Kipnis, D. (1976). *The powerholders*. Chicago: University of Chicago Press.

Kuhn, T. (1962). *The structure of scientific revolutions.* Chicago: University of Chicago Press.

Laird, J. (1998). Family-centered practice in the postmodern era. In C. Franklin and P. S. Nurius (Eds.), *Constructivism in practice: Methods and challenges.* Milwaukee: Families International Inc.

May, R. (1972). *Power and innocence.* New York: Dell.

Ornstein, R. E. and Sobel, D. S. (1987). *The healing brain.* New York: Simon and Schuster.

Polanyi, M. (1958). *Personal knowledge.* Chicago: University of Chicago Press.

Rappaport, J. (1981). In praise of paradox: A social policy of empowerment over prevention. *American Journal of Community Psychology, 9:* 1-23.

Rotter, J. (1972). *Applications of a social learning theory of personality.* New York: Holt, Rinehart and Winston.

Saleebey, D. (1979). The tension between research and practice: Assumptions of the experimental paradigm. *Clinical Social Work Journal, 7:* 267-284.

Saleebey, D. (1996). *The strengths perspective in social work practice.* White Plains, NY: Longman.

Sampson, E. E. (1983). *Justice and the critique of pure psychology.* New York: Plenum.

Sands, R.G. and Nuccio, K. (1992). Postmodern feminist theory and social work. *Social Work, 37:* 489-494.

Schon, C. (1983). *The reflective practitioner.* New York: Basic.

Sennett, R. and Cobb, J. (1972). *The hidden injuries of class.* New York: Alfred A. Knopf.

Van Den Bergh, N. and Cooper, L. B. (Eds.) (1986). *Feminist visions for social work.* Silver Spring, MD: National Association of Social Workers.

Walker, L. E. (1984). *The battered women syndrome.* New York: Springer.

Weick, A. (1981). Reframing the person-in-environment perspective. *Social Work, 26:* 140-143.

Weick, A. (1983). A growth-task model of human development. *Social Casework, 64:* 131-137.

Weick, A. (1987). Reconceptualizing the philosophical perspective of social work. *Social Service Review, 61:* 218-230.

Witkin, S. (1995). Family social work: A critical constructionist perspective. *Journal of Family Social Work, 1:* 33-46.

Chapter 12

Changing Women's Narratives: Taking Back the Discourse

Joan Laird

Night after night my mother would talk-story until we fell asleep. I couldn't tell where the stories left off and the dreams began. . . . At last I saw that I too had been in the presence of great power, my mother talking-story. . . . She said I would grow up a wife and a slave, but she taught me the song of the warrior woman, Fa Mu Lan. I would have to grow up a warrior woman.

Maxine Hong Kingston (1975, p. 24)

INTRODUCTION

Gender, we have learned, is socially constructed. The meanings of being male and being female are fashioned, in varying cultures, through language, social discourse, the stories we tell about ourselves, and the stories that are told about us. These sociocultural stories tell us what we are like and what we are to be like, how we are to think, with whom we should choose to be, and even how we do and should speak. In reciprocal and circular fashion, these narratives both reinforce what already is and create it anew, as we speak our lives within the constraints of prevailing public discourses.

Portions of this chapter have been excerpted from J. Laird (1993). Women's silences—women's secrets. In E. Imber-Black (Ed.), *Secrets in family therapy* (pp. 243-267). New York: W.W. Norton. Reprinted by permission of W.W. Norton & Co.

The stories in the larger sociocultural surroundings provide the contextual repertoire we draw upon to construct our autobiographies, the life narratives that we build and revise as we construct, deconstruct, and reconstruct ourselves. The shape of these self-narratives is influenced in particular by the prevailing folklores in our families and other important groups, that is, by the unique ways our families and other primary reference groups have translated larger social constructions into prescriptions for living.

Clearly the relationship between the personal and the social story is an interactive one. Larger social discourses are constructed from what Geertz (1983) calls "local knowledges," and these larger social discourses, in turn, provide contexts in which local knowledges may flourish or, conversely, become extinct or go underground. Local knowledges—sets of ideas, explanations, and interpretations about the world—gradually take hold and may gain increasing numbers of adherents. These local knowledges/stories, as they become part of the surrounding discourse, guide our everyday words, thoughts, and actions. They shape the lives of women in very powerful ways, guiding and constraining their speech and even their thoughts.

For example, the popular idea that women encourage sexual exploitation on the part of men is one of the many "stories" that has kept generations of women silent about their experiences of harassment, molestation, and rape. The Anita Hill–Clarence Thomas episode demonstrates just how influential this set of ideas is and how difficult it is to dislodge it. Similarly, we now have a prevailing social discourse, reinforced by a largely white-male dominated fashion industry, that dictates women's own body images (Faludi, 1991). In the social construction of beauty, women must be extraordinarily thin and, paradoxically, voluptuous. Anorexia and other eating disorders, as well as the current popularity of silicone breast implants, at least in part, may be interpreted in the context of these larger social stories that prescribe and proscribe women's bodies.

Of course, a remarkably intimate relationship exists between knowledge and gender and between power and gender (Goodrich, 1991). One of the most powerful lessons of feminist research over the past two decades has been that ways of knowing and speaking are gendered and are socially reproduced through mothering (Chodorow, 1978), education (Belenky et al., 1986), story and folklore (Laird, 1989), ritual (Imber-Black, 1989; Laird, 1988), the popular media, and in the arts—indeed, in all of the contexts in which our lives are defined. It is white, middle- and upper-class males who largely control the making of local knowledges and of social discourse and social meanings. The making of women's narratives and women's silences, then, cannot be explored without constant attention to issues of gender and power and to how these forces operate in the constituting of women's lives.

The language of the mental health professions, which I would call "stories" or "local knowledges," has also had enormous influence in shaping the public's ideas about people and about individual and family functioning. For example, widespread "depression" among women is rarely termed "oppression," which is more difficult to "treat." Instead of directly naming the molestation and violence that men commit against women, we tend to name the effects on women, directing attention to women's symptomatology and away from the original offenses and offenders. Thus, many women sexually abused as children are now termed "borderline personality disorder" or "multiple personality disorder" or "anorexic." In the process, attention is diverted from the offenders. What might be better storied as wife beating is named "marital discord," "spouse abuse," or "family violence." Such euphemisms, argues Lamb (1991), implicate mental health professionals in a powerful obfuscation of language, which masks gender oppression and detours social solutions to massive social problems. Furthermore, storying these experiences as problems in individual and family functioning is one way the mental health field ensures its own perpetuation and expands its influence over thought, language, and the social construction of gender.

In this chapter, I examine how the story metaphor can provide a tool for both understanding and transforming women's lives. I am particularly interested in how woman can and cannot use their voices, how women's language is constituted and perceived, how women are silenced, how they can and do resist oppression through finding their voices and using their silences in strengthening ways, how they can and do transform their stories and thus themselves.

Two examples of the relationship between public discourse and individual story and the impact of that relationship on women are used—the incest story and the lesbian story. In each case, I look at some of the ways that women have been silenced as well as some of the ways that they have begun to restory their lives and to influence the larger public story.

Many postmodern thinkers argue that the self is constituted through the narratives we construct to explain our lived experiences, through the self bearing witness to the self, through a mutually affirming sharing of stories with others with like experiences, and through the narratives others construct about us (Bauman, 1986; Bruner, 1986; Gergen and Gergen, 1983; Polkinghorne, 1988). Story, then, or restorying, is an important pathway to change. Just as gaining the power to influence social discourse and social meanings can bring about change on the societal level, so the restorying process on the individual or family level offers powerful potential for change, not only for the individuals involved but in initiating and strengthening alternative local knowledges. For example, as the women's movement has helped to shape our consciousness concerning the patriarchal nature of the traditional family, so many individual women, strengthened by feminism, have restoried and restructured their family lives in very important ways.

Similarly, the clinical context can offer an opportunity for the reshaping of women's personal and familial narratives and thus for the beginnings of new local knowledges. Throughout this chapter, questions for social work clinicians are generated. I end with some suggestions regarding how restorying can be applied to a formulation for clinical practice that builds on women's strengths and helps women to take more charge of their own meaning making. This restorying phenomenon, I argue, is one of the major ways that clinical practice and the collaborative helping relationship contain transformative power.

STORY, KNOWLEDGE, AND POWER

In the era of the "scientific" paradigm, sometimes called logical positivism, we were told that our task, as scientists, scholars, and professionals, was to discover, measure, test, prove, validate, generalize and be accountable for something "out there," to tease out the "truth," the real story. In the postmodern era of constructionism, constructivism, and deconstructionism, another view of "reality," or rather a different way to think about reality, has gained favor across many disciplines of scholarship. In this story, it is the narrative itself, not the raw data "out there," that assumes primary importance. Edward Bruner (1986), an anthropologist, frames this view as follows:

It is not that we initially have a body of data, the facts, and we then must construct a story or theory to account for them. Instead . . . the narrative structures we construct are not secondary narratives about data but primary narratives that establish what is to count as new data. New narratives yield new vocabulary, syntax, and meaning in our ethnographic accounts; they define what constitute the data of those accounts. (p. 143)

Bauman (1986), a linguist, makes a similar point when he argues that the fact or fiction, historical truth or mythical truth dichotomies are not useful. He suggests that perhaps events are not the raw materials from which we construct our stories but rather the reverse, that events may be abstractions from narrative. "It is the structures of signification in narrative that give coherence to events in our understanding, that enable us to construct in the interdependent process of narration and interpretation a coherent set of interrelationships that we call an event" (Bauman, 1986, p. 5).

Polkinghorne (1988), a cognitive psychologist, argues that historical narratives are a test of the capacity of a culture's fictions to endow real events with the kinds of meaning patterns that its stories have fashioned from imagined events. Historical narratives transform a culture's collection of past happenings (its first-order references) by "shaping them into a second-order pattern of meaning" (p. 62). Stories or narratives (terms I use interchangeably here), then, are not simply reflections about real events, but they are themselves *constitutive* of those events; events gain meaning only when they are storied. Thus stories are extremely powerful categories for individual and social meaning making and action. There is, then, an intimate relationship between story, knowledge, and power (White and Epston, 1990).

Indeed, Foucault (1980), as discussed in White and Epston (1990), argues that power and knowledge are inseparable. Through those "knowledges" that claim to hold "truth" or "objective reality" we are ". . . judged, condemned, classified, . . . destined to a certain mode of living or dying, as a function of the true discourses which are the bearers of the specific effects of power" (Foucault, 1980, p. 94). Tomm, in the foreword to White and Epston (1990), describes the knowledge/power relationship as follows:

. . . our personal identities are constituted by what we "know" about ourselves and how we describe ourselves as persons. But what we know about ourselves is defined, for the most part, by the cultural practices (of describing, labeling, classifying, evaluating, segregating, excluding, etc.) in which we are embedded. As human beings in language, we are, in fact, all subjugated by invisible social "controls" of presuppositional linguistic practices and implicit sociocultural patterns of coordination. In other words, if family members, friends, neighbors, coworkers, and professionals think of a person as "having" a certain characteristic or problem, they exercise "power" over him or her by "performing" this knowledge with respect to that person. Thus, in the social domain, knowledge and power are inextricably interrelated. (Tomm, 1990, p. viii)

This interrelationship is, of course, highly complex. One of the problems with constructivist epistemology or philosophy, as MacKinnon and Miller (1987) so aptly point out, is that it is often assumed that we all participate equally in the construction of social knowledge. Knowledge making, or what I call storying or myth making, is not a value-free or influence-free endeavor. It is a political process. Clearly, all stories are not equal. Foucault argues, however, that we are *all* caught up in a web of power/knowledge. Indeed, it is not possible *not* to exercise power/knowledge, as "we are simultaneously undergoing the effects of power and exercising this power in relation to others" (quoted in White and Epston, 1990, p. 22). Various groups gain dominance by controlling social discourses, by qualifying particular knowledges and sanctifying them. There are, of course, significant differences, both overt and covert, in the power particular groups have to ensure that certain narratives will prevail. This is the case in our families, in our communities, in our society, and in the world. Language does not simply mirror society; it is used to construct and maintain various distinctions and inequalities, in the case at hand, between men and women.

WOMEN, LANGUAGE, AND STORY

Women's lives have been largely defined and described by men. Furthermore, women's language has been defined, interpreted, and demeaned by men and by women themselves. For women are also influenced by the larger social discourse that defines them. The contemporary feminist movement and important work in women's studies has taught us well how women's lives have been measured with yardsticks designed by and for men and have been found wanting (see, e.g., Chodorow, 1978; Gilligan, 1982). Women learn to regard themselves according to the prevailing story for their lives, to gauge their performances against available socially constructed stories. A few examples make the point.

Belenky and her colleagues (1986), in their interviews with some 100 women of differing ages, educations, and social classes, found that many women feel "voiceless" and unheard in educational contexts that do not value women's ways of learning and knowing, contexts in which "truth" is sought through objective, rational search rather than through intuition, self-understanding, and connection. Throughout *his*tory, a meaning-making process (Spence, 1983) dominated by men, women have often been denied their stories which, as Heilbrun (1988) points out, deprives them of the narratives by which they might take control of their own lives. For Heilbrun, to gain the right to tell one's own story is contingent upon the ability to act in the public domain. Women's storying, in contrast to men's, has been limited largely to the family, a domestic or largely private storytelling context. In revisiting the autobiographies of a number of famous women, Heilbrun concludes that "male power has made certain stories unthinkable" for women (1988, p. 44). Women who do not make their lives contingent upon their husbands or children, who seek adventures or quests independently of men, have few stories to follow, for "lives do not serve as models; only stories do that" (Heilbrun, 1988, p. 37). Conway (1983) notes the narrative flatness in which women of the Progressive Era in the United States, such as Jane Addams or Ida Tarbell, wrote their lives. In their public stories, their autobiographies, they portray themselves as feminine—as intuitive, passive, and nurturing. Their causes and their successes occur almost fortuitously, accidentally, not as the result of a conscious vision or purposeful quest. Other notable women, if they are grandiose enough to follow a vision and to describe it without qualification, risk public ridicule (Laird, 1986). Their literature or their science or their psychology may be storied as faulty and sentimental (or, if it is terribly good, perhaps someone else wrote or invented it). Such women are often described as having failed as mothers, as promiscuous and, to place the final nails in the coffin, as unfeminine, manly, or perhaps even lesbian. Such women, it is implied, are not real women.

Certain storying *genres* have also excluded women. Written language, until the invention of the novel, was largely the province of men. In Eastern European Jewish culture, for example, women spoke Yiddish, the spoken language of the commoner, but were forbidden Hebrew, the language of writing and of the scholar (Zborowski and Herzog, 1952). (One colleague told me the story of her grandmother, who confessed on her deathbed that as a child she had secretly learned Hebrew by peeking in through the window of the boy's "shul." Never in her life had she dared to tell anyone of her hidden power).

Women have also been excluded from other forms of public storying. For example, until recently the female comedian was a rare occurrence, limited to situation comedy and domestic humor. The public storyteller, the community humorists, have been men whose humor is frequently about women. Jewish mothers, mothers-in-law in general, and wives are particular targets. (I have never heard a joke about Jewish fathers and fathers-in-law are rarely targeted). In this age of measuring success through Nielson ratings and sound bites, it is men who largely control the stories, the images, and the icons that we are bombarded with daily on television and in print. These popular "stories" often portray women benignly as creatures who clean and need to be cleaned, and less benignly as sexual objects and targets for violence. The popular media is, according to the title of a powerful film commentary, "still killing us softly."

Certainly there are exceptions. Although many television series feature stereotyped women who act silly and hysterical, several recent programs have featured women who are strong, courageous, and competent—women who are more androgynous, who learn how to speak in clearer and more assertive voices, who take firm positions, and who can act with bravery in dangerous situations. Nor are women's lives necessarily contingent on those of men. Some of today's heroines are single or, as *Murphy Brown* did, are breaking the code of silencing of solo mothers. The 1990s also brought the "out-ing" of the first woman who is lesbian both in real life and in her *Ellen* persona. Although this program was canceled not long after this most controversial event, it represented a major breakthrough for its time. In Hollywood, too, several films of the 1990s, such as *Thelma & Louise* or the lesbian films *Bound* and *When Night Is Falling* feature women who, like Hong Kingston's woman warrior, face the contradictions between the choice of wife and slave or woman warrior.

As the old couple said to the young woman who followed the bird up the mountain: "You can go to pull sweet potatoes, or you can stay with us and learn how to fight barbarians and bandits" (Kingston, 1975, p. 27). The woman warrior learns to not let menstrual days interrupt her training; she learns that motherhood and warriorhood seem not to mix, that she must put off having children for a few more years. "No husband of mine will say, 'I could have been a drummer, but I had to think of the wife and kids. You know how it is.' Nobody supports me at the expense of his own adventure" (Kingston, 1975, p. 57).

Women-Talk

Women, in their historical assignment to the domestic sphere, have clearly had a far less powerful role than men in the development of the public, collective stories that in turn shape domestic stories. Folklores, local knowledges, take shape and gain sanction in communities (Kirshenblatt-Gimblett, 1970, 1987). Not only have women had less access to the powerful shaping sources for social definitions of gender as well as to certain discourse genres, but those ways of speaking identified as "women's talk" have frequently been demeaned and less valued. Women as talkers have been variously labeled gossips, chatterboxes, or nags (Coates, 1986). Their speech, in various studies of and commentaries on language, has been seen as vacuous and restricted, full of useless adverbs and hyperbole; women have been said to be expert in the use of euphemism (Lakoff, 1975). Yet, said Rousseau, their writing lacks eloquence and passion. "They may show great wit but never any soul" (Quoted in Coates, 1986, p. 28). Women have been said to have much more restricted vocabularies, yet to talk too much. As one old English proverb would have it, "Many women, many words; many geese, many turds." Another old English proverb suggests the ideal: "Silence is the best ornament of a woman."

Men, on the other hand, are in charge of eloquence. One has only to attend a university faculty meeting, a meeting of the legislature, or a corporate board gathering today to observe that oratory eloquence, in the best tradition of the Roman Senate, is still the province of men. Our national debating societies, such as the U.S. Congress or the Supreme Court, serve as public forums featuring the voices of men, as prevailing public discourse is made and remade. It is male voices that determine women's lives and even women's bodies, as men consider whether women will have the right to control the use of their own bodies.

Coates (1986), in a study of historic folk linguistic beliefs about sex differences in language, articulates the "androcentric rule":

> Men will be seen to behave linguistically in a way that fits the writer's view of what is desirable or admirable; women on the other hand will be blamed for any linguistic state or development which is regarded by the writer as negative or reprehensible. (p. 15)

Many scholars of language, in the past fifteen to twenty years, have turned their attention to the study of the relationships between gender and language, to the study of male and female voices. Similar to one of the central arguments in feminist theory itself (Are men and women *really* so very different from each other?), it is not clear whether women's language (voice) is fundamentally very different from that of men or is only stereotyped and reinforced as different. But for our purposes here, three points should be stressed. First, what is important is the fact that women's language and women's storying are perceived and marked as different or "other" to the unmarked language and storying of men (Andersen, 1988; Coates, 1986; Graddol and Swann, 1989). Second, women have less access to the shaping of local knowledges and the larger social discourses that define them as women, to themselves and to others. And third, women are represented, and thus created and recreated, very differently than men in and by language.

> There is a Chinese word for the female I—which is "slave." Break the women with their own tongues. (Kingston, 1975, p. 56)

LANGUAGE AND THE MENTAL HEALTH PROFESSIONS

A series of professional "movements" has defined women's lives in the past century. For example, the medicalization of birthing restoried birthing from a process in which women were expert into one which transferred both definition and process into the hands/instruments of men. Women were now told to lie down, take drugs, play a passive role, and remove themselves from the company of other women (Rich, 1976). The home-economics movement turned wives and mothers into household scientists, dedicated to full-scale and full-time war against household dirt, to scientific housekeeping, to the artful making of a haven for men to escape from the difficult and sometimes cruel world of industry (Mintz and Kellogg, 1988). The mental-hygiene movement extended and reinforced the notion of mothering as a self-conscious, scientific process in which mothers became entirely responsible not only for the physical but also for the emotional lives of their children.

Mother-wife blaming has been an important part of almost every major school of developmental and clinical theory, including family theory and therapy (Luepnitz, 1988). In fact, some argue that the blaming of women and the assignment of "responsibility" for individual and family development to women is an essential part of preserving and extending the influence of the mental health professions. To be "womanly," argued Chesler (1972) in her groundbreaking book, is to risk hospitalization for mental illness.

The storying of women's physical and mental health also illustrates the intimate connections between story, knowledge, and power. The power assumed by and granted to "professionals" to pathologize women's experiences of oppression extends even to women's abilities to define and understand their own bodies. Many women, even in contemporary times, have grown up without ever knowing the proper terms for their own genital parts; they cannot speak of important parts of themselves (Lerner, 1988).

As professionals, it is difficult for us to extricate ourselves from the cultural/linguistic surroundings that shape what we see and hear. We, too, influence and are influenced by our professional languages, which make possible what we see and hear or do not see and hear. For example, depending on our favorite human behavior theories, the behavior of an angry, hostile, and rebellious fourteen-year-old girl toward her single-parent mother may be seen as part of normal development, as the consequence of turmoil and loss following an acrimonious divorce, as the girl's faulty object relations, as a result of the mother's lack of sensitivity or firmness, or as faulty family structure or communication. Rarely do clinicians consider the powerful issues of gender oppression that shape the lives of mother, daughter, the relationship between them, and the larger social stories that condition their thoughts and actions. For example, perhaps the daughter struggles against identifying with her mother, who is overworked, undervalued, and depressed about her own life circumstances. Perhaps the mother sees her family as incomplete and herself as an inadequate parent, helpless without the strong voice or authority of a male in the home. How we see and hear affects even the contexts we will create for possible stories to take shape.

In the next sections, two stories, that of the incest victim/survivor and that of the contemporary lesbian, serve to extend the story metaphor and to further examine women's strengths in a context of unequal power.

The Incest Story

Throughout history, women have been denied their own experiences in ways that have for many proved destructive to their mental health and their survival, in ways that have silenced their stories. Many of these experiences have to do with violence, as children and as adults, at the hands of men, from sexual harassment to battering, from rape to murder. Men's violence against women, not only during the rape and pillage of war but in everyday family and community life, has until recently been unspeakable, in the sense of being unable to be spoken. Not only have victimizer and victim alike maintained silence, but so has the world around them, protecting patriarchal definitions and power arrangements in the society and in the family.

The silence and secrecy of these experiences cannot be understood without reference to the larger social contexts and the social discourses or culturally agreed-upon sets of meanings that direct interpretations by layperson and professional alike. The story of the battered woman was not only silenced by her husband but could not be heard by her neighbors or the police or the judge, while the raped woman often found that *she* had become the target of social blame and approbation. As Anita Hill showed us recently, even a successful, well-educated African-American attorney did not believe, some eighteen years ago, that she could speak of what she describes as repeated experiences of sexual harassment by her supervisor without endangering her own career. Although these kinds of stories are being told today, the Hill-Thomas encounter provides a dramatic example both of the personal costs of breaking silence and of the ways in which one narrative generates multiple meanings, some far from the narrator's own meanings and intentions, all reflecting, among other things, personal and political agendas and ideologies as well as community expectations for moral behavior. Each new "reading" of the text generates new possibilities for meaning. Even so, to break the silence is not necessarily to be heard. As Senator Edward Kennedy remarked to Anita Hill's corroborating witnesses, "These gentlemen cannot hear you because they do not wish to hear you."

When women do try to fight back, as the Hill-Thomas incident demonstrates, the backlash can be powerful. In a public double-binding process, Professor Hill was excoriated on the one hand for her years of silence, for not leaving the scene of the crime (and no one asks why it is *she* who should do the leaving), for failing to repeat to her friends the graphic language allegedly used by Judge Thomas, and on the other hand for speaking out, for viciously smearing a respected man, for destroying his life and his family, for seeking personal fame and money. Interestingly, the great majority of both men and women seem to have aligned with Thomas, with his story, reflecting the power of prevailing patriarchal discourse concerning gender, sexuality, and violence. The metamessage was displayed in the context itself, the all-white male Senate Judiciary Committee vividly reinforcing our understandings about who controls the spoken word, who makes the rules for social discourse, and demonstrating the precarious future for any woman who does not know when to hold her tongue.

For the victimizer, the offender, the perpetrator (or whatever gender-neutral words are used to describe the violent person, most frequently a male), secrecy is often enforced through threats of retribution. For the victim, denied her story, the pain may be so unspeakable that it can only be repressed, expressed through extreme dissociation and even body desecration. Women who have been battered or whose children have been molested by fathers, stepfathers, brothers, or by more transient men passing through their families help to maintain the silence and to protect the family from outside encroachment.

They do this for reasons of fear, shame, and guilt, because they are afraid their families will disintegrate and they will lose the only identity that seems possible, because they have learned to disbelieve in themselves and to be reliant on men, because they do not wish to give up their homes or the only lives for which they have been readied. Many such women are poor already or are dependent on men's incomes, ill prepared for the poverty and despair that can accompany single parenthood. Some blame themselves: They must have asked for it. They deserved it. They did not protect their daughters. Why, we rarely ask, should women be in the position of having to defend their daughters from their daughters' fathers?

The abusers not only enforce a code of secrecy and silence but, in Scarry's (1985) sense, they "shatter" the language of pain; that is, like other torturers or killers or men who must kill in war, they detach the pain from its referent. For example, many fathers or stepfathers who abuse their children not only fail to recognize the moral failure of their role as parent or the destruction of the parent-child relationship but fail to recognize the severe emotional and even physical pain they are inflicting on their own children (Gordon, 1989; Herman, 1981). In what may be one of the more perverse efforts in modern times to shape a social discourse in order to protect such power injustices, some writers and researchers have greatly minimized the effects of child sexual molestation (e.g., Kinsey et al., 1953), while others have attempted to redefine it as a natural phenomenon pleasurable to the child and positive for her development (Nobile, 1977; Pomeroy, 1976; Ramey, 1979).

The spoken and the unspoken constitute each other. As Linda Gordon (1989) has shown in her fascinating historical study documenting the shaping of social discourse around child sexual abuse, a number of special social categories of language and social institutions to support these social definitions were created to reconstitute the abuse of female children as female sexual delinquency. In a blaming-the-victim solution, father and the privacy and sanctity of home and family were protected from encroachments by the state through the creation of a huge complex for institutionalizing young girls. Also, by constructing the concept of the "town pervert" or the "dirty old man," the occasional deviant, the practice of fathers sexually exploiting their own daughters remained an unspoken part of the social discourse. And for those who were the victims, the lack of language became a lack of consciousness, in extreme cases to the point where young females learned to deny their own experiences, sometimes turning upon their self-hated and "soiled" bodies in self-destructive ways. For others, the more well-meaning and benign among us, it is simply too troubling or too painful to think about such acts, for they shatter our images of our culture and the institution of family; they imply profound and difficult commitments to change.

But what of the social workers and other mental health professionals, the clinicians who have worked with the victims of male violence? Immersed like everyone else in prevailing larger cultural discourses/"knowledges," professionals have helped to support, indeed to create and define, one of the most hostile of silences in human experience. Here the power of the expert has been used to reinforce the subjugation of the least powerful, women and children. The long conspiracy of silence in Freudian thought about incest and other forms of sexual abuse and its interpretation as female fantasy served to keep generations of therapists focused on children's and women's symptoms (Herman, 1981; Masson, 1984). This story, this local knowledge, this psychology of women, gained great power over the decades, helping to shape a larger social discourse that defined women as seething with repressed sexual wishes, incompletely developed, and "hysterical." The psychoanalytic interpretation fit neatly with the discourse of patriarchy; in recursive fashion it became such a powerful "truth" that women learned to deny their own experiences or to blame themselves for having been violated by others.

The problem with this storying process is, of course, that it constructs a plot in which the central character is a "sick" woman in need of rescue and help from a "doctor" (sometimes disguised as a social worker). This is not to suggest that victimized women do not need help, but rather to point out that the storying metaphor has great power in redefining the experience and in prescribing the "treatment." Not only are women seen as deficient, defective, and diseased, defined by the effects of their denied experiences as "borderlines," "multiples," or "anorexics," but the very language used serves to divert attention from the social context that allows and indeed promotes such exploitation.

Family therapists, when they wrote about family violence at all, with their language of systems, form, pattern, structure, and game, continued and reinforced the code of silence, ignoring power differentials in the family and in the world, and even shifting major responsibility for the sexual abuse of their children and their own battering by their husbands to the wife/mother or to the marital interaction (see, e.g., Gutheil and Avery, 1977; Matchotka, Pittman, and Flomenhaft, 1967). Only as the heightened consciousness generated by the women's movement slowly fostered a changing psychology of women and a new sociology of the family did psychodynamic and systemic clinicians begin to scrutinize prevailing clinical models for their gender biases and their blind spots to violence against women.

Recently, women have begun to develop new "local knowledges." These local knowledges, which begin with the storying of individual experiences, are, in turn, reshaping the larger public discourse. Courageous women from all walks of life are speaking out, from former Miss Americas to leading comedians to mental hospital patients. They are speaking and writing, in public forums and in their autobiographies, of their physical and sexual abuse as children and their battering as adults. In the process, they are rewriting their lives, healing themselves through ritual and restorying (Winslow, 1990), in self-help movements (Bass and Davis, 1988), and in therapy. Some publicly confront their abusers (see, e.g., Randall, 1987, 1991). Some see the bearing witness phenomenon as unseemly, a public breaking of a private rule, while others are countering with a powerful backlash that seeks once again to reinforce the norms of patriarchy (Faludi, 1991).

But it is unlikely such women will be easily silenced again. Women have learned that silence, although at times necessary for self-protection and survival, can be costly. The costs of silence, in fact, can be so great that the story one creates to make sense of the world denies the self and validates social interpretations of personhood that are demeaning and distorted. To break the silence, to tell the story, implies a taking charge of one's own herstory, developing a revised story that is congruent with one's lived experience. It means "going public," if only to one other person. It means placing responsibility for unhappiness and shame where it belongs. Sometimes it means confronting the abuser, making the violence *his* shame, not one's own. It means freeing oneself from past stories that are personally debilitating. It means writing a new self-narrative in which the self-definition is revised from that of "victim" to that of "survivor"

(Riessman, 1989). It means undermining the truth-making power of patriarchy.

As clinicians, captured by the discourse of patriarchy, for a long time we failed to see or to hear what often lay beyond children's and women's symptoms. And thus we failed to create a context in which women's realities might be validated and new, more life-affirming stories shaped. Some survivors are insisting now that we listen; they are speaking so loudly we cannot *not* hear. It is incumbent on every practitioner *always* to consider how the larger social context affects our own vision, always to wear our gender lenses, always to create a context in which alternative stories may emerge.

The Lesbian Story

Until relatively recently, the lesbian in this society, with rare exception, has led a life of invisibility and secrecy. Gay men and lesbians, in many cultures and throughout history, have faced everything from execution and murder to more subtle forms of overt and covert hostility and discrimination (Adam, 1987; Comstock, 1991; D'Emilio, 1983). Predominant metaphors and interpretations in public discourse about homosexuality have shifted over time from those of evil and sin to those of sexual perversion, mental illness, genetic aberration, and, most benignly, arrested psychosexual development.[1] However, sparked by the Stonewall riot of 1969, a spontaneous resistance ignited by a police raid of a gay bar in New York City and strengthened by the civil rights and women's movements, the gay rights movement gathered momentum throughout the late 1960s and 1970s. A growing number of "out" gays and lesbians today continue to resist oppression in its many guises and are actively restorying the gay and lesbian experience in public discourse. One important marker of progress was, of course, the 1973 removal of homosexuality as an illness or diagnosable condition per se from the American Psychiatric Association's *Diagnostic and Statistical Manual of Psychiatric Disorders* (DSM-II). Many mental health professionals today, however, continue to oppose that move and "treat" homosexuality as an illness or aberration that can be "cured."

Although gays and lesbians, by virtue of their sexual orientation, face similar kinds of oppression, lesbians risk double discrimination: They are considered sexually deviant, and they are women. If they are women of color, they face multiple prejudices. Lesbian lives, along with incest, have been, perhaps, one of the best kept secrets in American society. The lesbian must be silenced for she represents the most serious challenge possible to patriarchy, to men, and to manhood, a living threat to the norm of compulsory heterosexuality (Rich, 1980). That some women might choose or prefer to love and to spend their emotional and sexual lives with other women is unthinkable in patriarchal discourse. The lesbian's very existence gives testimony to the notion that women do not need men to become complete, to survive, to succeed, to live in families, to raise children. Heilbrun (1988) notes that being single, defined until very recently by society as a pathetic, deviant state, if not a source of mental illness, allowed many women to follow their own muses. Freed from the demands of marriage, homemaking, and child rearing, many famous women leaders over the past two centuries have been, at least as far as anyone knows, single women. Some have been mistresses to married men (love and sexuality without responsibility), while for many others, close and intimate friendships with other women have been at the center of their emotional lives. Although we do not know how many of these intimate connections between women were sexual or would be defined as lesbian in modern times, we do know that many women couples have lived together for most of their adult lives, sharing their dreams and household responsibilities (Faderman, 1981, 1991). Less fettered by rigid gender-role assignments, such women are freer to pursue their quests and to support each other's visions.

The space available here allows me to focus only on a very small piece of the lesbian story, a social and personal story that is in part about oppression, social approbation, silence, invisibility, shame, isolation, and suffering. But these are not the only parts to this larger story; they are simply the parts that can be and are told. What has not been told, even in the clinical research and practice literature, which has itself undergone profound changes in focus in just a few years, is a story of strength and resilience, a story of private satisfaction and public success.[2]

For a long period of time, the overriding focus in research on homosexuality was a search for "cause." While no one ever asked what "caused" heterosexuality, several generations of researchers attempted to find the sources of homosexuality in genetic or hormonal aberration, in arrested or incomplete psychosexual development, in faulty parenting, or sometimes in unfortunate social experiences. In the 1970s, after what seems now many years of a futile scholarly journey, researchers began to shift their attention to studying the mental, emotional, and social adjustments of gay men and, to a much lesser extent, lesbians. A number of studies have compared the mental health of gay men and lesbians to their heterosexual counterparts, repeatedly finding few if any links between sexual orientation and mental or emotional health or social adjustment.[3] Furthermore, as society has grudgingly begun to acknowledge that a significant number of lesbians and gay men have children, a phenomenon once considered *by definition* next to impossible, a growing number of researchers have turned their attention to the children of homosexuals (e.g., Golombok, Spencer, and Rutter, 1983; Green, 1978; Green et al., 1986; Kirkpatrick, Smith, and Roy, 1981; Paul, 1986). The sexual identity, sex-role behavior, sexual orientation, psychological health, and social adaptation of children of lesbians have been compared to children of heterosexual women.[4] Again, study after study attests that the sexual orientation of the mother does not seem to have significant influence on the development of children along the dimensions mentioned. If there are any differences of interest, children of lesbians seem more flexible and more comfortably androgynous.

These latter researchers are helping to construct a story that in turn may help to correct some of the widespread myths and misconceptions about the experiences of children in gay and lesbian families, myths that have resulted in extensive pain and tragedy. For example, lesbians repeatedly have been judged unfit parents in the courts and social agencies, simply by virtue of their sexual orientation. It remains extremely difficult for gay men or lesbians to adopt or to serve as foster parents (Ricketts and Achtenberg, 1987). Other gay men and lesbians have lost or been denied jobs where they might have contact with children, victims of various myths that raise the specter of sexual molestation or deviant influence.

Clinicians identified with and/or sympathetic to lesbians and lesbian issues and experienced in clinical work with this population have made important contributions in detailing the impact of social oppression, of homophobia, and familial disapproval on the life experiences of individual lesbians, lesbians in couple and family relationships, and children in lesbian families (see, e.g., Burch, 1982, 1985; Crawford, 1987; Hall, 1978; Krestan and Bepko, 1980; Loulan, 1986; Roth, 1985). Much of this literature, which constitutes the only "ethnography" of lesbian life available to our profession, explores the effects of stress and discrimination on individual and familial adjustment. Much attention is given to internalized homophobia and its insidious effects. Most clinical observers seem to agree that although some issues are unique to sexual orientation (for example, attempting to construct a strong, coherent identity and build a satisfying life in a world at worst hostile and at best tolerant of one's sexual orientation; the fact that in couple relationships both partners are women, which affects the nature and quality of the relationship and the kinds of problems that can emerge; the fact that children in lesbian families risk negative peer pressures and social humiliation), the issues that emerge are similar to those faced by all individuals and families (Blumstein and Schwartz, 1983).

Although these profound shifts in the research and clinical literature represent vital and important progress in documenting lesbian experience, another part of the lesbian story is not yet told. It seems to me that the trends described above fail to capture or communicate that part of the story that tends to appear only in the more radical women's literature, a story of strength, resilience, and astonishing success. Both the research and the clinical literature retain something of a "deficit" or at least defensive stance. Myths must be debunked and troubles linked to oppression. What we do not know enough about and do not hear about are the stories of our lesbian "goddesses" or even the stories of ordinary lesbians, many of whom, in an era of profound dissatisfaction in heterosexual marriage and a tragic degree of male violence against women, lead successful and enormously satisfying and stable lives, in or out of the proverbial closet. Such stories have much to teach us about women's strengths, about resilience, about growth through adversity, and about resistance to an oppressive culture of gender relations.

This is the case even in social work, which has perhaps been more tolerant than some professions. Many of the founding mothers and early leaders in social work, and in other "women's" professions, were single woman or women who spent their entire adult lives in live-in relationships with one or more longtime women companions. Julia Jessie Taft and Virginia Robinson, founders and leaders of the Pennsylvania School of Social Work, lived together for most of their adult lives, adopting and raising two children. Jane Addams, Charlotte Towle, Gordon Hamilton, and Florence Hollis, to mention a few other prominent social work leaders, all remained unmarried, sharing their personal lives and their professional dreams with intimate women companions.[5] We do not know whether these women would describe themselves as lesbians in the contemporary meaning of the term. What is clear is that they were "women-identified women," living in families with other women. The point I wish to make here is that these essential parts of their life herstories are largely unwritten and undertold; the personal and familial stories of these magnificent women-identified women, who might serve as models of strength for our young lesbian and other women-identified women students, are largely unavailable to the profession.

Some questions that must be asked are: How is it that lesbians and children of lesbians do so well in all of the comparative studies to date, *in spite of the fact* that they face constant confrontations with homophobia, considerable discrimination, and alienation often from their own families of origin? What can their life stories tell us about resilience? Where do their strengths come from? What can their experiences tell us about how heterosexual women and heterosexual families can resist the debilitating effects of heterosexism and patriarchy?

In my own recent ethnographic interviews with seventeen lesbians, one of the patterns that stands out is that, in this sample, almost all of the women seem "exceptional" in their own families. Whether working class or professional, well-off or marginal economically, urban, suburban, or rural, they dare to be different from family prescriptions, not just in the matter of sexual orientation but in their politics, their academic achievements, their career choices and successes, their lifestyles and family values, and their selection for health. For example, one woman, a maintenance worker in an apartment complex, is the only one of her eight siblings who is not actively alcoholic. After several trips to a mental hospital in her teens and young adulthood, provoked by efforts to "cure" her homosexuality and her own excessive alcohol and drug use, she became active in Alcoholics Anonymous and has been "dry" for many years. She now hopes to attend college.

Another woman, from a large and conservative Italian-American family, is the only female member of her sibling group to attend college, itself a violation of family prescriptions for daughters. She is a graduate of a prestigious woman's college, where she won five major academic awards, including Phi Beta Kappa. Her family will not allow her partner in their home and has been unable to participate in this young woman's many successes, a situation that she finds saddening but in many ways personally strengthening.

These women seem to me unusually thoughtful about their lives and their choices; they bring a remarkable level of "consciousness" not just to the "choice" of lesbianism but to all of their commitments. These successes emerge in the face of enforced silences, of certain kinds of exclusions from mainstream society.

Perhaps, as Herdt and Boxer (1992) note in their collection of essays on gay male culture in America, what we need to ask about is: What is authentic and strong in lesbian experience? "Coming out," in their view, is no longer simply a matter of emerging *from* silence and secrecy to an uncertain reception, a drop into a "well of loneliness," but an active entry *into* a legitimate culture, with its own symbols, language, myths, imagery, art, politics, groups, communities, and so on. Is there a lesbian culture that may be different from gay male culture? What does it look like? How accessible is it to women coming out today? What special perspectives might lesbian stories offer us, not only on sexuality but on human nature and the world? Without such knowledge, without such a context, our clinical lenses will have "deficit" distortions. We will tend to see only the pain, and the problems, and we will find it difficult to ask the kinds of questions that will truly affirm the impressive strengths to be found in lesbian women and families.

IMPLICATIONS FOR PRACTICE

Many other examples would suffice to portray how the public storying of women's lives by public myth makers, our primary purveyors of local knowledges that become writ large upon the screen, serves to define "good" or "healthy" womanliness and femininity and then to label as deficient the very actions women take to live out these stories.

What, then, are the implications for us as social workers and particularly as clinical practitioners? The work must begin with a sensitivity both to the ways "stories" are made and the ways in which they shape women's lives as well as a sensitivity to the ways in which women have been denied their own stories. If clinicians are to help women and their families, they must understand the ways in which the oppression of women has generated secrecy and silence. Otherwise, it is unlikely that the clinician can create the conversational spaces or continue the conversation in ways that the unspeakable can be voiced and its multiple meanings explored.

On the widest level, clinicians can miss no opportunity to bear witness, to insist on public storying of the atrocities women have experienced. This storying process needs to go on in the schools, in agencies, in the media, and in governmental settings.

Furthermore, as a profession largely shaped by women, we must make better efforts to claim our own history, both in terms of its many contributions and the ways that the lives of our female ancestors may inform and inspire our own. In other words, we need to know our own stories and to take charge of our own storying and myth making, essential to the process of developing influential local knowledges, of using the power of discourse for change.

On the clinical level, recent work in the family therapy field offers the potential for radical change in the ways we think about theory, about prevailing notions of the worker-client relationship, and about how change occurs. In relation to theory, the social constructivist movement is depriviledging theories of human behavior in favor of a stance in which there are no certainties, only ideas, meanings, and interpretations of those meanings (Andersen, 1987; Anderson and Goolishian, 1988, 1992; Hoffman, 1990). The clinician's interpretations of the meanings of various behaviors or events in the client's life are no more privileged than those of the client herself.

Mirroring the "glasnost" phenomenon, the hierarchical nature of the clinical relationship is shifted. In the process, the clinician as expert is depowered; she begins from a "not-knowing" rather than a "knowing" stance (Anderson and Goolishian, 1992); she becomes a respectful facilitator of conversation and a collaborator in a search for new meanings. The clinician's task is to create a conversational space in which the only goal is to continue the conversation long enough for the problems, which are defined as existing "in language," to be redefined or "relanguaged" in a way that loosens their control over the client's life. Laird (1989) describes this restorying process in relation to women's lives and issues as taking charge of one's own narratives, while White and Epston (1990) speak of "narrative means to therapeutic ends." In both of these works, therapy becomes a quest for loosening the control of disaffirming stories and searching for alternative stories that better fit one's "lived" experience. In this kind of work, the therapeutic stance of the clinician is that of the interested stranger/ethnographer whose skill lies in creating a context in which the most fruitful conversations can take place, one that will allow for the voices of the silent and the silenced to be heard.

Although I believe that constructivist models have the potential for correcting many of the disempowering aspects of the therapeutic process and for allowing women's stories to surface and to be heard, several cautionary notes must be sounded. First, these theories and models that seem sociopolitically neutral themselves have emerged during an era of political conservatism that has affected the mental health professions. Are constructivist approaches just another way of perpetuating the patriarchal status quo (MacKinnon and Miller, 1987)? One possibility is that we could be lulled into thinking that everyone has equal power to shape his or her own story, forgetting that we must always be sensitive to the fact that our individual stories take shape in a powerful sociopolitical context. As social workers we have an obligation to be alert to the larger social stories that constrain individual and family narratives.

In my view, it is not possible to create neutral conversational spaces from a "not knowing" position, as Anderson and Goolishian (1992) would have it. Like the ethnographer, we may be successful in bracketing or even abandoning our prior theories with their constraining lenses, but there is never anything "neutral" about the choices we make as therapists regarding when to speak or remain silent. Our own narratives are not neutral. They are, among other things, shaped by gender for, as Goldner (1985) and others have argued, gender is a central organizing category for human experience. Both men and women need special help in connecting their gendered personal silences with their public oppressions. Although it may be true, as many constructivist clinicians imply, that the social context is always embedded in the individual narrative, the narratives of clinician and client alike are shaped and constrained by their own gendered experiences. The clinician who is not particularly sensitive to gendered silences may not be able to create the conversational spaces in which the unsaid may be recognized or spoken or alternative stories generated.

Clinicians must be alert to the differential ways that men and women story their lives, as well as to the silence and secrecy. Storying is gendered; gender differences may be connected to oppression, to differential exposures to "knowing" or the opportunity to shape "knowledges," to different linguistic styles, to different potentialities in trying to present a coherent self to the self and to others. As clinicians, we must be aware of our own gendered narratives and how they shape and constrain what we hear and what do not hear, what we ask and what we do not ask.

Finally, it should be noted that, in spite of recent interest in the phenomenon of "disclosure," clinical work takes place in a conversational context in which we as clinicians reveal very little and expect others to reveal a great deal. This inequality in and of itself creates a certain kind of silent power, for the clinician is then always a stranger, always mysterious. If we give up the power in our silence, what then do we have to offer that may be different from the very powerful "story sharing" aspects of the many self-help movements, which, if nothing else, have helped so many women to bear witness?

These and other questions must be raised as we search for ways to help women take back their own narratives.

> I musn't feel bad that I haven't done as well as the swordswoman did; after all no bird called me, no wise old people tutored me. I have no magic beads. . . . I've looked for the bird. . . . But I am useless, one more girl who couldn't be sold. When I visit the family now, I wrap my American successes around me like a private shawl; I *am* worthy of eating the food. From afar I can believe my family loves me fundamentally. They only say, "When fishing for treasures in the flood, be careful not to pull in girls," because that is what one says about daughters. . . and I had to get out of hating range. I once read in an anthropology book that Chinese say: "Girls are necessary too"; I have never heard the Chinese I know make that concession. The swordswoman and I are not so dissimilar. May my people understand the resemblance soon so that I can return to them. (Kingston, 1975, pp. 58-62)

NOTES

1. Browning (1984) reviews and challenges these various understandings of homosexuality. However, what goes around comes around. At the present time we are seeing a renewed interest in genetic explanations. See, for example, the article "Born or Bred: The Origins of Homosexuality," in *Newsweek*, February 24, 1992, pp. 46-63.

2. Although stories of strength and resilience are rare in the clinical literature, in recent years lesbians have been, sometimes joyously, writing the stories of their lives and telling their lives in music, literature, film, and other media. See, for example, Barrett, 1990; Hall Carpenter Archives, 1989; Lesbian History Group, 1989; Penelope and Wolfe, 1980/1989.

3. Throughout the 1960s and 1970s, a large number of studies was conducted, using personality assessment measures, to determine if gay men and lesbians were less healthy than their heterosexual counterparts. See Hart and colleagues (1978) and Mannion (1981) for reviews of these studies, which are methodologically flawed and have contradictory results. Lesbians actually do better than nonlesbian women on many of the measures. Evelyn Hooker (1957) was the first to demonstrate that trained professionals could not differentiate the projective test results on nonpatient homosexual men from those of heterosexual men, a study that was influential in undermining the popularity of "adjustment" research.

4. Although most of the mental health research is focused on gay men, most of the research on children of homosexuals has compared lesbian mothers with single-parent heterosexual mothers. Most studies fail to take into account whether a co-parent is involved with child rearing in either type of family. There is much less information in general on gay male parenting, although a recent book by Bozett (1987) helps to correct this deficit. See Patterson (1992) for an excellent and thorough review of the literature on children of lesbian and gay parents.

5. This information comes to me from informal conversations with women social work leaders who knew these women well or, in the case of those long gone, knew other women who knew them well. Rarely are these parts of women's lives "storied" in published accounts of their works or their lives.

REFERENCES

Adam, B. D. (1987). *The rise of a gay and lesbian movement*. Boston: Twayne Publishers.

Andersen, R. (1988). *The power and the word*. London: Paladin Grafton Books.

Andersen, T. (1987). The reflecting team: Dialogue and meta-dialogue in clinical work. *Family Process, 26:* 415-428.

Anderson, H. and Goolishian, H. (1988). Human systems as linguistic systems: Preliminary and evolving ideas about the implications for clinical theory. *Family Process, 27:* 371-393.

Anderson, H. and Goolishian, H. (1992). The client is the expert: A not-knowing approach to therapy. In K. Gergen and S. McNamee (Eds.), *Inquiries in social construction* (pp. 25-39). Newbury Park, CA: Sage.

Barrett, M. B. (1990). *Invisible lives: The truth about millions of women-loving women.* New York: Harper and Row.

Bass, E. and Davis, L. (1988). *The courage to heal: A guide for women survivors of sexual abuse.* New York: Harper and Row.

Bauman, R. (1986). *Story, performance, and event: Contextual studies of oral narrative.* Cambridge: Cambridge University Press.

Belenky, M. F., Clinchy, B. M., Goldberger, N. R., and Tarule, J. M. (1986). *Women's ways of knowing: The development of self, voice, and mind.* New York: Basic Books.

Blumstein, P. and Schwartz, P. (1983). *American couples: Money, work, sex.* New York: William Morrow.

Born or bred: The origins of homosexuality (1992). *Newsweek*, February 24, 46-53.

Bozett, F. W. (Ed.) (1987). *Gay and lesbian parents.* New York: Praeger.

Browning, C. (1984). Changing theories of lesbianism: Challenging the stereotypes. In T. Darty and S. Potter (Eds.), *Women-identified women.* Palo Alto, CA: Mayfield Publishing Company.

Bruner, E. (1986). Ethnography as narrative. In V. Turner and E. Bruner (Eds.), *The anthropology of experience.* Chicago: University of Illinois Press.

Burch, B. (1982). Psychological merger in lesbian couples: A joint ego psychological and systems approach. *Family Therapy, 9:* 201-277.

Burch, B. (1985). Another perspective on merger in lesbian relationships. In L. B. Rosewater and L. E. A. Walker (Eds.), *Handbook of feminist therapy* (pp. 100-109). New York: Springer.

Chesler, P. (1972). *Women and madness.* New York: Avon.

Chodorow, N. (1978). *The reproduction of mothering: Psychoanalysis and the sociology of gender.* Berkeley: University of California Press.

Coates, J. (1986). *Women, men and language: A sociolinguistic account of sex differences in language.* London: Longman.

Comstock, G. D. (1991). *Violence against lesbians and gay men.* New York: Columbia University Press.

Conway, J. (1983). Convention versus self-revelation: Five types of autobiography by women of the Progressive Era. Paper for Project on Women and Social Change, Smith College, Northampton, MA. June 13.

Crawford, S. (1987). Lesbian families: Psychosocial stress and the family building process. In Boston Lesbian Psychologies Collective (Eds.), *Lesbian psychologies: Explorations and challenges* (pp. 195-215). Urbana: University of Illinois Press.

D'Emilio, J. (1983). *Sexual politics, sexual communities: The making of a homosexual minority in the United States.* Chicago: University of Chicago Press.

Faderman, L. (1981). *Surpassing the love of men: Romantic friendship and love between women from the Renaissance to the present.* New York: William Morrow.

Faderman, L. (1991). *Odd girls and twilight lovers: A history of lesbian life in twentieth-century America.* New York: Columbia University Press.

Faludi, S. (1991). *Backlash: The undeclared war against American women.* New York: Crown Publishers.

Foucault, M. (1980). *Power/knowledge: Selected interviews and other writings.* New York: Pantheon Books.

Geertz, C. (1983). *Local knowledge: Further essays in interpretive anthropology.* New York: Basic Books.

Gergen, K. and Gergen, M. (1983). Narratives of the self. In T. R. Sarbin and K. E. Scheibe (Eds.), *Studies in social identity* (pp. 254-273). New York: Praeger.

Gilligan, C. (1982). *In a different voice: Psychological theory and women's development.* Cambridge, MA: Harvard University Press.

Goldner, V. (1985). Feminism and family therapy. *Family Process, 24:* 31-47.

Golombok, S., Spencer, A., and Rutter, M. (1983). Children in lesbian and single-parent households: Psychosocial and psychiatric appraisal. *Journal of Child Psychology and Psychiatry, 24*: 552-572.

Goodrich, T. J. (Ed.) (1991). *Women and power: Perspectives for family therapy.* New York: Norton.

Gordon, L. (1989). *Heroes of their own lives: The politics and history of family violence* (pp. 204-249), New York: Penguin Books.

Graddol, D. and Swann, J. (1989). *Gender voices.* Oxford: Basil Blackwell, Ltd.

Green, R. (1978). Sexual identity of 37 children raised by homosexual or transsexual parents. *American Journal of Orthopsychiatry, 135:* 692-697.

Green, R., Mandel, J. B., Hotvedt, M. E., Gray, J., and Smith, L. (1986). Lesbian mothers and their children: A comparison with solo parent heterosexual mothers and their children. *Archives of Sexual Behavior, 15:* 167-183.

Gutheil, T. and Avery, N. (1977). Multiple overt incest as family defense against loss. *Family Process, 16:* 106-116.

Hall Carpenter Archives, Lesbian Oral History Group (1989). *Inventing ourselves: Lesbian life stories.* London and New York: Routledge.

Hall, M. (1978). Lesbian families: Cultural and clinical issues. *Social Work, 23:* 380-385.

Hart, M., Roback, H., Tittler, B., Weitz, L., Walston, B., and McKee, E. (1978). Psychological adjustment of nonpatient homosexuals: Critical review of the research. *Journal of Clinical Psychiatry, 39:* 604-608.

Heilbrun, C. (1988). *Writing a woman's life.* New York: Ballantine Books.

Herdt, G. and Boxer, A. (1992). Introduction: Culture, history, and life course of gay men. In G. Herdt (Ed.), *Gay culture in America: Essays from the field* (pp. 1-28). Boston: Beacon Press.

Herman, J. L. (1981). *Father-daughter incest.* Cambridge: Harvard University Press.

Hoffman, L. (1990). Constructing realities: An art of lenses. *Family Process, 29:* 1-12.

Hooker, E. (1957). The adjustment of the male overt homosexual. *Journal of Projective Techniques, 21:* 18-31.

Imber-Black, E. (1989). Rituals of stabilization and change in women's lives. In M. McGoldrick, C. Anderson, and F. Walsh (Eds.), *Women in families: A framework for family therapy* (pp. 451-469). New York: Norton.

Kingston, M. (1975). *The woman warrior: Memoirs of a girlhood among ghosts.* New York: Vintage Books.

Kinsey, A. C., Pomeroy, W. B., Martin, C. E., and Gebhard, P. H. (1953). *Sexual behavior in the human female.* Philadelphia: Saunders.

Kirkpatrick, M., Smith, C., and Roy, R. (1981). Lesbian mothers and their children: A comparative study. *American Journal of Orthopsychiatry, 51:* 545-551.

Kirshenblatt-Gimblett, B. (1970). Culture shock and narrative creativity. In R.M. Dorson (Ed.), *Folklore in the modern world.* The Hague: Mouton Publishers.

Kirshenblatt-Gimblett, B. (1987). The folk culture of Jewish immigrant communities. In M. Rischin (Ed.), *The Jews of North America.* Detroit: Wayne State University Press.

Krestan, J. and Bepko, C. (1980). The problem of fusion in the lesbian relationship. *Family Process, 19:* 277-289.

Laird, J. (1986). Women, family therapists, and other mythical beasts. *American Family Therapy Association Newsletter, 25* (Fall): 32, 35.

Laird, J. (1988). Women and ritual. In E. Imber-Black, J. Roberts, and R. Whiting (Eds.), *Rituals in families and family therapy* (pp. 331-362). New York: Norton.

Laird, J. (1989). Women and stories: Restorying women's self-constructions. In M. McGoldrick, C. Anderson, and F. Walsh (Eds.), *Women in families: A framework for family therapy* (pp. 428-449). New York: Norton.

Lakoff, R. (1975). *Language and woman's place.* New York: Harper and Row.

Lamb, S. (1991). Acts without agents: An analysis of linguistic avoidance in journal articles on men who batter women. *American Journal of Orthopsychiatry, 61:* 250-57.

Lerner, H. (1988). *Women in therapy.* New York: Jason Aronson.

Lesbian History Group (1989). *Not a passing phase: Reclaiming lesbians in history 1840-1985.* London: The Women's Press.

Loulan, J. (1986). Psychotherapy with lesbian mothers. In T. S. Stein and C. J. Cohen (Eds.), *Contemporary perspectives on psychotherapy with lesbians and gay men.* New York: Plenum Medical Book Company.

Luepnitz, D. A. (1988). *The family interpreted: Feminist theory in clinical practice.* New York: Basic Books.

MacKinnon, L. and Miller, D. (1987). The new epistemology and the Milan approach: Feminist and sociopolitical considerations. *Journal of Marital and Family Therapy, 13:* 139-155.

Macthotka, P., Pittman, F., and Flomenhaft, K. (1967). Incest as a family affair. *Family Process, 6:* 98-116.

Mannion, K. (1981). Psychology and the lesbian: A critical review of the research. In S. Cox (Ed.), *Female psychology* (pp. 256-274). New York: St. Martin's.

Masson, J. (1984). *The assault on truth: Freud's suppression of the seduction theory.* New York: Farrar, Straus, and Giroux.

Mintz, S. and Kellogg, S. (1988). *Domestic revolutions: A social history of American family life.* New York: The Free Press.

Nobile, P. (1977). Incest: The last taboo. *Penthouse,* December: 117-118, 126, 157-158.

Patterson, C. J. (1992). Children of lesbian and gay parents. *Child Development, 63:* 1025-1042.

Paul, J. (1986). *Growing up with a gay, lesbian, or bisexual parent: An exploratory study of experiences and perceptions.* Unpublished doctoral dissertation, University of California at Berkeley, Berkeley, CA.

Penelope, J. and Wolfe, S. J. (1980/1989). *The original coming out stories.* Freedom, CA: The Crossing Press.

Polkinghorne, D. (1988). *Narrative knowing and the human sciences.* Albany: State University of New York Press.

Pomeroy, W. (1976). Incest: A new look. *Forum,* November.

Ramey, J. (1979). Dealing with the last taboo. *SIECUS Report, 7* (May): 1-2, 6-7.

Randall, M. (1987). *This is about incest.* Ithaca, NY: Firebrand Books.

Randall, M. (1991). *Walking to the edge: Essays of resistance.* Boston: South End Press.

Rich, A. (1976). *Of woman born: Motherhood as experience and institution.* New York: Norton.

Rich, A. (1980). Compulsory heterosexuality and lesbian existence. *Signs, 5:* 631-660.

Ricketts, W. and Achtenberg, R. (1987). The adoptive and foster gay and lesbian parent. In F. W. Bozett (Ed.), *Gay and lesbian parents* (pp. 89-111). New York: Praeger.

Riessman, C. K. (1989). From victim to survivor: A woman's narrative reconstruction of marital sexual abuse. *Smith College Studies in Social Work, 59:* 232-251.

Roth, S. (1985). Psychotherapy with lesbian couples: Individual issues, female socialization, and the social context. *Journal of Marital and Family Therapy, 11:* 273-286.

Scarry, E. (1985). *The body in pain: The making and unmaking of the world.* New York: Oxford University Press.

Spence, D. (1983). *Narrative truth and historical truth: Meaning and interpretation in psychoanalysis.* New York: Norton.

Tomm, K. (1990). Foreword. In M. White and D. Epston, *Narrative means to therapeutic ends* (pp. vii-xi). New York: Norton.

White, M. and Epston, D. (1990). *Narrative means to therapeutic ends.* New York: Norton.

Winslow, S. (1990). The use of ritual in incest healing. *Smith College Studies in Social Work, 61:* 27-41.

Zborowski, M. and Herzog, E. (1952). *Life is with people: The culture of the shtetl.* New York: Schocken Books.

Index